Pediatric Gastroenterology

Editor

ROBERT J. SHULMAN

GASTROENTEROLOGY CLINICS OF NORTH AMERICA

www.gastro.theclinics.com

Consulting Editor
ALAN L. BUCHMAN

December 2018 • Volume 47 • Number 4

ELSEVIER

1600 John F. Kennedy Boulevard • Suite 1800 • Philadelphia, Pennsylvania, 19103-2899
http://www.theclinics.com

GASTROENTEROLOGY CLINICS OF NORTH AMERICA Volume 47, Number 4
December 2018 ISSN 0889-8553, ISBN-13: 978-0-323-64328-3

Editor: Kerry Holland
Developmental Editor: Sara Watkins

Gastroenterology Clinics of North America (ISSN 0889-8553) is published quarterly by Elsevier Inc., 360 Park Avenue South, New York, NY 10010-1710. Months of issue are March, June, September, and December. Business and Editorial Offices: 1600 John F. Kennedy Blvd., Suite 1800, Philadelphia, PA 19103-2899. Customer Service Office: 6277 Sea Harbor Drive, Orlando, FL 32887-4800. Periodicals postage paid at New York, NY and additional mailing offices. Subscription prices are $350.00 per year (US individuals), $100.00 per year (US students), $659.00 per year (US institutions), $383.00 per year (Canadian individuals), $220.00 per year (Canadian students), $809.00 per year (Canadian institutions), $458.00 per year (international individuals), $220.00 per year (international students), and $809.00 per year (international institutions). Foreign air speed delivery is included in all *Clinics* subscription prices. All prices are subject to change without notice. **POSTMASTER:** Send address changes to *Gastroenterology Clinics of North America*, Elsevier Health Sciences Division, Subscription Customer Service, 3251 Riverport Lane, Maryland Heights, MO 63043. **Telephone: 1-800-654-2452 (U.S. and Canada); 314-447-8871 (outside U.S. and Canada). Fax: 314-447-8029. E-mail: journalscustomerservice-usa@elsevier.com (for print support); journalsonlinesupport-usa@elsevier.com (for online support).**

Reprints. For copies of 100 or more, of articles in this publication, please contact the Commercial Reprints Department, Elsevier Inc., 360 Part Avenue South, New York, New York 10010-1710. Tel. 212-633-3874, Fax: 212-633-3820, E-mail: reprints@elsevier.com.

Gastroenterology Clinics of North America is also published in Italian by Il Pensiero Scientifico Editore, Rome, Italy; and in Portuguese by Interlivros Edicoes Ltda., Rua Commandante Coelho 1085, 21250 Cordovil, Rio de Janeiro, Brazil.

Gastroenterology Clinics of North America is covered in *MEDLINE/PubMed (Index Medicus), Excerpta Medica, Current Contents/Clinical Medicine, Science Citation Index, ISI/BIOMED,* and *BIOSIS.*

Contributors

CONSULTING EDITOR

ALAN L. BUCHMAN, MD, MSPH
Medical Director, Health Care Services Corporation; and Professor of Clinical Surgery and Medical Director, Intestinal Rehabilitation and Transplant Center, University of Illinois at Chicago, Chicago, Illinois, USA

EDITOR

ROBERT J. SHULMAN, MD
Professor of Pediatrics, Baylor College of Medicine, Children's Nutrition Research Center, Texas Children's Hospital, Houston, Texas, USA

AUTHORS

MAISAM ABU-EL-HAIJA, MD
Pediatric Gastroenterology, Hepatology and Nutrition, Cincinnati Children's Hospital Medical Center, Cincinnati, Ohio, USA

NEIL W. ANDERSON, MD
Division of Laboratory and Genomic Medicine, Assistant Medical Director of Microbiology, Assistant Professor of Laboratory Medicine, Barnes Jewish Hospital, Washington University School of Medicine in St. Louis, St Louis, Missouri, USA

RACHEL A. ANNUNZIATO, PhD
Associate Dean for Strategic Initiatives, Associate Professor, Psychology, Fordham College at Rose Hill, Fordham University, Bronx, New York, USA

OSVALDO BORRELLI, MD, PhD
Neurogastroenterology and Motility Unit, Department of Pediatric Gastroenterology, Great Ormond Street Hospital, London, United Kingdom

HAYLEY A. BRAUN, MPH
Division of Gastroenterology, Hepatology and Nutrition, Department of Pediatrics, Emory University School of Medicine, Atlanta, Georgia, USA

CHARLES A. CARTER, BS, PharmD, MBA
Associate Professor of Clinical Research, College of Pharmacy & Health Sciences, Campbell University, Buies Creek, North Carolina, USA

BRUNO P. CHUMPITAZI, MD, MPH
Associate Professor, Department of Pediatrics, Baylor College of Medicine, Houston, Texas, USA

EILEEN CROWLEY, MD
Cell Biology Program, Division of Gastroenterology, Hepatology and Nutrition, Inflammatory Bowel Disease Center, The Hospital for Sick Children, IBD Clinical Research Fellow, Department of Pediatric Gastroenterology, Hepatology and Nutrition, SickKids, Toronto, Ontario, Canada; School of Medicine, Conway Institute, University College Dublin, Dublin, Ireland

CATHERINE DEGEETER, MD
Clinical Assistant Professor, Division of Gastroenterology, Hepatology, Pancreatology, and Nutrition, Stead Family Department of Pediatrics, University of Iowa Health Care, Iowa City, Iowa, USA

CLAIRE DUNPHY, MA
Doctoral Student, Clinical Psychology, Department of Psychology, Fordham University, Bronx, New York, USA

MATTHEW D. EGBERG, MD, MPH, MMSc
Assistant Professor, Department of Pediatrics, The University of North Carolina at Chapel Hill, Chapel Hill, North Carolina, USA

SARAH A. FAASSE, MD
Division of Gastroenterology, Hepatology and Nutrition, Department of Pediatrics, Emory University School of Medicine, Atlanta, Georgia, USA

NICOLE Y. FATHEREE, BBA
Research Coordinator, Department of Pediatrics, Division of Gastroenterology, Hepatology, and Nutrition, The University of Texas Health Science Center at Houston McGovern Medical School, Houston, Texas, USA

WALLACE GLEASON, MD
Professor, Department of Pediatrics, Division of Gastroenterology, Hepatology, and Nutrition, The University of Texas Health Science Center at Houston McGovern Medical School, Houston, Texas, USA

STEFANO GUANDALINI, MD
Division of Gastroenterology, Hepatology and Nutrition, Department of Pediatrics, The University of Chicago, Chicago, Illinois, USA

AJAY S. GULATI, MD
Associate Professor, Departments of Pediatrics and Pathology, The University of North Carolina at Chapel Hill, Chapel Hill, North Carolina, USA

MICHAEL D. KAPPELMAN, MD, MPH
Professor, Departments of Pediatrics and Epidemiology, The University of North Carolina at Chapel Hill, Chapel Hill, North Carolina, USA

JULIE KHLEVNER, MD
Assistant Professor, Department of Pediatrics, Columbia University Vagelos College of Physicians and Surgeons, New York, New York, USA

MARY W. LENFESTEY, MD
Pediatric Gastroenterology Fellow, Department of Pediatrics, University of Florida, Gainesville, Florida, USA

YUYING LIU, PhD, MEd
Associate Professor, Department of Pediatrics, Division of Gastroenterology, Hepatology, and Nutrition, The University of Texas Health Science Center at Houston McGovern Medical School, Houston, Texas, USA

MARK E. LOWE, MD, PhD
Pediatric Gastroenterology, Hepatology and Nutrition, Washington University School of Medicine in St. Louis, St Louis, Missouri, USA

PETER L. LU, MD, MS
Division of Gastroenterology, Hepatology and Nutrition, Assistant Professor, Department of Pediatrics, Nationwide Children's Hospital, Columbus, Ohio, USA

TU MAI, MD
Pediatric Gastroenterology Fellow, Department of Pediatrics, Division of Gastroenterology, Hepatology, and Nutrition, The University of Texas Health Science Center at Houston McGovern Medical School, Houston, Texas, USA

MARK J. MANARY, MD
Department of Pediatrics, Washington University at St. Louis, St Louis, Missouri, USA; School of Public Health and Family Medicine, College of Medicine, Blantyre, Malawi; United States Department of Agriculture/Agricultural Research Service, Children's Nutrition Research Center, Houston, Texas, USA

KARA GROSS MARGOLIS, MD
Associate Professor, Department of Pediatrics, Columbia University Vagelos College of Physicians and Surgeons, New York, New York, USA

PATRICK McKIERNAN, MD
Division of Gastroenterology, Hepatology and Nutrition, UPMC Children's Hospital of Pittsburgh, Pittsburgh, Pennsylvania, USA

PETER C. MELBY, MD
Center for Tropical Diseases, Division of Infectious Diseases, Department of Internal Medicine, University of Texas Medical Branch, Galveston, Texas, USA

HAYAT M. MOUSA, MD
Division of Gastroenterology, Hepatology and Nutrition, Professor, Department of Pediatrics, University of California, San Diego, Rady Children's Hospital, San Diego, California, USA

ALEIXO MUISE, MD, PhD, FRCPC
Professor, Departments of Biochemistry and Pediatrics, Institute of Medical Science, University of Toronto, Clinician-Scientist, Division of Gastroenterology, Hepatology and Nutrition, Senior Scientist, Cell Biology Program, Research Institute, The Hospital for Sick Children, University of Toronto, Co-Director, SickKids, Inflammatory Bowel Disease Centre, Toronto, Ontario, Canada

JOSEF NEU, MD
Professor, Department of Pediatrics, University of Florida, Gainesville, Florida, USA

YEJI PARK, MS
Department of Pediatrics, Columbia University Vagelos College of Physicians and Surgeons, New York, New York, USA

MARCELLA PESCE, MD
Neurogastroenterology and Motility Unit, Department of Pediatric Gastroenterology, Great Ormond Street Hospital, London, United Kingdom; Department of Clinical Medicine and Surgery, 'Federico II' University of Naples, Naples, Italy

GEOFFREY A. PREIDIS, MD, PhD
Section of Gastroenterology, Hepatology, and Nutrition, Department of Pediatrics, Baylor College of Medicine, Texas Children's Hospital, Houston, Texas, USA

JON MARC RHOADS, MD
Director and Professor, Department of Pediatrics, Division of Gastroenterology, Hepatology, and Nutrition, The University of Texas Health Science Center at Houston McGovern Medical School, Houston, Texas, USA

EFSTRATIOS SALIAKELLIS, MD, PhD
Neurogastroenterology and Motility Unit, Department of Pediatric Gastroenterology, Great Ormond Street Hospital, London, United Kingdom

EYAL SHEMESH, MD
Chief, Division of Behavioral and Developmental Health, Professor of Pediatrics and Psychiatry, Department of Pediatrics, Kravis Children's Hospital, Icahn School of Medicine at Mount Sinai, New York, New York, USA

CAITLIN SHNEIDER, BA
Clinical Research Coordinator, Center for Translational Science, Children's National Medical Center, Washington, DC, USA

JAMES E. SQUIRES, MD, MS
Division of Gastroenterology, Hepatology and Nutrition, UPMC Children's Hospital of Pittsburgh, Pittsburgh, Pennsylvania, USA

PHILLIP I. TARR, MD
Chief, Division of Gastroenterology, Hepatology and Nutrition, Melvin E. Carnahan Professor of Pediatrics, Department of Pediatrics, Washington University School of Medicine in St. Louis, St Louis, Missouri, USA

NIKHIL THAPAR, BM, MRCP(UK), FRCPCH, PhD
Neurogastroenterology and Motility Unit, Department of Pediatric Gastroenterology, Great Ormond Street Hospital, Stem Cells and Regenerative Medicine, UCL Institute of Child Health, London, United Kingdom

GRACE E. THAXTON, BS
Department of Microbiology and Immunology, The University of Texas Medical Branch at Galveston, Galveston, Texas, USA

MIRANDA A.L. VAN TILBURG, PhD
Associate Professor of Clinical Research, College of Pharmacy & Health Sciences, Campbell University, Buies Creek, North Carolina, USA; Adjunct Professor, Department of Medicine, Division of Gastroenterology and Hepatology, The University of North Carolina at Chapel Hill, Chapel Hill, North Carolina, USA; Affiliate Associate Professor, School of Social Work, University of Washington, Seattle, Washington, USA

MIRIAM B. VOS, MD, MSPH
Division of Gastroenterology, Hepatology and Nutrition, Assistant Professor, Department of Pediatrics, Emory University School of Medicine, Atlanta, Georgia, USA

Contents

Diet plays a significant role for children with functional abdominal pain disorders. A large majority of these children identify at least 1 food that exacerbates their symptoms. Malabsorbed carbohydrates may have both direct and microbiome-mediated physiologic effects. There are several factors associated with carbohydrate symptom generation, including (1) the amount ingested, (2) ingestion with a meal, (3) small intestinal enzymatic activity, (4) consuming the carbohydrate with microorganisms capable of breaking down the carbohydrate, (5) the gut microbiome, and (6) host factors. Therapies include carbohydrate (single and/or comprehensive) restriction, selective prebiotic and/or enzyme supplementation. Fiber supplementation may also be beneficial.

This article provides an overarching view of what is currently known about the physiology of the brain–gut axis in both health and disease and how these concepts apply to irritable bowel syndrome, the most common functional gastrointestinal disorder in pediatrics.

Pediatric pancreatitis is an emerging field with an increasing incidence of disease. Management of pediatric pancreatitis is understudied and, therefore, extrapolated from adult studies (although the etiologies are different). There is evidence that feeding is safe in mild acute pancreatitis in children without increased pain or length of stay. Studies are needed to predict course of the disease, disease severity, and risk of chronic pancreatitis in children.

Inflammatory bowel disease (IBD) is a chronic inflammatory disorder of the gastrointestinal tract, of which ulcerative colitis and Crohn's disease are the 2 most prevailing entities. Very early onset IBD (VEO-IBD) children diagnosed with IBD under age 6 years. Although the etiology of IBD is mostly unknown, it involves a complex interaction among host genetics, microbiota, environmental factors, and aberrant immune responses. Advances in the understanding of the genetic contribution, which appears to be much more significant in younger children, gives us a useful insight into the pathogenesis and potential future therapeutic targets in IBD.

The gastrointestinal (GI) system provides digestive, absorptive, neuro-endocrine, and immunologic functions to support overall health. If normal development is interrupted, a variety of complications and disease can arise. This article explores normal development of the GI tract and specific clinical challenges pertinent to preterm and term infants. Specific topics include abnormal motility, gastroesophageal reflux, current feeding recommendations for preterm infants, effects of parenteral nutrition, and the relationship between the GI tract and the immune system.

Multiplex nucleic acid testing is increasingly used to diagnose childhood gastroenteritis. The advantages of this disruptive technology include rapidity, sensitivity, and ability to detect pathogenic viruses, bacteria, and parasites simultaneously. The drawbacks are its capacity to identify organisms of uncertain clinical significance in North American children, cost, and inability to provide viable bacteria for strain typing by public health authorities. However, this technology will certainly improve our knowledge of the causes of human gut infections. As data emerge, physicians should interpret results cautiously, and, most important, consider the context of the presentation before making clinical decisions based on the readouts.

The volume of research into the pathogenesis and treatment of malnutrition has increased markedly over the past ten years, providing mechanistic insights that can be leveraged into more effective treatment options. These discoveries have been driven by several landmark studies employing metabolomics, metagenomics, and new preclinical models. This review highlights some of the most important recent findings, focusing in particular on the emerging roles of prenatal and perinatal factors, protein deficiency, impaired gut barrier function, immune deficiency, and the intestinal microbiome.

including novel drugs, electrical pacing, and manipulation of fecal microbiota, as well as stem cell and gene therapy.

Food allergies are on the rise, for reasons that are not fully understood. However, there is a tendency to overestimate their frequency, mostly based on parents' reports or on the assumption that a positive skin or blood IgE test implies the existence of clinically relevant allergy. It is imperative to base food allergy diagnosis on well-defined criteria, avoiding "alternative" tests that are available to the general public. Non-celiac gluten sensitivity is a misnomer and should be abandoned in favor of non-celiac wheat intolerance, an entity suffering from lack of biomarkers and still not convincingly described in children.

Pediatric patients with inflammatory bowel disease (IBD) stand to benefit from quality improvement (QI) due to the chronic nature of the disease, frequent interaction with the health care system, and exposure to high-risk treatments. The use of QI in health care has led to significant improvements in quality and reliability of care. Despite these advances, significant deficits in providing high-quality pediatric IBD care persist. This article describes a brief history of health care QI, identifies gaps and challenges in delivery of quality pediatric IBD care, highlights several IBD QI initiatives, and concludes with future directions for improving pediatric IBD outcomes.

Pediatric cholestasis often results from mechanical obstruction of the biliary tract or dysfunction in the processes of forming and excreting bile. Various genetic defects with resulting molecular inaccuracies are increasingly being recognized, often with specific clinical characteristics. Identifying of the molecular abnormality can enable implementation of timely, appropriate treatment in some affected individuals and provide prognostic indicators for both families and care teams.

Stable intake of an immunosuppressant medication regimen is essential for posttransplant survival in the vast majority of cases. And yet, many patients are nonadherent (do not take their medications as prescribed), and suffer consequences ranging from rejection to morbidity and mortality. We review the evidence related to monitoring of adherence to medications, and intervention strategies. Our aim is to provide a baseline from which readers may approach behavioral aspects of posttransplant care. This review may also help readers in designing clinical programs for routine monitoring of adherence, and inform the choice of intervention when adherence falls below a certain threshold.

Pediatric nonalcoholic fatty liver disease is an increasingly prevalent disease, but its pathophysiology is not fully elucidated, diagnosis is difficult and invasive, and therapeutic options are limited. This article addresses the recent advancements made in understanding the pathophysiology of nonalcoholic fatty liver disease, the development of less invasive diagnostic modalities, and emerging therapeutic options, including ongoing clinical trials in children.

GASTROENTEROLOGY CLINICS OF NORTH AMERICA

Foreword

Pediatric Gastroenterology: Not Just Dealing with Little Adults

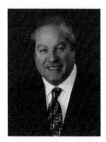

Alan L. Buchman, MD, MSPH
Consulting Editor

The practice of pediatric gastroenterology has grown substantially since its first appearance as a subspecialty in the 1960s in Europe and Australia. Yes, North America lagged behind a little, although many advances in the field have been discovered and promoted by clinicians and investigators in North America. Some diseases are limited to children, while others only begin with childhood and may often have different manifestations and associated psychosocial issues that are not apparent in their adult counterparts. Pediatric gastroenterologists place an emphasis on nutrition, which is obviously important to growth and development. This is an area where procedure-oriented adult gastroenterologists can learn something important that also affects their patients, from the pediatric counterparts. Pediatric gastroenterology has flourished as a subspecialty in recent years, with formal recognition of the subspecialty through board examination in 1990. Now rarely is the adult gastroenterologist needed to see a child with inflammatory bowel disease or to perform an endoscopic retrograde cholangiopancreatography. Harry Shwachman, Marvin Ament, Emmanuel Lebenthal, Bill Balistreri, Harry Greene, Barbara Kirsner, Bill Klish, Alan Walker, and the Guest Editor of this issue of *Gastroenterology Clinics of North America*, Rob Shulman, all deserve special credit for developing and enhancing training programs specific to pediatric gastroenterology.

Dr Shulman has assembled a talented list of thought leaders that cover the breadth of pediatric gastroenterology who have provided contemporary reviews on important

Gastroenterol Clin N Am 47 (2018) xiii–xiv
https://doi.org/10.1016/j.gtc.2018.07.018
0889-8553/18/© 2018 Published by Elsevier Inc.

gastro.theclinics.com

and/or emerging topics in the field, including functional and neuropathic disorders, inflammatory bowel disease, infections, nutrition, liver disease, and transplantation.

Alan L. Buchman, MD, MSPH
Intestinal Rehabilitation and Transplant Center
Department of Surgery
University of Illinois at Chicago
Suite 402 CSB, MC 958
840 South Wood Street
Chicago, IL 60612, USA

E-mail address:
buchman@uic.edu

Preface

Pediatric Gastroenterology

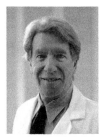

Robert J. Shulman, MD
Editor

It is an honor and a privilege to have helped bring this issue of *Gastroenterology Clinics of North America* to you. Pediatric gastroenterology continues to grow as a vibrant field, helping to improve the health of children through advances in clinical medicine and research. This issue reflects both of these areas. Ever-improving molecular techniques are helping to define new disorders and clarify existing ones, and pointing the way to new therapies; these advances are reflected in the topics presented here.

The articles are written by experts in their respective fields who have extensive experience in clinical management of the diseases/disorders described and are also key researchers—pushing the boundaries of our understanding of the pathogenesis of these ailments. Importantly, they are also excellent writers, and I believe you will find the articles engaging and clearly written. It certainly was a great learning experience for me, and I believe it will be for you as well.

I am greatly indebted to the authors for their willingness to contribute their time and expertise not only to this issue of *Gastroenterology Clinics of North America* but also to the field of pediatric gastroenterology. My hope is that they not only will impart new knowledge to us but also inspire others to join in the pursuit of expanding that knowledge so that all of us can do better by our patients.

The topics cover the gamut of problems commonly encountered in pediatric gastroenterology practice. Each article outlines the clinical presentation and most up-to-date management and treatment strategies. In addition, our current understanding of the cause of each disorder is outlined with implications for future treatments. Controversies in management, when present, also are discussed.

The articles are a mirror of pediatric gastroenterology in the early twenty-first century and reflect how far we have come and where we need to go as we strive to move the field of pediatric medicine forward, while maintaining what makes medicine special: the touch of empathy from practitioner to patient, in the face of forces that, at times, make that more and more difficult.

Gastroenterol Clin N Am 47 (2018) xv–xvi
https://doi.org/10.1016/j.gtc.2018.07.017
0889-8553/18/© 2018 Published by Elsevier Inc.

Finally, I want also to thank Dr Alan Buchman for the invitation to edit this issue, and Kerry Holland and Sara Watkins at Elsevier for their efforts in bringing this issue to fruition.

Robert J. Shulman, MD
Baylor College of Medicine
Children's Nutrition Research Center
Texas Children's Hospital
1100 Bates Street
Houston, TX 77030, USA

E-mail address:
rshulman@bcm.edu

Update on Dietary Management of Childhood Functional Abdominal Pain Disorders

Bruno P. Chumpitazi, MD, MPH

KEYWORDS

- Irritable bowel syndrome • Diet • Dyspepsia • FODMAP • Microbiome • Fiber

KEY POINTS

- Diet plays a significant role for many children with functional abdominal pain disorders; most identify at least one food that exacerbates their symptoms.
- Malabsorbed carbohydrates have both direct and microbiome-mediated physiologic effects.
- Factors associated with whether a malabsorbed carbohydrate will exacerbate symptoms include the amount ingested, whether ingestion is with a meal, small intestinal enzymatic activity, consuming the carbohydrate with microorganisms capable of breaking it down, the gut microbiome, and host factors.
- Therapies addressing carbohydrate malabsorption include carbohydrate restriction, selective prebiotic supplementation, and enzyme supplementation.
- Fiber supplementation may be beneficial in children with functional abdominal pain disorders; psyllium was recently identified in a study of children with irritable bowel syndrome to decrease abdominal pain frequency.

INTRODUCTION

Functional bowel disorders (also termed disorders of the brain-gut axis) affect up to 20% of the world's adult and pediatric population.[1] Based on the latest Rome IV classification, pediatric functional bowel disorders associated with abdominal pain include functional dyspepsia (which may be associated with postprandial fullness, early satiation, epigastric pain), irritable bowel syndrome (IBS) in which the abdominal pain is associated with defecation and/or changes in frequency of stool or stool form, abdominal migraine, and functional abdominal pain not otherwise specified.[1] Children with these disorders (as compared with healthy controls) have a decreased overall quality of life.[2]

Disclosure Statement: Support was provided by NIH K23 DK101688 and NIH R03 DK117219.
Department of Pediatrics, Baylor College of Medicine, 6701 Fannin Street, MWT 1010.03, Houston, TX, USA
E-mail address: chumpita@bcm.edu

Gastroenterol Clin N Am 47 (2018) 715–726
https://doi.org/10.1016/j.gtc.2018.07.001
0889-8553/18/© 2018 Elsevier Inc. All rights reserved.

Abbreviations	
FODMAP	Fermentable oligosaccharides, disaccharides, monosaccharides, and polyols
IBS	Irritable bowel syndrome

Functional bowel disorder etiology is attributed to several potential factors. These may include early life stress, psychosocial distress (eg, somatization), postinfectious physiology, low-grade gut inflammation, gut microbiome abnormalities (dysbiosis), genetics, visceral hypersensitivity, and diet.[3] Diet plays a significant role in the majority of children with functional bowel disorders; up to 93% identify at least one food and/or food type as being associated with a worsening in gastrointestinal symptoms.[4–6] In adolescents with IBS, gastrointestinal symptoms associated with diet occurred on more than 3 days per week.[6] Subjects with functional bowel disorders (as compared with healthy controls) avoid foods more frequently and self-implement additional dietary strategies including modification (eg, removing ingredients) of the foods they eat.[4–6]

Despite the common clinical experience of diet being associated with worsening gastrointestinal symptoms, there are several challenges. One clinical challenge is that children with functional bowel disorders may perceive a wide variety of foods as being potential culprits; however, they do not uniformly identify the same food culprits. The most common culprit foods in children with functional gastrointestinal disorders include: spicy foods, cow's milk, pizza, fried foods, deep-fried foods, fast foods, sodas, cheese and ice cream and salsa.[4] In one study of children with IBS, the most frequently identified food culprit (dairy) was identified by only approximately one-third of the subjects.[5] This finding is not unique to children with functional bowel disorders; adults with IBS also identify a wide variety of potential culprit foods and do not consistently identify a single food or food type as being a culprit.[7] An additional clinical challenge relates to strength of the association of a potential food culprit and subsequent symptom generation. When asked to rate symptom correlation (rarely, sometimes, often, or always) when eating a presumed symptom inducing food, children with functional bowel disorders do not consistently identify the same foods as either often or always causing their gastrointestinal symptoms.[4] This lack of an absolute association with symptoms with perceived culprit foods may explain the high percentage of children with functional bowel disorders consuming a potential culprit food based on 24-hour dietary recall.[4] Despite these clinical challenges, dietary intervention studies in children with functional bowel disorders have demonstrated efficacy (discussed elsewhere in this article).

CARBOHYDRATE MALABSORPTION

Malabsorption of individual carbohydrates (such as lactose) have been proposed to worsen gastrointestinal symptoms in children with abdominal pain-related functional bowel disorders for several decades.[8,9] More recently, potential carbohydrates that may be malabsorbed and exacerbate gastrointestinal symptoms have been grouped together. Investigators at Monash University in Australia termed such carbohydrates fermentable oligosaccharides, disaccharides, monosaccharides, and polyols (FODMAP). FODMAP carbohydrates traditionally include lactose, fructose, galactans, fructans, and polyols. Common sources of FODMAP carbohydrates, their general structure, and factors related to their propensity for malabsorption may be found in **Table 1**.

One randomized, double-blind, placebo-controlled trial in adults with IBS found significantly higher symptom severity scores with fructose, fructans, or a

Table 1
Type and sources of fermentable oligosaccharides disaccharides monosaccharides and polyols

Carbohydrate	Structure	Factors Related to Malabsorption	Common Food Examples
Lactose	Disaccharide	Lactase enzyme expression diminishes over time in majority of world's population	Cow's milk, cheese and other dairy products
Fructose	Monosaccharide	Passive absorption related to GLUT2 and GLUT5 transporters	Apples, pears, honey
Fructans	Oligosaccharide made of fructose polymers	Lack of human hydrolases; poorly absorbed	Wheat, onions, rye
Galactans	Oligosaccharide composed of galactose polymers	Lack of human hydrolases; poorly absorbed	Beans, legumes, asparagus
Sorbitol	Sugar alcohol	Lack of human hydrolases; passive absorption	Apricots, cherries, pears

combination of fructose and fructans the two versus glucose (placebo).[10] A double-blind, placebo-controlled, crossover trial identified a subset of children with IBS who were particularly sensitive (increase abdominal pain frequency) when challenged with fructans.[11]

Physiologic Effects of Malabsorbed Carbohydrates

Malabsorbed carbohydrates have a direct physiologic effect on the gastrointestinal tract; these effects include both increased osmotic activity (particularly in the small bowel) and fermentation with gas production.[12] These physiologic effects subsequently lead to gut luminal distention. In those with functional bowel disorders, this luminal distention may lead to symptoms such as abdominal pain, bloating, flatus, and changes in bowel habits (**Fig. 1**).

Although FODMAP carbohydrates are grouped together, each malabsorbed carbohydrate may have a more pronounced physiologic effect in 1 area (eg, small bowel water

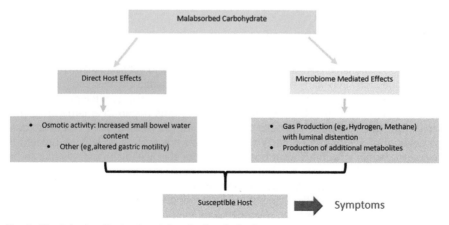

Fig. 1. Physiologic effects of malabsorbed carbohydrates.

content) versus another. Using MRI, fructose has been shown to significantly increase small bowel water content in both healthy adults and those with IBS.[12,13] The increase in small bowel water content is greater with fructose as compared with fructans. In contrast, fructans increase the overall hydrogen production and luminal (particularly colonic) gas distention in both health adults and adults with IBS. This gas production effect is greater with fructans as compared with fructose.[12,13] Though these physiologic changes may occur following ingestion of a malabsorbed carbohydrate, when comparing adults with IBS versus healthy controls, the amount of both small bowel water content increase and colonic distention that occurred did not differ.[13]

Other mechanisms, although not well-elucidated, may therefore also play a role in carbohydrate malabsorption-related exacerbation in those with functional bowel disorders. Fermentation of carbohydrates by the gut microbiome leads to the creation of several metabolites, including short chain fatty acids. Short chain fatty acids may have physiologic effects, including alteration of local ion secretion, changes in colonic motility, and activation of colonic mast cells.[14] Mast cells and their mediators (including histamine) have been associated with increased visceral nociception in both adults and children with functional bowel disorders.[15,16] Potential support for this mechanism can be found in a randomized, controlled trial in adults with IBS demonstrating urinary metabolite profiles that differed between those who were instructed to follow a low FODMAP diet and those who were instructed to follow a high FODMAP diet.[17] In those assigned to a low FODMAP diet, the amount of histamine decreased significantly after the dietary intervention.[17] Further studies are needed to investigate additional potential carbohydrate-related mechanisms in childhood functional bowel disorders.

Factors Related to Carbohydrate Malabsorption and Subsequent Gastrointestinal Symptom Exacerbation

Several factors may play a role in determining whether a FODMAP carbohydrate will exacerbate symptoms. These include (1) the amount of carbohydrate ingested, (2) ingestion of the carbohydrate with a meal, which in turn affects transit time to the colon, (3) small intestinal enzymatic (eg, lactase for lactose ingestion) activity, (4) whether the meal contains microorganisms with enzymes capable of breaking down the carbohydrate, (5) colonic microbiome at time of carbohydrate ingestion and subsequent adaptation response to one's diet, and (6) host factors such as the presence or absence of either low-grade gut inflammation and/or visceral hypersensitivity.

Amount of Carbohydrate Ingested

Although primarily derived from adult studies, data on lactose intolerance has clearly identified a relationship between the amount ingested and subsequent symptom generation. One study in healthy adults with lactose maldigestion challenged the subjects with different lactose amounts (0, 2, 6, 12, and 20 g).[18] The subjects tolerated doses of up to 6 g (representing 120 mL of milk), but symptoms began to emerge at 12 g.[18] Similar findings were noted in adults challenged with increasing quantities of lactose; the severity of symptoms primarily depended on the amount of lactose present.[19] However, certain individuals with possible functional bowel disorders seemed to be more sensitive.[19] The exact amount of lactose required to induce symptoms in children with functional bowel disorders is unknown.

Beyond lactose, the relationship between the amount of carbohydrate ingested and subsequent symptoms has been demonstrated. Increasing amounts of fructose have been shown to worsen gastrointestinal symptoms in children with functional abdominal pain.[9] Similarly in adults with IBS, increasing the amount of ingested fructose and fructans is associated with more severe gastrointestinal symptoms.[10]

Ingestion of the Carbohydrate with a Meal/Transit Time

The ingestion of a potentially malabsorbed carbohydrate with a meal may increase the amount threshold required for symptom induction. One study in adults with lactose intolerance found the symptom dosage threshold increased up to 18 g of lactose when other nutrients were concomitantly ingested.[20] Another study found that the severity of symptoms after lactose ingestion was decreased with consumption of food.[21] Moreover, based on breath hydrogen production, lactose given with a meal had a more prolonged overall transit time before reaching the colon.[21]

Meals composed of various carbohydrates may have variable effects on absorption. This has been seen in particular with fructose. Concomitant ingestion of fructose with glucose seems to facilitate fructose absorption through GLUT5.[22] However, the concomitant ingestion of fructose and sorbitol can worsen overall fructose absorption and decrease the amount of fructose required to cause symptoms.[23] Further studies evaluating meals of various carbohydrate compositions in children with functional bowel disorders are needed.

Small Intestinal Enzyme Activity

To facilitate absorption, small intestinal enzymatic activity is required to hydrolyze carbohydrates larger than monosaccharides. For example, lactose is hydrolyzed by the enzyme lactase. Lactase is a β-galactosidase found on the tips of the villi of the small intestine, which hydrolyzes lactose into 2 monosaccharides: galactose and glucose. These monosaccharides are then absorbed by the small intestine. In humans, lactase activity is at its peak at the time of birth. However, lactase activity begins to decrease in early childhood in approximately 70% of humans, so that by adulthood lactase activity is very low or undetectable.[24] Approximately 30% of the world's population has lactase persistence, whereby lactase activity remains beyond weaning and into adulthood.[25] Those with lactase persistence are able to continue to hydrolyze lactose well. Lactase persistence is a genetic trait that has been associated with at least 5 independent functional single nucleotide variants in a regulatory region upstream of the lactase gene.[26] In children undergoing endoscopy, lactase activity and lactase messenger RNA expression from duodenal biopsies correlated strongly with one of the single nucleotide variant (−13910) genotypes.[27]

Beyond lactose, decreased intestinal enzymatic activity may be involved in the malabsorption of other carbohydrates in those with functional bowel disorders. Sucrose and starch are normally easily hydrolyzed and absorbed in the small intestine through the activity of sucrase-isomaltase and maltase-glucoamylase.[28] However, in children with functional abdominal pain disorders undergoing upper endoscopy, small intestinal carbohydrate enzyme deficiencies related to sucrose (sucrase activity) and/or starch (maltase activity) digestion have been identified in 20% or more of these patients.[29,30] Further studies elucidating the potential role of sucrose and/or starch malabsorption in children with functional bowel disorders are needed.

Similar to lactase deficiency, sucrose/starch small intestinal enzyme deficiencies may have a genetic component. In 1 adult IBS study, functional variants in the sucrase-isomaltase gene were associated with an increased risk of IBS.[31] In a recently published abstract, children with functional bowel disorders (vs a large population reference database) were found to have an increased prevalence of pathogenic sucrase-isomaltase gene variants.[32] Whether these genetic components are associated with sucrose and/or starch malabsorption remains to be determined.

Meal Contains Microorganisms with Enzymes Capable of Breaking Down the Carbohydrate

Microorganisms have the capacity to metabolize carbohydrates, and many microorganisms can metabolize carbohydrates that humans cannot.[33] Subjects who were fed dairy-based yogurts with viable microbial cultures containing β-galactosidase activity (vs pasteurized yogurts) have demonstrated fewer signs of lactose malabsorption.[34] A recent systematic review identified 8 probiotic strains that have been studied to ameliorate lactose intolerance either alone or within milk-related products.[35] Of these strains. *Bifidobacterium animalis* seemed to be the most researched and effective strain.[35]

Colonic Microbiome at the Time of Carbohydrate Ingestion and Subsequent Dietary Adaptation

The gut microbiome seems to have a potential role within the paradigm of carbohydrate malabsorption and subsequent development of gastrointestinal symptoms. Within a randomized, double-blind, crossover trial of a low FODMAP versus a traditional American childhood diet in children with IBS, those children who had a 50% decrease in abdominal pain frequency on the low FODMAP diet (responders) had a different microbiome composition as compared with those who did not achieve this level of improvement.[36] Specifically, responders were enriched in both saccharolytic bacteria (including *Faecalibacterium prausnitzii*, Bacteroides, and Ruminococcaceae) and 2 Kyoto Encyclopedia of Genes and Genomes orthologues related to carbohydrate metabolism.[36] Although with mixed results, studies in adults with IBS have also identified microbiome composition as a potential predictor of response to a low FODMAP diet.[37,38]

Changes in the gut microbiome related to either chronic carbohydrate malabsorption or carbohydrate restriction may also play a role. In a small study of adults with lactose intolerance, lactose supplementation for 10 days both increased fecal microbiome β-galactosidase activity and decreased lactose-related gastrointestinal symptoms.[18] In children and adults with IBS, FODMAP restriction has been found to alter gut microbiome composition.[17,39,40] In addition, FODMAP restriction alters fecal and urinary metabolite profiles.[17,39] The relationship of these gut microbiome-related changes and relationship to gastrointestinal symptoms remains to be determined.

Host Factors

Host factors may also play a role in symptom generation in those with functional bowel disorders. Adults with lactose intolerance (vs those who did not develop gastrointestinal symptoms after malabsorbing lactose) had increased low-grade small bowel and colonic inflammation (including increased mast cells).[41] Although an association of carbohydrate intolerance and low-grade gut inflammation has not been made in children, children with IBS (vs healthy controls) were found to have increased fecal calprotectin (a marker of inflammation).[42]

Visceral hypersensitivity may also play a role in determining whether a host develops symptoms with carbohydrate malabsorption. Increased visceral hypersensitivity was identified in adults with functional bowel disorders who developed symptoms after ingesting lactose and lactulose.[41,43] Children with functional bowel disorders may also have increased visceral hypersensitivity.[44]

Carbohydrate Malabsorption-Related Therapies in Children with Functional Bowel Disorders

Carbohydrate malabsorption-related therapies in patients with functional bowel disorders often attempt to address 1 or more of the factors delineated that are associated with subsequent symptom generation.

Single Carbohydrate Restriction Trials

Although lactose restriction for children with functional bowel disorders may be commonly used in the clinical practice setting, the majority of studies supporting this practice are uncontrolled.[45] The only 2 randomized, controlled trials evaluating the need for lactose restriction in children with functional abdominal pain were negative.[45]

In comparison, fructose restriction alone is more strongly supported than for lactose. One prospective, randomized, controlled trial in children with abdominal pain related functional bowel disorders compared a 2 week fructose-restricted diet with no dietary intervention.[46] Those on the fructose-restricted diet had less severe pain. However, they did not have a decrease in pain frequency. The authors found that the improvement on the restricted fructose diet occurred irrespective of results from fructose hydrogen breath testing.[46]

Low Fermentable Oligosaccharides, Disaccharides, Monosaccharides, and Polyols Diet

As an alternative strategy to restricting single carbohydrates in children with functional bowel disorders, the entire group of FODMAP carbohydrates may be restricted simultaneously. A restricted (or low) FODMAP diet occurs in 3 phases: comprehensive FODMAP restriction, FODMAP reintroduction (during which individual FODMAP carbohydrates are used to determine which specific FODMAP carbohydrates are associated with symptoms), and FODMAP diet personalization (during which the subject tailors the low FODMAP diet to primarily avoid the FODMAP triggers that have been previously identified).[47] Working with a registered dietitian is strongly recommended to help provide appropriate education (eg, alternatives to FODMAP carbohydrates) and guide personalization of the participant's diet.

Several randomized, controlled studies in adults with IBS have demonstrated efficacy of a low FODMAP diet.[17,40] The studies have included both those that provided the foods to subjects and those that relied on dietitian education to follow the low FODMAP diet. In children with IBS, a randomized, double-blind, crossover study found that a low FODMAP diet decreased abdominal pain frequency.[36]

Selective Prebiotic Supplementation

In a randomized, double-blind, multisite, placebo-controlled trial, adults with lactose intolerance were challenged with either a short chain galactooligosaccharide or placebo.[48] The short chain galactooligosaccharide increased the relative abundance of lactose-fermenting Bifidobacterium, Faecalibacterium, and Lactobacillus, which correlated with improved clinical lactose tolerance.[48] Whether similar strategies can be used for other malabsorbed carbohydrates remains to be determined.

Enzyme Supplementation

Enzyme therapy to help prevent a carbohydrate from being malabsorbed has been trialed for several decades, primarily with lactose. In adults with either lactose intolerance or IBS, the addition of exogenous β-galactosidases (from various microorganisms) to ameliorate lactose intolerance after a lactose challenge has been shown to be successful.[49,50] Similarly in children with lactose intolerance enrolled in a randomized trial, subjects given lactase (vs placebo) had a decrease in clinical symptoms.[51]

Enzyme supplementation has also been used as a strategy for other malabsorbed carbohydrates. In adults with fructose intolerance, the addition of xylose isomerase (which may convert fructose to glucose) during a fructose challenge both decreased breath hydrogen production and ameliorated symptoms.[52] In adults with IBS who were sensitive to galactans, full dose (300 galactosidic units), α-galactosidase (vs either one-half of a dose or placebo) coingestion with a diet high in galactans ameliorated gastrointestinal symptoms.[53] Similar enzyme supplementation trials using these and/or other enzymes in children with functional bowel disorders are needed.

FIBER SUPPLEMENTATION

Insufficient dietary fiber intake has been associated with childhood functional bowel disorders.[54,55] Dietary fiber is composed of both soluble (water is able to be absorbed) and insoluble components. Soluble fiber, therefore, has the ability to maintain hydration of the stool.[56] Insoluble fiber may have the potential ability to mechanically stimulate and/or irritate the gut mucosa and this may induce a laxative effect through secretion of mucus and water, resulting in more rapid colonic transit.[56] The distinction regarding the classification of fiber is important as insoluble fiber (eg, bran) has been shown to exacerbate gastrointestinal symptoms in adults with IBS.[57]

Studies related to fiber supplementation in childhood abdominal pain-related functional bowel disorders have reported mixed results. In a double-blind, randomized, controlled trial in children with functional abdominal pain disorders, Feldman and colleagues[58] identified 10 g of corn fiber supplementation for 2 weeks was significantly more effective than placebo in decreasing abdominal pain frequency. Using a randomized, 4-week, double-blind, parallel design in children with Rome III abdominal pain-related functional bowel disorders, Romano and colleagues[59] demonstrated partially hydrolyzed guar gum (5 g/d) was significantly more effective than placebo in improving in gastrointestinal symptoms. Shulman and colleagues,[60] in the largest fiber supplementation study in children with IBS to date, reported that psyllium fiber (6 g for ages 7–11 years and 12 g for ages 12–17 years) was significantly more effective at reducing abdominal pain frequency. The psyllium benefit occurred irrespective of several physiologic measures that were assessed including gut microbiome composition.[60] Psyllium is a soluble fiber with high viscosity that is able to maintain its gellike property, thereby decreasing its fermentation by microorganisms while providing for increased water-holding capacity and regulation of stool form.[56]

In contrast with the studies suggesting that fiber supplementation is helpful in childhood functional abdominal pain disorders, 2 other randomized, placebo-controlled studies did not demonstrate any benefit; one used psyllium (ispaghula husk) and the other glucomannan.[61,62]

SUMMARY

A large majority of children with functional bowel disorders have food induced symptoms. Malabsorbed carbohydrates may have both direct and microbiome-mediated physiologic effects. Several factors are associated with carbohydrate symptom generation including (1) the amount ingested, (2) ingestion with a meal, (3) small intestinal enzymatic activity, (4) carbohydrate consumption with microorganisms capable of breaking down the carbohydrate, (5) the gut microbiome, and (6) host factors. Several therapies may address carbohydrate malabsorption induced symptoms. These therapies include dietary restriction of an individual offending carbohydrate or a more comprehensive restriction approach as seen in the low FODMAP diet. Additional approaches may include selective prebiotic, probiotic, and/or enzyme supplementation. Fiber supplementation may also be beneficial in children with functional bowel disorders.

REFERENCES

1. Hyams JS, Di Lorenzo C, Saps M, et al. Functional disorders: children and adolescents. Gastroenterology 2016;150:1456–68.
2. Varni JW, Lane MM, Burwinkle TM, et al. Health-related quality of life in pediatric patients with irritable bowel syndrome: a comparative analysis. J Dev Behav Pediatr 2006;27(6):451–8.
3. Chumpitazi BP, Shulman RJ. Underlying molecular and cellular mechanisms in childhood irritable bowel syndrome. Mol Cell Pediatr 2016;3(1):11.
4. Carlson MJ, Moore CE, Tsai CM, et al. Child and parent perceived food-induced gastrointestinal symptoms and quality of life in children with functional gastrointestinal disorders. J Acad Nutr Diet 2014;114(3):403–13.
5. Chumpitazi BP, Weidler EM, Lu DY, et al. Self-perceived food intolerances are common and associated with clinical severity in childhood irritable bowel syndrome. J Acad Nutr Diet 2016;116(9):1458–64.
6. Reed-Knight B, Squires M, Chitkara DK, et al. Adolescents with irritable bowel syndrome report increased eating-associated symptoms, changes in dietary composition, and altered eating behaviors: a pilot comparison study to healthy adolescents. Neurogastroenterol Motil 2016;28(12):1915–20.
7. Bohn L, Storsrud S, Tornblom H, et al. Self-reported food-related gastrointestinal symptoms in IBS are common and associated with more severe symptoms and reduced quality of life. Am J Gastroenterol 2013;108(5):634–41.
8. Barr RG, Levine MD, Watkins JB. Recurrent abdominal pain of childhood due to lactose intolerance. N Engl J Med 1979;300(26):1449–52.
9. Gomara RE, Halata MS, Newman LJ, et al. Fructose intolerance in children presenting with abdominal pain. J Pediatr Gastroenterol Nutr 2008;47(3):303–8.
10. Shepherd SJ, Parker FC, Muir JG, et al. Dietary triggers of abdominal symptoms in patients with irritable bowel syndrome: randomized placebo-controlled evidence. Clin Gastroenterol Hepatol 2008;6(7):765–71.
11. Chumpitazi BP, McMeans AR, Vaughan A, et al. Fructans exacerbate symptoms in a subset of children with irritable bowel syndrome. Clin Gastroenterol Hepatol 2018;16(2):219–25.e1.
12. Murray K, Wilkinson-Smith V, Hoad C, et al. Differential effects of FODMAPs (fermentable oligo-, di-, mono-saccharides and polyols) on small and large intestinal contents in healthy subjects shown by MRI. Am J Gastroenterol 2014;109(1):110–9.
13. Major G, Pritchard S, Murray K, et al. Colon hypersensitivity to distension, rather than excessive gas production, produces carbohydrate-related symptoms in individuals with irritable bowel syndrome. Gastroenterology 2017;152(1):124–33.e2.
14. Depoortere I. Taste receptors of the gut: emerging roles in health and disease. Gut 2014;63(1):179–90.
15. Barbara G, Wang B, Stanghellini V, et al. Mast cell-dependent excitation of visceral-nociceptive sensory neurons in irritable bowel syndrome. Gastroenterology 2007;132(1):26–37.

16. Di Nardo G, Barbara G, Cucchiara S, et al. Neuroimmune interactions at different intestinal sites are related to abdominal pain symptoms in children with IBS. Neurogastroenterol Motil 2014;26(2):196–204.

17. McIntosh K, Reed DE, Schneider T, et al. FODMAPs alter symptoms and the metabolome of patients with IBS: a randomised controlled trial. Gut 2017;66(7): 1241–51.

18. Hertzler SR, Savaiano DA. Colonic adaptation to daily lactose feeding in lactose maldigesters reduces lactose intolerance. Am J Clin Nutr 1996;64:232–6.

19. Gudmand-Hoyer E, Simony K. Individual sensitivity to lactose in lactose malabsorption. Am J Dig Dis 1977;22(3):177–81.

20. Shaukat A, Levitt MD, Taylor BC, et al. Systematic review: effective management strategies for lactose intolerance. Ann Intern Med 2010;152(12):797–803.

21. Martini MC, Savaiano DA. Reduced intolerance symptoms from lactose consumed during a meal. Am J Clin Nutr 1988;47(1):57–60.

22. Shepherd SJ, Gibson PR. Fructose malabsorption and symptoms of irritable bowel syndrome: guidelines for effective dietary management. J Am Diet Assoc 2006;106(10):1631–9.

23. Rumessen JJ, Gudmand-Hoyer E. Functional bowel disease: malabsorption and abdominal distress after ingestion of fructose, sorbitol, and fructose-sorbitol mixtures. Gastroenterology 1988;95(3):694–700.

24. Deng Y, Misselwitz B, Dai N, et al. Lactose intolerance in adults: biological mechanism and dietary management. Nutrients 2015;7(9):8020–35.

25. Curry A. Archaeology: the milk revolution. Nature 2013;500(7460):20–2.

26. Liebert A, Lopez S, Jones BL, et al. World-wide distributions of lactase persistence alleles and the complex effects of recombination and selection. Hum Genet 2017;136(11–12):1445–53.

27. Baffour-Awuah NY, Fleet S, Montgomery RK, et al. Functional significance of single nucleotide polymorphisms in the lactase gene in diverse US patients and evidence for a novel lactase persistence allele at -13909 in those of European ancestry. J Pediatr Gastroenterol Nutr 2015;60(2):182–91.

28. Robayo-Torres CC, Quezada-Calvillo R, Nichols BL. Disaccharide digestion: clinical and molecular aspects. Clin Gastroenterol Hepatol 2006;4(3):276–87.

29. Karnsakul W, Luginbuehl U, Hahn D, et al. Disaccharidase activities in dyspeptic children: biochemical and molecular investigations of maltase-glucoamylase activity. J Pediatr Gastroenterol Nutr 2002;35(4):551–6.

30. El-Chammas K, Williams SE, Miranda A. Disaccharidase deficiencies in children with chronic abdominal pain. JPEN J Parenter Enteral Nutr 2015;41(3):463–9.

31. Henstrom M, Diekmann L, Bonfiglio F, et al. Functional variants in the sucrase-isomaltase gene associate with increased risk of irritable bowel syndrome. Gut 2016;67(2):263–70.

32. Chumpitazi BP, Lewis JD, Elser H, et al. Prevalence of known congenital sucrase-isomaltase deficiency gene mutations in children with functional abdominal pain and/or functional diarrhea [abstract]. Gastroenterol 2017;152(5):S646.

33. Flint HJ, Scott KP, Duncan SH, et al. Microbial degradation of complex carbohydrates in the gut. Gut Microbes 2012;3(4):289–306.

34. Martini MC, Smith DE, Savaiano DA. Lactose digestion from flavored and frozen yogurts, ice milk, and ice cream by lactase-deficient persons. Am J Clin Nutr 1987;46(4):636–40.

35. Oak SJ, Jha R. The effects of probiotics in lactose intolerance: a systematic review. Crit Rev Food Sci Nutr 2018;1–9 [Epub ahead of print].

36. Chumpitazi BP, Cope JL, Hollister EB, et al. Randomised clinical trial: gut micro-biome biomarkers are associated with clinical response to a low FODMAP diet in children with the irritable bowel syndrome. Aliment Pharmacol Ther 2015;42(4): 418–27.
37. Halmos EP, Christophersen CT, Bird AR, et al. Diets that differ in their FODMAP content alter the colonic luminal microenvironment. Gut 2015;64(1):93–100.
38. Bennet SMP, Bohn L, Storsrud S, et al. Multivariate modelling of faecal bacterial profiles of patients with IBS predicts responsiveness to a diet low in FODMAPs. Gut 2018;67(5):872–81.
39. Chumpitazi BP, Hollister EB, Oezguen N, et al. Gut microbiota influences low fermentable substrate diet efficacy in children with irritable bowel syndrome. Gut Microbes 2014;5(2):165–75.
40. Halmos EP, Power VA, Shepherd SJ, et al. A diet low in FODMAPs reduces symp-toms of irritable bowel syndrome. Gastroenterology 2014;146(1):67–75.e5.
41. Yang J, Fox M, Cong Y, et al. Lactose intolerance in irritable bowel syndrome pa-tients with diarrhoea: the roles of anxiety, activation of the innate mucosal immune system and visceral sensitivity. Aliment Pharmacol Ther 2014;39(3):302–11.
42. Shulman RJ, Eakin MN, Czyzewski DI, et al. Increased gastrointestinal perme-ability and gut inflammation in children with functional abdominal pain and irrita-ble bowel syndrome. J Pediatr 2008;153(5):646–50.
43. Le Neve B, Brazeilles R, Derrien M, et al. Lactulose challenge determines visceral sensitivity and severity of symptoms in patients with irritable bowel syndrome. Clin Gastroenterol Hepatol 2015;14(2):226–33, e1-3.
44. Di Lorenzo C, Youssef NN, Sigurdsson L, et al. Visceral hyperalgesia in children with functional abdominal pain. J Pediatr 2001;139(6):838–43.
45. Chumpitazi BP, Shulman RJ. Dietary carbohydrates and childhood functional abdominal pain. Ann Nutr Metab 2016;68(Suppl 1):8–17.
46. Wirth S, Klodt C, Wintermeyer P, et al. Positive or negative fructose breath test re-sults do not predict response to fructose restricted diet in children with recurrent abdominal pain: results from a prospective randomized trial. Klin Padiatr 2014; 226(5):268–73.
47. Whelan K, Martin LD, Staudacher HM, et al. The low FODMAP diet in the manage-ment of irritable bowel syndrome: an evidence-based review of FODMAP restric-tion, reintroduction and personalisation in clinical practice. J Hum Nutr Diet 2018; 31(2):239–55.
48. Azcarate-Peril MA, Ritter AJ, Savaiano D, et al. Impact of short-chain galactooli-gosaccharides on the gut microbiome of lactose-intolerant individuals. Proc Natl Acad Sci U S A 2017;114(3):E367–75.
49. Solomons NW, Guerrero AM, Torun B. Effective in vivo hydrolysis of milk lactose by beta-galactosidases in the presence of solid foods. Am J Clin Nutr 1985;41(2): 222–7.
50. Lisker R, Solomons NW, Perez Briceno R, et al. Lactase and placebo in the man-agement of the irritable bowel syndrome: a double-blind, cross-over study. Am J Gastroenterol 1989;84:756–62.
51. Medow MS, Thek KD, Newman LJ, et al. Beta-galactosidase tablets in the treat-ment of lactose intolerance in pediatrics. Am J Dis Child 1990;144(11):1261–4.
52. Komericki P, Akkilic-Materna M, Strimitzer T, et al. Oral xylose isomerase de-creases breath hydrogen excretion and improves gastrointestinal symptoms in fructose malabsorption - a double-blind, placebo-controlled study. Aliment Phar-macol Ther 2012;36(10):980–7.

53. Tuck CJ, Taylor KM, Gibson PR, et al. Increasing symptoms in irritable bowel symptoms with ingestion of galacto-oligosaccharides are mitigated by alpha-galactosidase treatment. Am J Gastroenterol 2018;113(1):124–34.

54. Huang RC, Palmer LJ, Forbes DA. Prevalence and pattern of childhood abdominal pain in an Australian general practice. J Paediatr Child Health 2000;36(4): 349–53.

55. Paulo AZ, Amancio OM, de Morais MB, et al. Low-dietary fiber intake as a risk factor for recurrent abdominal pain in children. Eur J Clin Nutr 2006;60(7):823–7.

56. McRorie JW Jr. Evidence-based approach to fiber supplements and clinically meaningful health benefits, part 2: what to look for and how to recommend an effective fiber therapy. Nutr Today 2015;50(2):90–7.

57. Hebden JM, Blackshaw E, D'Amato M, et al. Abnormalities of GI transit in bloated irritable bowel syndrome: effect of bran on transit and symptoms. Am J Gastroenterol 2002;97(9):2315–20.

58. Feldman W, McGrath P, Hodgson C, et al. The use of dietary fiber in the management of simple, childhood, idiopathic, recurrent abdominal pain. Results in a prospective, double-blind, randomized, controlled trial. Am J Dis Child 1985;139: 1216–8.

59. Romano C, Comito D, Famiani A, et al. Partially hydrolyzed guar gum in pediatric functional abdominal pain. World J Gastroenterol 2013;19(2):235–40.

60. Shulman RJ, Hollister EB, Cain K, et al. Psyllium fiber reduces abdominal pain in children with irritable bowel syndrome in a randomized, double-blind trial. Clin Gastroenterol Hepatol 2017;15(5):712–9.e4.

61. Christensen MF. Recurrent abdominal pain and dietary fiber. Am J Dis Child 1986; 140(8):738–9.

62. Horvath A, Dziechciarz P, Szajewska H. Glucomannan for abdominal pain-related functional gastrointestinal disorders in children: a randomized trial. World J Gastroenterol 2013;19(20):3062–8.

Brain–Gut Axis
Clinical Implications

Julie Khlevner, MD, Yeji Park, MS, Kara Gross Margolis, MD*

KEYWORDS

- Enteric nervous system • Brain–gut axis • Brain–gut–microbiome axis
- Irritable bowel syndrome • Serotonin

KEY POINTS

- The brain–gut axis is a complex, bidirectional network consisting of reflex loops that ensure homeostatic control of gastrointestinal function and is impacted by the enteric microbiome.
- Serotonin is a critical mediator of the gut–brain development, which impacts the enteric microbiome, and may be a common node linking the brain–gut–microbiome axis.
- Irritable bowel syndrome is diagnosed by gastrointestinal symptomatology, and is often accompanied by mood, anxiety and/or somatoform disorders.
- Therapies targeting serotonin receptors have been shown to be useful in some cases of irritable bowel syndrome.
- Novel approaches to irritable bowel syndrome and other brain–gut axis conditions should consider holistic treatment of the central nervous system and the intestine and may involve modulation of serotonergic signaling.

INTRODUCTION

The importance of the gastrointestinal (GI) tract in human disease was first raised by Hippocrates m more than 2000 years ago. His statement, that "all disease begins in the gut," however, has only recently garnered significant interest. Although GI dysfunction has been reported to accompany an increasing number of central nervous system (CNS) disorders, there is emerging evidence to suggest that intestinal dysfunction may occur before the CNS manifestations and/or be a contributing factor to CNS disease.

The relationship between the brain and the intestine, termed the "brain–gut axis," begins during development and persists throughout life. It is what is thought to specifically link the emotional and cognitive centers of the brain with intestinal functions.[1–3]

Disclosure Statement: Support was provided by NIH RO1 NS015547-34. Department of Defense PR160365 NIH K08 DK093786 for Kara Gross Margolis.
Department of Pediatrics, Columbia University College of Physicians and Surgeons, 630 West 168th Street, PH 17, New York, NY 10032, USA
* Corresponding author.
E-mail address: kjg2133@cumc.columbia.edu

Abbreviations	
CNS	Central nervous system
CRF	Corticotropin-releasing factor
ENS	Enteric nervous system
fMRI	Functional MRI
FODMAP	Fermentable oligosaccharides, disaccharides, monosaccharides and polyols
GI	Gastrointestinal
HPA	Hypothalamic–pituitary–adrenal
5-HT$_3$	Serotonin 4
5-HT$_4$	Serotonin 4
IBS	Irritable bowel syndrome
IBS-D	Diarrhea-predominant irritable bowel syndrome
TCAs	Tricyclic antidepressants

This axis regulates homeostatic functions that were classically thought to be exclusively gut-centric or brain-centric. In the intestine, these functions include sensation and motility. In the CNS, these roles evolve around the control of behavior, cognition, and mental health. Thus, when either system is abnormal disease states emerge that can affect both systems.

In this article, we provide an overarching review of what is currently known about the physiology of the brain–gut axis in both health and disease and how these concepts apply to irritable bowel syndrome (IBS), the most researched gut–brain axis condition in neurogastroenterology.

THE PHYSIOLOGY OF BRAIN–GUT AXIS COMMUNICATION

The autonomic nervous system is the portion of the peripheral nervous system that is largely responsible for the body's reflexive, physiologic control. The autonomic nervous system is divided into the sympathetic, parasympathetic, and enteric nervous systems (ENS). The ENS is the subdivision of the autonomic nervous system that directly controls the GI tract.[4] The ENS consists of more than 100 million neurons that are organized into highly complex microcircuits that can function independent from the CNS and spinal cord.[5] Although the ENS has the ability to act autonomously, it does not usually do so. ENS communication with the CNS is continuous and bidirectional (**Fig. 1**). This communication normally occurs through the peripheral nervous system and sympathetic nervous system, via the vagus nerve and prevertebral ganglia, respectively.[4]

Abnormalities in brain–gut communication are one way that brain–gut axis disease may arise. There is also evidence to suggest that they may arise from common defects in developmental pathways of the CNS and ENS. In fact, the ENS is described as a second brain because of its many similarities with the CNS. Virtually every class of neurotransmitter found in the CNS is also detected in the ENS.[5] Further, the development of the ENS shows numerous parallels with that of the CNS.[6] Environmental and/or genetic influences on CNS development and function might, therefore, also affect these parameters in the ENS. Of these factors, serotonin (5-hydroxytryptamine [5-HT]) has been demonstrated to play important roles in development and function of the CNS and ENS and, as discussed elsewhere in this article, may modulate critical factors contributing to the development of brain–gut axis conditions like IBS.

An additional group of mediators that facilitate brain–gut interactions originate from the hypothalamic–pituitary–adrenal (HPA) axis (**Fig. 2**). The HPA axis is part of the limbic system, which is a brain area predominantly involved in emotional responses. HPA axis activation can be initiated by stressors and/or systemic

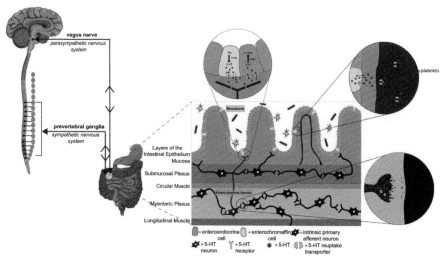

Fig. 1. Communication between the enteric nervous system (ENS) and central nervous system (CNS, brain and spinal cord) is bidirectional and continuous. The gut and the brain communicate via the parasympathetic nervous system through afferent sensory pathways of the vagus nerve and via the sympathetic nervous system through efferent motor pathways of the prevertebral ganglia. The brain–gut axis is also modulated by the enteric microbiota. The microbiota can modulate the CNS directly via the vagus nerve and/or indirectly by influencing the ENS and by production of metabolites that cross the blood brain barrier. Serotonin (5-HT) is important for brain–gut communication as both a neurotransmitter in the ENS and CNS, as well as a hormone present throughout the circulation. 5-HT is synthesized by tryptophan hydroxylase 1 (TPH1) in enterochromaffin (EC) cells, TPH2 in neurons, and is inactivated after reuptake primarily by the serotonin reuptake transporter (SERT). 5-HIAA, 5-hydroxyindoleacetic acid; 5-HT, 5-hydroxytryptamine; MAO, monoamine oxidase; TPH, tryptophan hydroxylase; Trp, tryptophan.

proinflammatory cytokines that induce secretion of corticotropin-releasing factor (CRF) from the hypothalamus. CRF secretion stimulates adrenocorticotropic hormone secretion from the pituitary gland that, in turn, leads to cortisol release from the adrenal glands. Cortisol is key in the stress response and may play an important role in IBS physiology.[7]

THE BRAIN–GUT AXIS IS MODULATED IN PART BY THE ENTERIC MICROBIOTA

The more than 1 billion organisms that inhabit the intestine influence human ENS and CNS development[8,9] and functions, including GI motility,[10–12] mood,[13] cognition, and learning.[14] This microbial population communicates directly with the CNS and ENS by way of the vagus nerve,[9,14–17] and/or by the production of active metabolites that directly influence enteric function. The microbiota can also act indirectly on the CNS by the production of metabolites that are carried in the blood and cross the blood–brain barrier.[18]

Enteric microbial manipulation may be a novel way to establish optimal neurodevelopment; evidence supports the idea that an infant's initial microbiome is influenced by its mother throughout the perinatal and breastfeeding periods and that it is this initial inoculation and subsequent development in early life that is crucial for healthy neurodevelopment.[1,19–21] The initiation of symbiosis during adolescence also seems to be a crucial step for optimal brain development and long-term mental health.[1,22,23]

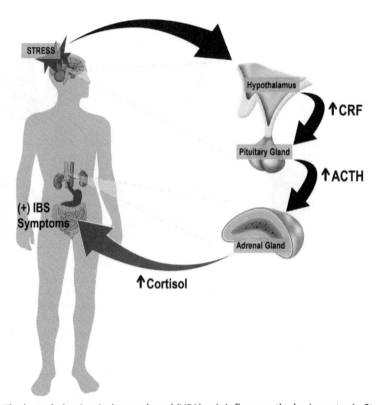

Fig. 2. The hypothalamic–pituitary–adrenal (HPA) axis influences the brain–gut axis. Stress can elicit an emotional response and hypothalamic activation. Activation of the hypothalamus induces the secretion of corticotropin-releasing factor (CRF). CRF activates the pituitary gland, and in response, adrenocorticotropic hormone is secreted. Adrenocorticotropic hormone (ACTH) acts on the adrenal gland to induce the secretion of cortisol. The increase in cortisol, a key hormone in stress response, acts on the gut to alter GI tract function, autonomic tone, visceral perception, and behavior, which all relate to irritable bowel syndrome (IBS).

SEROTONIN AS A CRITICAL MODULATOR OF THE BRAIN–GUT–MICROBIOME AXIS

There is significant evidence to suggest that serotonin may be an important link in the brain–gut axis. Serotonin and its primary inactivator, the serotonin reuptake transporter, are present in both the CNS and the ENS where they are critical mediators of development and function. During CNS development, serotonin is neurogenic and plays critical roles in cell division, migration, and differentiation.[16,17,24] CNS functions modulated by serotonin include mood (eg, depression and anxiety) and cognition.[19]

Despite its critical roles in CNS development and function, only approximately 3% of the body's serotonin is located in the CNS. The vast majority of serotonin (approximately 95%) is found in the intestine, where it is a multifunctional signaling molecule during fetal and throughout adult life.[25] Approximately 90% of enteric serotonin is located in the intestinal epithelium, in enterochromaffin cells, with the remainder located in neurons of the ENS. Two different isoforms of the same rate-limiting biosynthetic enzyme, tryptophan hydroxylase, are responsible for serotonin production in enterochromaffin cells and the ENS; tryptophan hydroxylase 1 is responsible for serotonin production in enterochromaffin cells and tryptophan hydroxylase 2 is in the ENS. Although it constitutes the minority of enteric serotonin, tryptophan hydroxylase 2-derived serotonin is most critical for ENS development, intestinal motility, permeability, and enteric epithelial growth and differentiation.[26–29]

There is evidence of interaction between serotonin and the enteric microbiome. Enteric bacteria and bacterial products, such as indigenous spore-forming bacteria and short chain fatty acids, have been demonstrated to modulate serotonin production.[12,17]

Based on its interactions with the CNS, ENS, and microbiome, serotonin may be a common node connecting the brain–gut–microbiome axis. In accordance with this notion, there are numerous links between the enteric microbiome, serotonin production, and changes in CNS and ENS function, demonstrated in both preclinical and clinical settings.[1,30–35]

THE BRAIN–GUT AXIS IN CLINICAL DISEASE: FOCUS ON IRRITABLE BOWEL DISEASE

The diagnosis of IBS relies on symptom-based criteria and is classified as constipation-predominant IBS or diarrhea-predominant IBS, mixed pattern, or unsubtyped.[36] Although individuals are diagnosed according to abdominal pain and bowel patterns, up to 50% of individuals also present with mood, anxiety, and/or somatoform disorders.[37,38] Further, it is this subset of individuals who often have a worse prognosis.[39]

Little is known regarding how and when brain–gut dysfunction originates in IBS. For many, abdominal pain begins in childhood and reflects learned illness behaviors.[40] Other childhood instances are triggered by CNS-based precipitants such as trauma, stress, abuse, or maternal neglect.[41] Patients with history of early adverse life events not only have increased odds of having IBS, but also experience an increase in disease severity.[42] The increased susceptibly may result from brain remodeling; exposure to childhood adversity resulting in alterations in emotional regulation and salience regions in the CNS, as detected by functional MRI (fMRI).[43] The CNS, however, is not always the precipitating factor; 50% of patients present after an intestinal trigger (eg, acute gastroenteritis and abdominal surgery).[44,45]

The gut–brain connection in IBS is further manifest in the abdominal pain sensation that is critical to its diagnosis. Some individuals with IBS demonstrate increased engagement of endogenous pain faciliatory mechanisms and decreased levels of endogenous pain inhibitory mechanism in brain regions associated with visceral afferent processing and emotional arousal, including the left dorsal anterior cingulate gyrus and the bilateral anterior insulae.[46] A metaanalysis of adult studies that evaluated brain response to rectal balloon distension by fMRI reported differences between healthy control subjects and patients with IBS in these brain regions[47] and a more consistent activation in regions associated with stress and arousal circuits and endogenous pain modulation.[48] In a separate study, patients with IBS with a history of abuse reported increased pain and anxiety with rectal distension accompanied by similar fMRI changes.[49] Interestingly, the stress and arousal circuit demonstrated in human subjects by fMRI share significant homology with the stress circuit related to CRF-CRF1 receptor signaling in rodents, potentially implicating the HPA axis as a facilitator of brain–gut axis communication.[50]

Findings in pediatric studies have largely mirrored those in adults.[51–53] Children exhibit an increased activation in perceptual brain regions during pain,[54] a high rate of psychiatric comorbidities,[51] and a significant association between psychiatric comorbidity and worse outcomes.[52]

As a mediator of gut–brain development and function, serotonin may play important roles in the brain and intestinal manifestations of IBS.[55] Serotonin modulates all GI functions implicated in IBS pathology, including motility, secretion, and visceral hypersensitivity.[56] Further, alterations in enteric mucosal and blood serotonin signaling have been demonstrated in children with IBS.[57] Serotonin regulates GI motility, at least in part, by binding to the serotonin 4 receptor ($5-HT_4$), which is located on both enteric neurons and intestinal epithelial cells.[25] Serotonin can affect pain pathways by binding to serotonin 3 ($5-HT_3$) receptors on intrinsic primary afferent neurons.[58]

Irritable Bowel Syndrome: Therapeutic Targets

Pharmacologic therapies targeted to the brain–gut axis in IBS have focused on the HPA axis, the microbiome and the serotonergic system. Nonpharmacologic holistic therapies are targeted toward diet, neurostimulation, cognitive–behavioral therapy, and hypnosis.

Pharmacologic therapies for irritable bowel syndrome

Serotonergic agents The physiology involved in the generation of IBS symptoms is thought to include modulation of $5-HT_4$ and/or $5-HT_3$.[56] By enhancing intestinal secretion, peristalsis, and GI transit, $5-HT_4$ agonists have been most successful in treating constipation-predominant IBS.[25,56] The initial class of $5-HT_4$ agonists (eg, cisapride) bound to cardiac potassium channels independent of their prokinetic activities, resulting in adverse events, including death. The more recently developed $5-HT_4$ agonists (eg, prucalopride, velusetrag) demonstrate greater GI specificity and are successful in treating symptoms in constipation-predominant IBS without evidence of cardiac injury.[59] These newer agonists, however, are either not currently available in the United States or are in clinical trials. The 5HT4 agonists have also been suggested as an effective target for depression.[60]

The $5-HT_3$ antagonists decrease intestinal pain sensation and slow transit.[56] The selective $5-HT_3$ antagonist, alosetron, showed efficacy for IBS-D,[61] although instances of severe constipation and ischemic colitis[62] led to its restriction for women with severe IBS-D who have not responded to conventional therapies.[63] Other $5-HT_3$ antagonists have not been introduced in the United States for similar safety concerns.

Antidepressants Antidepressants (tricyclic antidepressants [TCAs] and selective serotonin reuptake inhibitors) were introduced for IBS management based on the recognition that depression and anxiety were frequent comorbidities.[37] Accordingly, studies suggest that these agents relieve visceral pain and stabilize mood.

TCAs are associated with a decrease in IBS symptoms compared with placebo in adults.[61] A double-blind, placebo-controlled study in adolescents with IBS showed that patients receiving amitriptyline had an improvement in overall quality of life and were more likely to experience a decrease in abdominal pain and diarrhea.[64] Unfortunately, another pediatric double-blind, placebo-controlled, randomized, controlled trial examining amitriptyline efficacy in children with IBS, functional abdominal pain, and functional dyspepsia did not support these findings.[65] Further, TCAs have dose-limiting anticholinergic side effects. Selective serotonin reuptake inhibitors have been found in some adult randomized, controlled trials to be associated with a reduction in IBS symptoms compared with placebo with a number needed to treat that is similar to TCAs.[66,67] Unfortunately, these findings have not been replicated in children with functional abdominal pain.[68]

BRAIN–GUT–MICROBIOME AXIS: ROLE OF PROBIOTICS AND DIET

Enteric microbial imbalance has been suggested to underlie the pathophysiology of IBS and comorbid psychiatric conditions.[69] Controlled clinical trials on IBS with coexistent mental health conditions report symptom improvement following enteric microbial manipulation.[70–72] Microbial manipulation has been attempted by use of probiotics, antibiotics and the low fermentable oligosaccharides, disaccharides, monosaccharides, and polyols (FODMAPs) diet.

Probiotics

Bacterial species that have been shown to improve symptom severity in adults and children with IBS include strains of *Bifidobacterium* and/or *Lactobacillus*[73–79] and VSL#3.[80,81] Probiotics may impact pain pathways by influencing brain signaling; *Bifidobacterium longum* NCC3001 was shown to reduce depressive symptoms in adults with IBS while decreasing responses to negative emotional stimuli in IBS-associated brain areas, including the amygdala and frontolimbic regions.[72]

Low Fermentable Oligosaccharides, Disaccharides, Monosaccharides, and Polyols Diet

A low FODMAP diet may result in decreased microbial fermentation, and decreased production of gas and osmotically active metabolites leading to improvement in bloating, flatulence, and pain.[82] Randomized controlled trails in children and adults demonstrate that the low FODMAP diet improves IBS symptoms, regardless of subtype.[83,84] Further, this diet is also associated with improvements in health-related quality of life, anxiety, and activity impairment for adults with IBS-D.[85]

NONPHARMACOLOGIC BRAIN–GUT THERAPIES FOR IRRITABLE BOWEL SYNDROME
Psychological Therapies

In a metaanalysis including 32 adult trials and more than 2000 patients, psychological therapies were more effective than control treatments (placebo, supportive therapy, physician's "usual management") for alleviating chronic abdominal pain in adults and children, with the most beneficial outcomes reported for cognitive behavioral therapy, hypnotherapy, multicomponent therapy, and dynamic psychotherapy.[86] Cognitive-behavioral therapy, hypnotherapy, and guided imagery are also beneficial in decreasing GI and psychiatric symptoms in pediatric IBS.[87] Although the precise mechanisms are largely unknown, psychotherapy may enhance inhibition of hyperactive stress and arousal circuits, thus repairing ineffective cortico–limbic–pontine pain modulation mechanisms observed in individuals with chronic abdominal pain.[88]

Neuromodulation

The external ear contains branches of 4 cranial nerves (V, VII, IX, and X) that project to brainstem nuclei, particularly the nucleus tractus solitarius, a "relay station" to brain structures involved in autonomic control and pain.[89] The percutaneous electrical nerve field stimulator has recently been approved by the US Food and Drug Administration as a noninvasive central pain pathway modulator; percutaneous electrical nerve field stimulator is thought to provide analgesia by providing electrical stimulation of the peripheral cranial neurovascular bundles in the external ear that modulate central pain pathways. In a randomized, controlled study, adolescents with abdominal pain-related functional gastrointestinal disorder who received percutaneous electrical nerve field stimulator experienced a greater reduction in pain with sustained effect.[90]

Placebo

A high proportion of adults and children with IBS respond to placebo.[91,92] It is likely that a multitude of mechanisms contribute to the placebo effects, including expectancy of treatment success[93] and involvement of endogenous opioids.[94]

SUMMARY AND FUTURE DIRECTIONS

Although considerable progress has been made in the understanding of the brain–gut axis in health and disease, the precise mechanisms underlying both normal brain–gut homeostasis and the pathophysiology in conditions like functional gastrointestinal disorders remain incompletely understood. This lack of understanding has limited the development of holistic therapies. Several targets are evolving based on current research; targets for somatostatin, opioid and neurokinin receptors,[95] present in both the CNS and intestine, as well as CRF1 receptors, that target the HPA axis[96] have been developed but most have not been trialed in clinical studies and those that have did not demonstrate efficacy.[97,98] Pharmacologic therapies may not be necessary in all cases; the strong association of IBS with childhood trauma may provide a role for preventative psychotherapy in this subset of patients. A more comprehensive understanding of how serotonin affects the interplay between the components of the brain–gut–microbiome axis is needed to decipher novel therapies and is an area of active investigation. It is critical, however, that research focused on brain–gut physiology be undertaken to develop novel therapies for IBS and other brain–gut axis disorders.

REFERENCES

1. Borre YE, O'Keeffe GW, Clarke G, et al. Microbiota and neurodevelopmental windows: implications for brain disorders. Trends Mol Med 2014;20:509–18.
2. Carabotti M, Scirocco A, Maselli MA, et al. The gut-brain axis: interactions between enteric microbiota, central and enteric nervous systems. Ann Gastroenterol 2015;28:203–9.
3. Furness JB, Callaghan BP, Rivera LR, et al. The enteric nervous system and gastrointestinal innervation: integrated local and central control. Adv Exp Med Biol 2014;817:39–71.
4. Costa M, Brookes SJ, Hennig GW. Anatomy and physiology of the enteric nervous system. Gut 2000;47(Suppl 4):iv15–9 [discussion: iv26].
5. Gershon MD. Developmental determinants of the independence and complexity of the enteric nervous system. Trends Neurosci 2010;33:446–56.
6. Brummelte S, Mc Glanaghy E, Bonnin A, et al. Developmental changes in serotonin signaling: implications for early brain function, behavior and adaptation. Neuroscience 2017;342:212–31.
7. Chang L. The role of stress on physiologic responses and clinical symptoms in irritable bowel syndrome. Gastroenterology 2011;140:761–5.
8. Obata Y, Pachnis V. The effect of microbiota and the immune system on the development and organization of the enteric nervous system. Gastroenterology 2016;151(5):836–44.
9. Sampson TR, Mazmanian SK. Control of brain development, function, and behavior by the microbiome. Cell Host Microbe 2015;17:565–76.
10. Zhao Y, Yu YB. Intestinal microbiota and chronic constipation. Springerplus 2016; 5:1130.
11. Quigley EM, Spiller RC. Constipation and the microbiome: lumen versus mucosa! Gastroenterology 2016;150:300–3.
12. Reigstad CS, Salmonson CE, Rainey JF 3rd, et al. Gut microbes promote colonic serotonin production through an effect of short-chain fatty acids on enterochromaffin cells. FASEB J 2015;29:1395–403.
13. Yarandi SS, Peterson DA, Treisman GJ, et al. Modulatory effects of gut microbiota on the central nervous system: how gut could play a role in neuropsychiatric health and diseases. J Neurogastroenterol Motil 2016;22:201–12.

14. Gareau MG. Microbiota-gut-brain axis and cognitive function. Adv Exp Med Biol 2014;817:357–71.
15. Forsythe P, Bienenstock J, Kunze WA. Vagal pathways for microbiome-brain-gut axis communication. Adv Exp Med Biol 2014;817:115–33.
16. Mayer EA, Knight R, Mazmanian SK, et al. Gut microbes and the brain: paradigm shift in neuroscience. J Neurosci 2014;34:15490–6.
17. Yano JM, Yu K, Donaldson GP, et al. Indigenous bacteria from the gut microbiota regulate host serotonin biosynthesis. Cell 2015;161:264–76.
18. Smith PA. The tantalizing links between gut microbes and the brain. Nature 2015; 526:312–4.
19. Francino MP. Early development of the gut microbiota and immune health. Pathogens 2014;3:769–90.
20. Thum C, Cookson AL, Otter DE, et al. Can nutritional modulation of maternal intestinal microbiota influence the development of the infant gastrointestinal tract? J Nutr 2012;142:1921–8.
21. Al-Asmakh M, Anuar F, Zadjali F, et al. Gut microbial communities modulating brain development and function. Gut Microbes 2012;3:366–73.
22. McVey Neufeld KA, Luczynski P, Seira Oriach C, et al. What's bugging your teen?-The microbiota and adolescent mental health. Neurosci Biobehav Rev 2016;70: 300–12.
23. Goyal MS, Venkatesh S, Milbrandt J, et al. Feeding the brain and nurturing the mind: linking nutrition and the gut microbiota to brain development. Proc Natl Acad Sci U S A 2015;112:14105–12.
24. Montiel-Castro AJ, Gonzalez-Cervantes RM, Bravo-Ruiseco G, et al. The microbiota-gut-brain axis: neurobehavioral correlates, health and sociality. Front Integr Neurosci 2013;7:70.
25. Gershon MD. 5-Hydroxytryptamine (serotonin) in the gastrointestinal tract. Curr Opin Endocrinol Diabetes Obes 2013;20:14–21.
26. Gross ER, Gershon MD, Margolis KG, et al. Neuronal serotonin regulates growth of the intestinal mucosa in mice. Gastroenterology 2012;143:408–17.e2.
27. Li Z, Chalazonitis A, Huang YY, et al. Essential roles of enteric neuronal serotonin in gastrointestinal motility and the development/survival of enteric dopaminergic neurons. J Neurosci 2011;31:8998–9009.
28. Margolis KG, Li Z, Stevanovic K, et al. Serotonin transporter variant drives preventable gastrointestinal abnormalities in development and function. J Clin Invest 2016;126:2221–35.
29. Margolis KG, Stevanovic K, Li Z, et al. Pharmacological reduction of mucosal but not neuronal serotonin opposes inflammation in mouse intestine. Gut 2014;63: 928–37.
30. Jenkins TA, Nguyen JC, Polglaze KE, et al. Influence of tryptophan and serotonin on mood and cognition with a possible role of the gut-brain axis. Nutrients 2016; 8(1) [pii:E56].
31. Kennedy PJ, Cryan JF, Dinan TG, et al. Kynurenine pathway metabolism and the microbiota-gut-brain axis. Neuropharmacology 2017;112(Pt B):399–412.
32. Mittal R, Debs LH, Patel AP, et al. Neurotransmitters: the critical modulators regulating gut-brain axis. J Cell Physiol 2017;232(9):2359–72.
33. Morris G, Berk M, Carvalho A, et al. The role of the microbial metabolites including tryptophan catabolites and short chain fatty acids in the pathophysiology of immune-inflammatory and neuroimmune disease. Mol Neurobiol 2017; 54(6):4432–51.

34. O'Mahony SM, Clarke G, Borre YE, et al. Serotonin, tryptophan metabolism and the brain-gut-microbiome axis. Behav Brain Res 2015;277:32–48.

35. Moloney RD, Johnson AC, O'Mahony SM, et al. Stress and the microbiota-gut-brain axis in visceral pain: relevance to irritable bowel syndrome. CNS Neurosci Ther 2016;22:102–17.

36. Hyams JS, Di Lorenzo C, Saps M, et al. Functional disorders: children and adolescents. Gastroenterology 2016;150:1456–68.

37. Van Oudenhove L, Levy RL, Crowell MD, et al. Biopsychosocial aspects of functional gastrointestinal disorders: how central and environmental processes contribute to the development and expression of functional gastrointestinal disorders. Gastroenterology 2016;150:1355–67.

38. Fond G, Loundou A, Hamdani N, et al. Anxiety and depression comorbidities in irritable bowel syndrome (IBS): a systematic review and meta-analysis. Eur Arch Psychiatry Clin Neurosci 2014;264:651–60.

39. Lackner JM, Brasel AM, Quigley BM, et al. The ties that bind: perceived social support, stress, and IBS in severely affected patients. Neurogastroenterol Motil 2010;22:893–900.

40. Mayer EA, Tillisch K. The brain-gut axis in abdominal pain syndromes. Annu Rev Med 2011;62:381–96.

41. Halland M, Almazar A, Lee R, et al. A case-control study of childhood trauma in the development of irritable bowel syndrome. Neurogastroenterol Motil 2014;26: 990–8.

42. Park SH, Videlock EJ, Shih W, et al. Adverse childhood experiences are associated with irritable bowel syndrome and gastrointestinal symptom severity. Neurogastroenterol Motil 2016;28:1252–60.

43. Gupta A, Mayer EA, Acosta JR, et al. Early adverse life events are associated with altered brain network architecture in a sex- dependent manner. Neurobiol Stress 2017;7:16–26.

44. Sykes MA, Blanchard EB, Lackner J, et al. Psychopathology in irritable bowel syndrome: support for a psychophysiological model. J Behav Med 2003;26: 361–72.

45. Rosen JM, Adams PN, Saps M. Umbilical hernia repair increases the rate of functional gastrointestinal disorders in children. J Pediatr 2013;163:1065–8.

46. Wilder-Smith CH, Schindler D, Lovblad K, et al. Brain functional magnetic resonance imaging of rectal pain and activation of endogenous inhibitory mechanisms in irritable bowel syndrome patient subgroups and healthy controls. Gut 2004;53:1595–601.

47. Tillisch K, Mayer EA, Labus JS. Quantitative meta-analysis identifies brain regions activated during rectal distension in irritable bowel syndrome. Gastroenterology 2011;140:91–100.

48. Phillips ML, Gregory LJ, Cullen S, et al. The effect of negative emotional context on neural and behavioural responses to oesophageal stimulation. Brain 2003; 126:669–84.

49. Ringel Y, Drossman DA, Leserman JL, et al. Effect of abuse history on pain reports and brain responses to aversive visceral stimulation: an FMRI study. Gastroenterology 2008;134:396–404.

50. Mayer EA, Bradesi S, Chang L, et al. Functional GI disorders: from animal models to drug development. Gut 2008;57:384–404.

51. Iovino P, Tremolaterra F, Boccia G, et al. Irritable bowel syndrome in childhood: visceral hypersensitivity and psychosocial aspects. Neurogastroenterol Motil 2009;21:940-e74.

52. Di Lorenzo C, Youssef NN, Sigurdsson L, et al. Visceral hyperalgesia in children with functional abdominal pain. J Pediatr 2001;139:838–43.
53. Van Ginkel R, Voskuijl WP, Benninga MA, et al. Alterations in rectal sensitivity and motility in childhood irritable bowel syndrome. Gastroenterology 2001;120:31–8.
54. Huang JS, Terrones L, Simmons AN, et al. Pilot study of functional magnetic resonance imaging responses to somatic pain stimuli in youth with functional and inflammatory gastrointestinal disease. J Pediatr Gastroenterol Nutr 2016;63:500–7.
55. Gershon MD, Tack J. The serotonin signaling system: from basic understanding to drug development for functional GI disorders. Gastroenterology 2007;132:397–414.
56. Mawe GM, Hoffman JM. Serotonin signalling in the gut–functions, dysfunctions and therapeutic targets. Nat Rev Gastroenterol Hepatol 2013;10:473–86.
57. Faure C, Patey N, Gauthier C, et al. Serotonin signaling is altered in irritable bowel syndrome with diarrhea but not in functional dyspepsia in pediatric age patients. Gastroenterology 2010;139:249–58.
58. Gershon MD. Review article: serotonin receptors and transporters – roles in normal and abnormal gastrointestinal motility. Aliment Pharmacol Ther 2004; 20(Suppl 7):3–14.
59. Jadallah KA, Kullab SM, Sanders DS. Constipation-predominant irritable bowel syndrome: a review of current and emerging drug therapies. World J Gastroenterol 2014;20:8898–909.
60. Samuels BA, Mendez-David I, Faye C, et al. Serotonin 1A and serotonin 4 receptors: essential mediators of the neurogenic and behavioral actions of antidepressants. Neuroscientist 2016;22:26–45.
61. Ford AC, Moayyedi P, Lacy BE, et al. American College of Gastroenterology monograph on the management of irritable bowel syndrome and chronic idiopathic constipation. Am J Gastroenterol 2014;109(Suppl 1):S2–26 [quiz: S27].
62. Chang L, Chey WD, Harris L, et al. Incidence of ischemic colitis and serious complications of constipation among patients using alosetron: systematic review of clinical trials and post-marketing surveillance data. Am J Gastroenterol 2006; 101:1069–79.
63. Tong K, Nicandro JP, Shringarpure R, et al. A 9-year evaluation of temporal trends in alosetron postmarketing safety under the risk management program. Ther Adv Gastroenterol 2013;6:344–57.
64. Bahar RJ, Collins BS, Steinmetz B, et al. Double-blind placebo-controlled trial of amitriptyline for the treatment of irritable bowel syndrome in adolescents. J Pediatr 2008;152:685–9.
65. Saps M, Youssef N, Miranda A, et al. Multicenter, randomized, placebo-controlled trial of amitriptyline in children with functional gastrointestinal disorders. Gastroenterology 2009;137:1261–9.
66. Tack J, Broekaert D, Fischler B, et al. A controlled crossover study of the selective serotonin reuptake inhibitor citalopram in irritable bowel syndrome. Gut 2006;55: 1095–103.
67. Vahedi H, Merat S, Rashidioon A, et al. The effect of fluoxetine in patients with pain and constipation-predominant irritable bowel syndrome: a double-blind randomized-controlled study. Aliment Pharmacol Ther 2005;22:381–5.
68. Roohafza H, Pourmoghaddas Z, Saneian H, et al. Citalopram for pediatric functional abdominal pain: a randomized, placebo-controlled trial. Neurogastroenterol Motil 2014;26:1642–50.
69. Rhee SH, Pothoulakis C, Mayer EA. Principles and clinical implications of the brain-gut-enteric microbiota axis. Nat Rev Gastroenterol Hepatol 2009;6:306–14.

70. Moayyedi P, Ford AC, Talley NJ, et al. The efficacy of probiotics in the treatment of irritable bowel syndrome: a systematic review. Gut 2010;59:325–32.

71. Pirbaglou M, Katz J, de Souza RJ, et al. Probiotic supplementation can positively affect anxiety and depressive symptoms: a systematic review of randomized controlled trials. Nutr Res 2016;36:889–98.

72. Pinto-Sanchez MI, Hall GB, Ghajar K, et al. Probiotic Bifidobacterium longum NCC3001 reduces depression scores and alters brain activity: a pilot study in patients with irritable bowel syndrome. Gastroenterology 2017;153:448–59.e8.

73. O'Mahony L, McCarthy J, Kelly P, et al. Lactobacillus and Bifidobacterium in irritable bowel syndrome: symptom responses and relationship to cytokine profiles. Gastroenterology 2005;128:541–51.

74. Whorwell PJ, Altringer L, Morel J, et al. Efficacy of an encapsulated probiotic Bifidobacterium infantis 35624 in women with irritable bowel syndrome. Am J Gastroenterol 2006;101:1581–90.

75. Gawronska A, Dziechciarz P, Horvath A, et al. A randomized double-blind placebo-controlled trial of Lactobacillus GG for abdominal pain disorders in children. Aliment Pharmacol Ther 2007;25:177–84.

76. Francavilla R, Miniello V, Magista AM, et al. A randomized controlled trial of Lactobacillus GG in children with functional abdominal pain. Pediatrics 2010;126:e1445–52.

77. Horvath A, Dziechciarz P, Szajewska H. Meta-analysis: Lactobacillus rhamnosus GG for abdominal pain-related functional gastrointestinal disorders in childhood. Aliment Pharmacol Ther 2011;33:1302–10.

78. Giannetti E, Maglione M, Alessandrella A, et al. A mixture of 3 Bifidobacteria decreases abdominal pain and improves the quality of life in children with irritable bowel syndrome: a multicenter, randomized, double-blind, placebo-controlled, crossover trial. J Clin Gastroenterol 2017;51:e5–10.

79. Guglielmetti S, Mora D, Gschwender M, et al. Randomised clinical trial: Bifidobacterium bifidum MIMBb75 significantly alleviates irritable bowel syndrome and improves quality of life–a double-blind, placebo-controlled study. Aliment Pharmacol Ther 2011;33:1123–32.

80. Yoon JS, Sohn W, Lee OY, et al. Effect of multispecies probiotics on irritable bowel syndrome: a randomized, double-blind, placebo-controlled trial. J Gastroenterol Hepatol 2014;29:52–9.

81. Guandalini S, Magazzu G, Chiaro A, et al. VSL#3 improves symptoms in children with irritable bowel syndrome: a multicenter, randomized, placebo-controlled, double-blind, crossover study. J Pediatr Gastroenterol Nutr 2010;51:24–30.

82. Staudacher HM, Whelan K. The low FODMAP diet: recent advances in understanding its mechanisms and efficacy in IBS. Gut 2017;66:1517–27.

83. Halmos EP, Power VA, Shepherd SJ, et al. A diet low in FODMAPs reduces symptoms of irritable bowel syndrome. Gastroenterology 2014;146:67–75.e5.

84. Chumpitazi BP, Cope JL, Hollister EB, et al. Randomised clinical trial: gut microbiome biomarkers are associated with clinical response to a low FODMAP diet in children with the irritable bowel syndrome. Aliment Pharmacol Ther 2015;42:418–27.

85. Eswaran S, Chey WD, Jackson K, et al. A diet low in fermentable Oligo-, Di-, and Monosaccharides and Polyols improves quality of life and reduces activity impairment in patients with irritable bowel syndrome and diarrhea. Clin Gastroenterol Hepatol 2017;15:1890–9.e3.

86. Ford AC, Quigley EM, Lacy BE, et al. Effect of antidepressants and psychological therapies, including hypnotherapy, in irritable bowel syndrome: systematic review and meta-analysis. Am J Gastroenterol 2014;109:1350–65 [quiz: 1366].
87. Rutten JM, Vlieger AM, Frankenhuis C, et al. Gut-directed hypnotherapy in children with irritable bowel syndrome or functional abdominal pain (syndrome): a randomized controlled trial on self exercises at home using CD versus individual therapy by qualified therapists. BMC Pediatr 2014;14:140.
88. Lackner JM, Lou Coad M, Mertz HR, et al. Cognitive therapy for irritable bowel syndrome is associated with reduced limbic activity, GI symptoms, and anxiety. Behav Res Ther 2006;44:621–38.
89. Frangos E, Ellrich J, Komisaruk BR. Non-invasive access to the vagus nerve central projections via electrical stimulation of the external ear: fMRI evidence in humans. Brain Stimul 2015;8:624–36.
90. Kovacic K, Hainsworth K, Sood M, et al. Neurostimulation for abdominal pain-related functional gastrointestinal disorders in adolescents: a randomised, double-blind, sham-controlled trial. Lancet Gastroenterol Hepatol 2017;2:727–37.
91. Camilleri M, Di Lorenzo C. Brain-gut axis: from basic understanding to treatment of IBS and related disorders. J Pediatr Gastroenterol Nutr 2012;54:446–53.
92. Kaptchuk TJ, Friedlander E, Kelley JM, et al. Placebos without deception: a randomized controlled trial in irritable bowel syndrome. PLoS One 2010;5:e15591.
93. Benedetti F, Pollo A, Lopiano L, et al. Conscious expectation and unconscious conditioning in analgesic, motor, and hormonal placebo/nocebo responses. J Neurosci 2003;23:4315–23.
94. Finniss DG, Benedetti F. Mechanisms of the placebo response and their impact on clinical trials and clinical practice. Pain 2005;114:3–6.
95. Bradesi S, Tillisch K, Mayer E. Emerging drugs for irritable bowel syndrome. Expert Opin Emerg Drugs 2006;11:293–313.
96. Mayer EA, Tillisch K, Bradesi S. Review article: modulation of the brain-gut axis as a therapeutic approach in gastrointestinal disease. Aliment Pharmacol Ther 2006;24:919–33.
97. Martinez V, Tache Y. CRF1 receptors as a therapeutic target for irritable bowel syndrome. Curr Pharm Des 2006;12:4071–88.
98. Sweetser S, Camilleri M, Linker Nord SJ, et al. Do corticotropin releasing factor-1 receptors influence colonic transit and bowel function in women with irritable bowel syndrome? Am J Physiol Gastrointest Liver Physiol 2009;296:G1299–306.

Pediatric Pancreatitis— Molecular Mechanisms and Management

Maisam Abu-El-Haija, MD[a], Mark E. Lowe, MD, PhD[b],*

KEYWORDS

- Pancreatitis • Children • Severe pancreatitis • Molecular pathways • Genetic testing

KEY POINTS

- Pediatric pancreatitis is an emerging field with an increasing incidence of disease.
- Management of pediatric pancreatitis is understudied and, therefore, extrapolated from adult studies (although the etiologies are different).
- There is evidence that feeding is safe in mild acute pancreatitis in children without increased pain or length of stay.
- Studies are needed to predict course of the disease, disease severity, and risk of chronic pancreatitis in children.

INTRODUCTION

With the publication of studies indicating an increased incidence of acute pancreatitis (AP) in children within the past 2 decades, there has been growing interest in studying pediatric pancreatitis.[1,2] The reported increase in incidence likely results from increased awareness.[2] In addition, there is greater appreciation of the role chronic pancreatitis (CP) plays in childhood and how it leads to increased admissions from repeated episodes of AP.[3,4] In a majority of cases, AP is a single episode, with a subset of 15% to 30% progressing to acute recurrent pancreatitis (ARP); and that is a risk for CP.[5]

MOLECULAR MECHANISMS OF PANCREATITIS
Acute Pancreatitis

The pathogenesis of AP remains enigmatic despite significant new knowledge gained over the past 25 years. Chiari proposed that after an inciting event pancreatitis

Disclosure Statement: M.E. Lowe is on the Board of Directors of the National Pancreas Foundation and receives royalties from Millipore BMH and UpToDate.
[a] Pediatric Gastroenterology, Hepatology and Nutrition, Cincinnati Children's Hospital Medical Center, 3333 Burnet Ave MLC 2010, Cincinnati, Ohio 45229, USA; [b] Pediatric Gastroenterology, Hepatology and Nutrition, Washington University School of Medicine, 660 South Euclid Avenue, MPRB 4th Floor, Campus Box 8208, St Louis, MO 63110, USA
* Corresponding author.
E-mail address: loweme2@upmc.edu

Gastroenterol Clin N Am 47 (2018) 741–753
https://doi.org/10.1016/j.gtc.2018.07.003
0889-8553/18/© 2018 Elsevier Inc. All rights reserved.

gastro.theclinics.com

Abbreviations	
AP	Acute pancreatitis
ARP	Acute recurrent pancreatitis
CASR	Calcium sensing receptor
CEL	Carboxyl ester lipase
CFTR	Cystic fibrosis transmembrane regulator
CP	Chronic pancreatitis
CPA1	Carboxypeptidase 1
CTRC	Chymotrypsin C
ER	Endoplasmic reticulum
NASPGHAN	North American Society for Pediatric Gastroenterology, Hepatology and Nutrition
PRSS1	Cationic trypsinogen gene
SPINK1	Serine protease inhibitor Kazal type 1
UPR	Unfolded protein response

occurred through autodigestion of the gland by prematurely activated digestive enzymes.[6] This theory remains the basis for much work on the molecular details of AP. The concept of a trigger or inciting event is common to all current models of the pathogenesis of AP. Sometimes, the initiating event is known. Medications, gallstones, trauma, endoscopic retrograde cholangiopancreatography, and alcohol are all well-defined triggers for AP. Many times, the initiating event is not known. Which cellular pathways contribute to pancreatitis after the initiating event and why a specific trigger results in AP in some patients but not in others remain vague.

Multiple studies have demonstrated that changes in calcium flux occur early in experimental models of AP.[7] The sources of calcium and downstream targets are currently active areas of investigation. Abundant evidence suggests that calcineurin is an important downstream target of increased intracellular calcium.[8,9] The calcineurin inhibitor, tacrolimus, protected against acinar cell injury in a model of experimental pancreatitis.[10]

Another early event in experimental and human AP is the formation of cytoplasmic vacuoles in acinar cells. The vacuoles appear to contain both zymogen and lysosomal enzymes and are likely autolysophagosomes.[11] Activation of trypsinogen to trypsin occurs in the vacuoles possibly through the action of cathepsin B. Most likely, lowering of the pH in the vacuoles is critical for this cleavage to occur.[12]

Even though it is implicated in formation of the vacuoles, autophagy's role in AP remains controversial. Evidence exists for a protective and harmful role of autophagy in experimental AP. In 1 study, inhibition of autophagy decreased pancreatic damage.[11] Another study provided evidence that autophagy is a protective response in that the process segregates and degrades activated digestive enzymes like trypsin.[13] In this study, inhibition of autophagy increased acinar cell death and up-regulation of autophagy decreased acinar cell injury. The role of autophagy in AP is yet to be further explored.

From current investigations, 2 main models of AP have emerged. The oldest are the trypsin-dependent models. Accordingly, the premature activation of trypsinogen to trypsin within the acinar cell results in acinar cell damage and triggering of an inflammatory response.[14] These models are attractive in that they make intuitive sense; intracellular activation of trypsinogen is observed in experimental models and genetic variants in the cationic trypsinogen gene, PRSS1, cause hereditary pancreatitis.[15] In vitro studies show that the most common genetic variant in PRSS1, p.R122H, shows increased trypsinogen activation.[16] Based on the role of PRSS1 in hereditary pancreatitis, several other genetic variants in genes related to trypsinogen or trypsin regulation, *SPINK1*, *CFTR*, and *CTRC* were found to increase risk for pancreatitis in candidate gene analysis of populations with CP. The role of genetic variants in the mechanisms leading to pancreatitis is evolving as more genetic studies emerge.

Despite the apparent support of these genetic variants for a trypsin-dependent model of pancreatitis, little direct evidence exists for the model. Mouse models of genetic variants have been contradictory and do not provide even weak support for premature trypsinogen activation in pancreatitis. Additionally, the extrapolation of results from genetic variants associated with CP to the pathogenesis of AP is speculative because the relationship of CP and AP has not been clearly defined.

Over the past 15 years, another model for the pathogenesis of AP has emerged— endoplasmic reticulum (ER) stress and the unfolded protein response (UPR).[17] Protein synthesis in the ER results in unfolded polypeptides that require other ER proteins to aid folding and modification. Along with the machinery for folding polypeptides into the proper conformation, the ER has pathways to remove polypeptides that do not fold correctly. When the burden of unfolded proteins increases in the ER, an ER stress response occurs and activates the adaptive, UPR. The response is a quality-control mechanism for restoring protein homeostasis in the ER. The UPR increases synthesis of ER proteins required for proper folding, increases degradation pathways to remove unfolded proteins, and decreases synthesis of other proteins, thereby returning protein homeostasis to a normal balance. When this response is overwhelmed, the UPR activates cell death and inflammatory programs and pancreatitis results. Pancreatic acinar cells synthesize more protein per weight than any other organ. This production makes acinar cells particularly susceptible to altered ER protein homeostasis.

Another attraction of the ER stress model is that many of the known triggers of AP, such as alcohol, smoking, metabolic disorders, and medications, can result in oxidative stress, which is a trigger for ER stress. Furthermore, many of the genetic variants associated with CP increase protein misfolding and activate ER stress pathways and the UPR.[18–20]

Regardless of the mechanism, another phenomenon of AP may play a role in disease progression and severity. In experimental AP, the secretory pathway of acinar cells is altered in a significant way. Normally, zymogen granules release their contents, digestive enzymes, at the apical surface that faces the duct lumen. During AP, zymogen granules release contents along the basolateral membranes where they may deliver digestive enzymes into the interstitial space.[21] The presence of digestive enzymes in the interstitial space may have several results. First, they may be transported into the bloodstream and be the source of elevated pancreatic enzymes in the serum during AP. Second, they may contribute to the pathogenesis of AP. For instance, interstitial trypsin may cleave protease-activated receptors and contribute to the inflammatory response. Pancreatic lipases may participate in causing fat necrosis, a risk factor for more severe disease.[22] Lipotoxicity is a potential mechanism for the increased AP severity in obese adults.[23]

Whether the underlying pathophysiology of AP is trypsin dependent, unmitigated ER stress, or a combination, it has become clear that the molecular details of AP are not simplistic. AP is a complex disorder influenced by interplay among environmental, genetic, and developmental elements. Each of these factors can contribute to susceptibility, progression, and severity of AP. A clear understanding of the pathogenesis will lead to improved therapies for severe pancreatitis and ARP.

Chronic Pancreatitis

The pathogenesis in CP likely overlaps with that of AP. Most adults and children have ARP prior to showing signs of CP.[24,25] With repeated injury to the pancreas, CP may develop overtime, through a fibroinflammatory process that leads to end organ damage.[26] Different immune pathways (macrophage activation, mast cell degranulation, T-lymphocyte activation, and the presence of stellate cells) have been postulated to play a role in the pathogenesis of CP.[27–29] Organ fibrosis, destruction, ductal changes, gland volume loss, and calcifications are late phenomena of CP.[30]

DIAGNOSIS
Acute Pancreatitis

A diagnosis of AP requires 2 of 3 criteria: compatible symptoms, which may vary by age; serum amylase or lipase greater than 3 times upper limit of normal; and imaging findings consistent with pancreatic inflammation, as previously published by the International Study for Pediatric Pancreatitis in Search for a Cure (INSPIRE) criteria.[30,31] The AP criteria are shown in **Box 1**.

Some patients go on to have repeated episodes of AP or ARP. As opposed to patients who have a prolonged course of AP with waxing and waning symptoms, patients with ARP must have complete resolution of pain and greater than a month without pain between episodes or AP. Typically, lipase and amylase return to normal levels between episodes. Patients with ARP do not have the irreversible features of CP.

Chronic Pancreatitis

The definition of CP is controversial and early diagnosis is problematic if not impossible.[32] Typically, CP has been defined as a persistent inflammatory disease of the pancreas characterized by chronic pain, loss of endocrine or exocrine function, and irreversible morphologic changes. In practice, this definition makes a diagnosis of early CP impossible and most patients are diagnosed after CP is well established. A recent group suggested that CP be defined mechanistically as a fibroinflammatory syndrome in patients with risk factors, such as genetic and environmental factors, contributing to a persistent inflammatory response to triggers of pancreatic injury or stress.[32] Although changing the way the mechanism is thought about, this definition does not improve the ability to diagnose CP. Currently, the diagnosis is made based on endoscopic ultrasound and/or other radiological (CT or magnetic resonant imaging (MRI)) changes in the gland and the presence of pain or loss of function.

Box 1
Criteria for acute pancreatitis diagnosis (meeting 2 of 3)

1. Clinical symptoms consistent with pancreatitis: epigastric abdominal pain, nausea, and vomiting

2. Serum lipase and or Serum amylase at or more than the 3 times upper limit of normal

3. Imaging findings of AP on ultrasound, CT, or MRI: edema in the pancreas, fat stranding, fluid collection, and others

Data from Kandula L, Lowe ME. Etiology and outcome of acute pancreatitis in infants and toddlers. J Pediatr 2008;152(1):106–10, 110.e1; and *From* Whitcomb DC, Frulloni L, Garg P, et al. Chronic pancreatitis: an international draft consensus proposal for a new mechanistic definition. Pancreatology 2016;16(2):218–24.

ETIOLOGY
Acute Pancreatitis

AP in adults is mainly due to alcohol and gallstone disease[33,34]; however, in children it results from a host of etiologies: systemic illness, viral, anatomic causes, gallstone, genetic risk factors, and trauma (**Fig. 1**). As with symptoms, the etiology varies with age (**Fig. 2**). Children less than 2 years of age are more likely to have trauma, systemic disease, and inborn errors of metabolism as etiologies than older children. Older children are more likely to have idiopathic and medication-associated etiologies. Biliary disease occurs in all age groups.

Acute Recurrent Pancreatitis and Chronic Pancreatitis

Somewhere between 15% and 30% of children have another discrete episode of AP.[5] In these cases, it is important to test for genetic risk factors, because they occur in more than two-thirds of children with recurrent AP.[25,36] Common genes involved in pancreatitis are PRSS1,[15,37] the serine protease inhibitor Kazal type 1 (SPINK1),[38,39] the cystic fibrosis transmembrane regulator (CFTR),[40,41] chymotrypsin C (CTRC),[42,43] and calcium sensing receptor (CASR) genes.[44] In the past few years, even more genes have been identified as risk factors for ARP and CP, including carboxypeptidase 1 (CPA1)[45] and carboxyl ester lipase (CEL).[46,47] The number of genetic risk variants makes the decision of how best to approach gene testing of great importance. For patients with a family history suggesting hereditary pancreatitis, *PRSS1* testing may be sufficient. For other patients, gene panels are appropriate and have a high yield. The most common commercial panels test for mutations in *PRSS1*, *CFTR*, *SPINK1*, and *CTRC*. Newer panels that screen for risk variants in additional genes are starting to become commercially available and may replace the smaller panels. The issues with the more extensive panels is they are more likely to identify genetic variants of unknown significance and they may be difficult to interpret. The best evidence for pathogenicity of risk variants is available for the genes in the 4 gene panels.

If genetic risk factors are present, patients are likely to progress to CP and should be followed closely. Family history of pancreatitis and genetic mutations

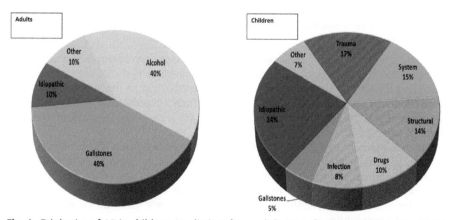

Fig. 1. Etiologies of AP in children are distinct from adult AP. *Left* adult AP etiologies, *Right* Children AP etiologies. A summary pooled from different pediatric and adult studies available prior to year 2014 is represented in the graph. (*Data from* Refs.[1,5,35]; and *Courtesy of* [Pie charts] Lindsey Hornung, MS, Cincinnati, Ohio.)

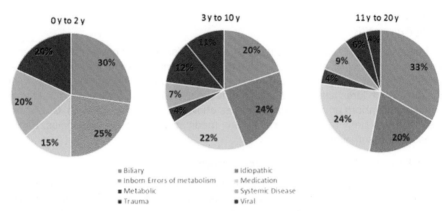

Fig. 2. Etiologies of AP varies by age. (*Reprinted by permission from* Springer Nature: Husain S, Srinath A. What's unique about acute pancreatitis in children: risk factors, diagnosis and management. Nat Rev Gastro Hepat 2017;14;336–72.)

are associated with earlier onset of disease.[48–50] ARP and CP have a significant disease burden for children and families,[3] making investigation into the etiology and progression of pancreatitis in children increasingly important. Genetics-related studies should focus not only on genetic mutations of patients with ARP and CP but also on their phenotypic manifestations of pancreatitis and course of the disease. Gene variants can have differential effects on the rate of progression and the phenotype of the disease. Thus, knowledge of genetic variants in a patient eventually helps the provider to counsel the family about the likely disease course, pain patterns, and progression to endocrine and exocrine insufficiency.[3,36]

The second most common risk factor that is involved in ARP and CP is anatomic or obstructive causes.[25] Other etiologies that contribute to ARP and CP in children include metabolic stressors, drugs, autoimmune, and others. Work-up for ARP should be tailored to investigate these risk factors, because finding a treatable cause may prevent the progression to CP[25] (**Box 2**).

MANAGEMENT OF PANCREATITIS
Acute Pancreatitis

Recently, the North American Society for Pediatric Gastroenterology, Hepatology and Nutrition (NASPGHAN) published management guidelines that can help providers in delivering care for AP patients.[51] A significant proportion of the recommendations were based on adult evidence given the limited studies in pediatrics. The NASPGHAN report highlights the need for pediatric studies to advance our knowledge on management of pediatric AP.

The management of AP in children remains supportive. Adequate hydration, pain control, and the institution of early nutrition are important facets of care. A focused effort to diagnose any treatable underlying cause, such as lipid disorders, gallstone disease, anatomic, calcium or renal imbalances, or traumatic duct injuries, should be undertaken.[5,52] Identification of treatable causes will minimize or eliminate the risk of ARP in in future.

An important issue in the management of AP is that management can vary widely even in the same institution.[53] Much of the variation occurred because different subspecialists, pediatricians, gastroenterologists, nephrologists, hematologists,

---

Box 2
Treatable chronic pancreatitis etiologies

Metabolic/toxic

- Hypercalcemia
- Hyperlipidemia
- Alcohol
- Smoking
- Medications

Autoimmune

- Autoimmune pancreatitis
- Celiac
- Inflammatory bowel disease

Obstructive

- Cholelithiasis
- Biliary sludge
- Biliary anomalies: divisum, choledochal cyst, anomalous insertion of the common bile duct
- Annular pancreas
- Duplication cyst
- Tumors
- Parasites

---

cardiologists and others cared for the patients depending on the presence or absence of underlying comorbid conditions.[53] Because of the variability, an admission order set was developed to standardize AP management following the best available evidence.[54] The order set facilitated the delivery of care as well as standardized the AP management. An initial study of the effect of a standard order set showed that a combination of early feeds and early aggressive fluid resuscitation with isotonic solutions (1.5–2 times maintenance rate) was associated with decreased length of hospital stay, ICU admissions, and severe pancreatitis complications.[54] To date, no data guide the choice of intravenous fluid in children. Either lactated Ringer solution or normal saline is appropriate.

Recent efforts to elucidate the role of nutrition in AP have been published. A study of children by Abu-El-Haija and colleagues[55] showed that feeds in the first 48 hours after presentation were feasible, safe, and not associated with increased lipase levels or worse pain. Importantly, the study showed that dietary fat did not affect the outcome in AP and efforts to provide a low-fat diet are unnecessary. Similar studies in adults also show that enteral feeding is safe and effective when introduced early in the course of AP.[56,57] "Resting" the pancreas is not appropriate in the overwhelming majority of patients with AP.

In terms of pain management, there is no medication that is superior to others in relieving the pain of AP.[58] An increasingly used approach to pain is to start with non-opioid medications for mild to moderate pain and escalate to opioids in cases of severe pain as needed to achieve the balance of adequate analgesia while minimizing the side effects of opioids.[58]

Chronic Pancreatitis

The management of AP episodes in patients with ARP or CP is similar to the management described previously. It is only when complications or end-stage disease develops that management differs. Patients with CP may develop strictures of the main pancreatic ducts or have pancreatic stones lodge in the duct. In these instances, therapeutic endoscopic techniques may be used.[59] The major issue with CP in both children and adults is chronic or frequent episodic pain.[3] Initial therapy for pain should begin with nonopioid medications, such as acetaminophen or nonsteroidal anti-inflammatory drugs. Frequently, gabapentin or amitriptyline is used as well. Too often patients require regular opioid dosing along with an opioid for break-through pain. The role of cognitive behavioral therapy and other nonmedication approaches to pain remains unclear although they are often tried. Pancreatic exocrine insufficiency is treated with pancreatic enzyme replacement therapy and endocrine insufficiency requires insulin under the supervision of an endocrinologist.[60] Patients with end-stage CP and poor quality of life can be referred for surgical therapy. Total pancreatectomy with islet cell autotransplant has become the preferred surgery for many patients, including children.[61] The experience at a large center indicates that children have pain relief and many are insulin independent after the surgery. In most, the quality of life improves.[62]

MANAGEMENT OF SEVERE PANCREATITIS

Although children with AP, with or without underlying ARP or CP, typically do well, up to 30% have severe disease, depending on the definition used.[63,64] Several scoring systems have been published to help identify children who will develop severe AP.[65–67] At present, no scoring system allows the reliable identification of children who will develop complications of AP, and further studies are required ideally classifying patients using the 2017 classification of mild, moderately severe, and severe AP.[65]

Complications can occur early or late in the course of pancreatitis.[68,69] Organ dysfunction or shock, peripancreatic fluid collections, and pancreatic necrosis typically occur early whereas organized pancreatic necrosis or walled-off necrosis, infected necrosis, and pseudocyst formation occur later in the course.[69] The lungs and kidneys are the most commonly involved organs. Pulmonary effusions, acute respiratory distress, or kidney failure may necessitate admission to an ICU. Care is identical to that for any patient with these complications. Death directly related to AP is rare in children and has been reported to range from 5% to 11%.[5] A recent survey of a large national database suggests the death rate is less than 1% from all AP cases in pediatrics.[4] When severe pancreatitis occurs in children, it is not clear what the best fluid management strategy or nutrition modality or even medications to stop the ongoing inflammatory cascade should be.

Both walled-off necrosis and pseudocysts can be managed conservatively and most resolve over time. Only when complications occur should intervention be considered. The most common complication of pseudocysts or walled-off necrosis is obstruction of a nearby organ, often the stomach. Infection and hemorrhage can also occur. In these cases, drainage of the collection for a pseudocyst and drainage with débridement for walled-off necrosis is warranted. Previously, open surgical therapy was the only option in children. Now, interventional radiology, endoscopic, and laparoscopic techniques have supplanted open surgical drainage.[70,71] In adults, a direct comparison of endoscopic and surgical step-up approaches was recently published.[72] Patients were randomized to endoscopic ultrasound-guided transluminal drainage with placement of pigtail stents followed by endoscopic débridement as needed or CT-guided or ultrasound-guided percutaneous catheter drainage followed by video-assisted retroperitoneal drainage as needed. The endoscopic approach reduced pancreatic fistulas, decreased length of hospital stay, and decreased costs, all with no difference in safety. Comparative studies for endoscopic, interventional, or surgical drainage are lacking in children. In general, however, endoscopic procedures, including endoscopic ultrasound, are safe and effective in children.[73]

SUMMARY

Pediatric pancreatitis is increasingly common at children's hospitals. Although most children do well, a subset has significant morbidity, especially if they develop severe pancreatitis or CP complications. Advancements in management are needed to optimize the outcomes from pancreatitis and its complications in pediatric pancreatitis.

REFERENCES

1. Lopez MJ. The changing incidence of acute pancreatitis in children: a single-institution perspective. J Pediatr 2002;140(5):622–4.
2. Morinville VD, Barmada MM, Lowe ME. Increasing incidence of acute pancreatitis at an American pediatric tertiary care center: is greater awareness among physicians responsible? Pancreas 2010;39(1):5–8.
3. Schwarzenberg SJ, Bellin M, Husain SZ, et al. Pediatric chronic pancreatitis is associated with genetic risk factors and substantial disease burden. J Pediatr 2015;166(4):890–6.e1.
4. Abu-El-Haija M, El-Dika S, Hinton A, et al. Acute pancreatitis admision trends: a national estimate through the kids' inpatient database. J Pediatr 2017;194: 147–51.e1.
5. Bai HX, Lowe ME, Husain SZ. What have we learned about acute pancreatitis in children? J Pediatr Gastroenterol Nutr 2011;52(3):262–70.
6. Chiari H. UberdieSelbstverdauung des menschlichen Pankreas. Zeitschrift für Heilkunde 1896;17:69096.
7. Sah RP, Saluja A. Molecular mechanisms of pancreatic injury. Curr Opin Gastroenterol 2011;27(5):444–51.
8. Husain SZ, Grant WM, Gorelick FS, et al. Caerulein-induced intracellular pancreatic zymogen activation is dependent on calcineurin. Am J Physiol Gastrointest Liver Physiol 2007;292(6):G1594–9.
9. Orabi AI, Wen L, Javed TA, et al. Targeted inhibition of pancreatic acinar cell calcineurin is a novel strategy to prevent post-ERCP pancreatitis. Cell Mol Gastroenterol Hepatol 2017;3(1):119–28.
10. Muili KA, Ahmad M, Orabi AI, et al. Pharmacological and genetic inhibition of calcineurin protects against carbachol-induced pathological zymogen activation and acinar cell injury. Am J Physiol Gastrointest Liver Physiol 2012;302(8): G898–905.
11. Hashimoto D, Ohmuraya M, Hirota M, et al. Involvement of autophagy in trypsinogen activation within the pancreatic acinar cells. J Cell Biol 2008;181(7): 1065–72.
12. Waterford SD, Kolodecik TR, Thrower EC, et al. Vacuolar ATPase regulates zymogen activation in pancreatic acini. J Biol Chem 2005;280(7):5430–4.
13. Grasso D, Ropolo A, Lo Re A, et al. Zymophagy, a novel selective autophagy pathway mediated by VMP1-USP9x-p62, prevents pancreatic cell death. J Biol Chem 2011;286(10):8308–24.

14. Sah RP, Dawra RK, Saluja AK. New insights into the pathogenesis of pancreatitis. Curr Opin Gastroenterol 2013;29(5):523–30.

15. Whitcomb DC, Gorry MC, Preston RA, et al. Hereditary pancreatitis is caused by a mutation in the cationic trypsinogen gene. Nat Genet 1996;14(2):141–5.

16. Teich N, Rosendahl J, Toth M, et al. Mutations of human cationic trypsinogen (PRSS1) and chronic pancreatitis. Hum Mutat 2006;27(8):721–30.

17. Pandol SJ, Gorelick FS, Lugea A. Environmental and genetic stressors and the unfolded protein response in exocrine pancreatic function - a hypothesis. Front Physiol 2011;2:8.

18. Kereszturi E, Szmola R, Kukor Z, et al. Hereditary pancreatitis caused by mutation-induced misfolding of human cationic trypsinogen: a novel disease mechanism. Hum Mutat 2009;30(4):575–82.

19. Szmola R, Sahin-Toth M. Pancreatitis-associated chymotrypsinogen C (CTRC) mutant elicits endoplasmic reticulum stress in pancreatic acinar cells. Gut 2010;59(3):365–72.

20. Szabo A, Xiao X, Haughney M, et al. A novel mutation in PNLIP causes pancreatic triglyceride lipase deficiency through protein misfolding. Biochim Biophys Acta 2015;1852(7):1372–9.

21. Gaisano HY, Gorelick FS. New insights into the mechanisms of pancreatitis. Gastroenterology 2009;136(7):2040–4.

22. Patel K, Trivedi RN, Durgampudi C, et al. Lipolysis of visceral adipocyte triglyceride by pancreatic lipases converts mild acute pancreatitis to severe pancreatitis independent of necrosis and inflammation. Am J Pathol 2015;185(3):808–19.

23. Navina S, Acharya C, DeLany JP, et al. Lipotoxicity causes multisystem organ failure and exacerbates acute pancreatitis in obesity. Sci Transl Med 2011;3(107):107ra110.

24. Yadav D, O'Connell M, Papachristou GI. Natural history following the first attack of acute pancreatitis. Am J Gastroenterol 2012;107(7):1096–103.

25. Kumar S, Ooi CY, Werlin S, et al. Risk factors associated with pediatric acute recurrent and chronic pancreatitis: lessons from INSPPIRE. JAMA Pediatr 2016; 170(6):562–9.

26. Jagannath S, Garg PK. Novel and Experimental Therapies in Chronic Pancreatitis. Dig Dis Sci 2017;62(7):1751–61.

27. Xue J, Sharma V, Habtezion A. Immune cells and immune-based therapy in pancreatitis. Immunol Res 2014;58(2–3):378–86.

28. Zimnoch L, Szynaka B, Puchalski Z. Mast cells and pancreatic stellate cells in chronic pancreatitis with differently intensified fibrosis. Hepatogastroenterology 2002;49(46):1135–8.

29. Schmitz-Winnenthal H, Pietsch DH, Schimmack S, et al. Chronic pancreatitis is associated with disease-specific regulatory T-cell responses. Gastroenterology 2010;138(3):1178–88.

30. Morinville VD, Husain SZ, Bai H, et al. Definitions of pediatric pancreatitis and survey of present clinical practices. J Pediatr Gastroenterol Nutr 2012;55(3):261–5.

31. Kandula L, Lowe ME. Etiology and outcome of acute pancreatitis in infants and toddlers. J Pediatr 2008;152(1):106–10, 110.e1.

32. Whitcomb DC, Frulloni L, Garg P, et al. Chronic pancreatitis: an international draft consensus proposal for a new mechanistic definition. Pancreatology 2016;16(2):218–24.

33. Yadav D, Whitcomb DC. The role of alcohol and smoking in pancreatitis. Nat Rev Gastroenterol Hepatol 2010;7(3):131–45.

34. Wang GJ, Gao CF, Wei D, et al. Acute pancreatitis: etiology and common pathogenesis. World J Gastroenterol 2009;15(12):1427–30.

35. Park AJ, Latif SU, Ahmad MU, et al. A comparison of presentation and management trends in acute pancreatitis between infants/toddlers and older children. J Pediatr Gastroenterol Nutr 2010;51(2):167–70.

36. Palermo JJ, Lin TK, Hornung L, et al. Genophenotypic analysis of pediatric patients with acute recurrent and chronic pancreatitis. Pancreas 2016;45(9): 1347–52.

37. Whitcomb DC, Preston RA, Aston CE, et al. A gene for hereditary pancreatitis maps to chromosome 7q35. Gastroenterology 1996;110(6):1975–80.

38. Pfutzer RH, Barmada MM, Brunskill AP, et al. SPINK1/PSTI polymorphisms act as disease modifiers in familial and idiopathic chronic pancreatitis. Gastroenterology 2000;119(3):615–23.

39. Witt H, Luck W, Hennies HC, et al. Mutations in the gene encoding the serine protease inhibitor, Kazal type 1 are associated with chronic pancreatitis. Nat Genet 2000;25(2):213–6.

40. Cohn JA, Friedman KJ, Noone PG, et al. Relation between mutations of the cystic fibrosis gene and idiopathic pancreatitis. N Engl J Med 1998;339(10):653–8.

41. Sharer N, Schwarz M, Malone G, et al. Mutations of the cystic fibrosis gene in patients with chronic pancreatitis. N Engl J Med 1998;339(10):645–52.

42. Rosendahl J, Witt H, Szmola R, et al. Chymotrypsin C (CTRC) variants that diminish activity or secretion are associated with chronic pancreatitis. Nat Genet 2008;40(1):78–82.

43. Masson E, Chen JM, Scotet V, et al. Association of rare chymotrypsinogen C (CTRC) gene variations in patients with idiopathic chronic pancreatitis. Hum Genet 2008;123(1):83–91.

44. Felderbauer P, Klein W, Bulut K, et al. Mutations in the calcium-sensing receptor: a new genetic risk factor for chronic pancreatitis? Scand J Gastroenterol 2006; 41(3):343–8.

45. Witt H, Beer S, Rosendahl J, et al. Variants in CPA1 are strongly associated with early onset chronic pancreatitis. Nat Genet 2013;45(10):1216–20.

46. Xiao X, Jones G, Sevilla WA, et al. A carboxyl ester lipase (CEL) mutant causes chronic pancreatitis by forming intracellular aggregates that activate apoptosis. J Biol Chem 2017;292(19):7744.

47. Fjeld K, Weiss FU, Lasher D, et al. A recombined allele of the lipase gene CEL and its pseudogene CELP confers susceptibility to chronic pancreatitis. Nat Genet 2015;47(5):518–22.

48. Giefer MJ, Lowe ME, Werlin SL, et al. Early-onset acute recurrent and chronic pancreatitis is associated with PRSS1 or CTRC gene mutations. J Pediatr 2017; 186:95–100.

49. Jalaly NY, Moran RA, Fargahi F, et al. An evaluation of factors associated with pathogenic PRSS1, SPINK1, CTFR, and/or CTRC genetic variants in patients with idiopathic pancreatitis. Am J Gastroenterol 2017;112(8):1320–9.

50. Pelaez-Luna M, Robles-Diaz G, Canizales-Quinteros S, et al. PRSS1 and SPINK1 mutations in idiopathic chronic and recurrent acute pancreatitis. World J Gastroenterol 2014;20(33):11788–92.

51. Abu-El-Haija M, Kumar S, Quiros JA, et al. The management of acute pancreatitis in the pediatric population: a clinical report from the NASPGHAN pancreas committee. J Pediatr Gastroenterol Nutr 2018;66(1):159–76.

52. Husain SZ, Morinville V, Pohl J, et al. Toxic-metabolic risk factors in pediatric pancreatitis: recommendations for diagnosis, management, and future research. J Pediatr Gastroenterol Nutr 2016;62(4):609–17.

53. Abu-El-Haija M, Palermo JJ, Fei L, et al. Variability in pancreatitis care in pediatrics: a single institution's survey report. Pancreas 2016;45(1):40–5.

54. Szabo FK, Fei L, Cruz LA, et al. Early enteral nutrition and aggressive fluid resuscitation are associated with improved clinical outcomes in acute pancreatitis. J Pediatr 2015;167(2):397–402.e1.

55. Abu-El-Haija M, Wilhelm R, Heinzman C, et al. Early enteral nutrition in children with acute pancreatitis. J Pediatr Gastroenterol Nutr 2016;62(3):453–6.

56. Kumar S, Gariepy CE. Nutrition and acute pancreatitis: review of the literature and pediatric perspectives. Curr Gastroenterol Rep 2013;15(8):338.

57. Li X, Ma F, Jia K. Early enteral nutrition within 24 hours or between 24 and 72 hours for acute pancreatitis: evidence based on 12 RCTs. Med Sci Monit 2014; 20:2327–35.

58. Abu-El-Haija M, Lin TK, Palermo J. Update to the management of pediatric acute pancreatitis: highlighting areas in need of research. J Pediatr Gastroenterol Nutr 2014;58(6):689–93.

59. Troendle DM, Fishman DS, Barth BA, et al. Therapeutic endoscopic retrograde cholangiopancreatography in pediatric patients with acute recurrent and chronic pancreatitis: data from the INSPPIRE (INternational Study group of Pediatric Pancreatitis: in search for a cuRE) study. Pancreas 2017;46(6):764–9.

60. Duggan SN. Negotiating the complexities of exocrine and endocrine dysfunction in chronic pancreatitis. Proc Nutr Soc 2017;76(4):484–94.

61. Kirchner VA, Dunn TB, Beilman GJ, et al. Total pancreatectomy with islet autotransplantation for acute recurrent and chronic pancreatitis. Curr Treat Options Gastroenterol 2017;15(4):548–61.

62. Bellin MD, Forlenza GP, Majumder K, et al. Total pancreatectomy with islet autotransplantation resolves pain in young children with severe chronic pancreatitis. J Pediatr Gastroenterol Nutr 2017;64(3):440–5.

63. Coffey MJ, Nightingale S, Ooi CY. Serum lipase as an early predictor of severity in pediatric acute pancreatitis. J Pediatr Gastroenterol Nutr 2013;56(6):602–8.

64. Szabo FK, Hornung L, Oparaji JA, et al. A prognostic tool to predict severe acute pancreatitis in pediatrics. Pancreatology 2016;16(3):358–64.

65. Abu-El-Haija M, Kumar S, Szabo F, et al. Classification of acute pancreatitis in the pediatric population: clinical report from the NASPGHAN pancreas committee. J Pediatr Gastroenterol Nutr 2017;64(6):984–90.

66. Debanto JR, Goday PS, Pedroso MR, et al. Acute pancreatitis in children. Am J Gastroenterol 2002;97(7):1726–31.

67. Grover AS, Kadiyala V, Banks PA, et al. The utility of the systemic inflammatory respsonse syndrome score on admission in children with acute pancreatitis. Pancreas 2017;46(1):106–9.

68. Balthazar EJ. Complications of acute pancreatitis: clinical and CT evaluation. Radiol Clin North Am 2002;40(6):1211–27.

69. Banks PA, Bollen TL, Dervenis C, et al. Classification of acute pancreatitis–2012: revision of the Atlanta classification and definitions by international consensus. Gut 2013;62(1):102–11.

70. Gurusamy KS, Pallari E, Hawkins N, et al. Management strategies for pancreatic pseudocysts. Cochrane Database Syst Rev 2016;(4):CD011392.

71. Shah A, Denicola R, Edirisuriya C, et al. Management of inflammatory fluid collections and walled-off pancreatic necrosis. Curr Treat Options Gastroenterol 2017; 15(4):576–86.
72. van Brunschot S, van Grinsven J, van Santvoort HC, et al. Endoscopic or surgical step-up approach for infected necrotising pancreatitis: a multicentre randomised trial. Lancet 2018;391(10115):51–8.
73. Nabi Z, Talukdar R, Reddy DN. Endoscopic management of pancreatic fluid collections in children. Gut Liver 2017;11(4):474–80.

Inflammatory Bowel Disease
What Very Early Onset Disease Teaches Us

Eileen Crowley, MD[a,b,c], Aleixo Muise, MD, PhD, FRCPC[d,e,f],*

KEYWORDS

- Very early onset • Inflammatory bowel disease • Monogenic disease
- Whole-exome sequencing • Targeted therapy • Personalized care

KEY POINTS

- Phenotypic and genotypic disease characteristics may be unique to children with very early onset inflammatory bowel disease (VEO-IBD), who may present with more severe disease due to a single gene defect.
- Pathway analysis of these gene defects allows us to learn more about the etiology of this disease.
- Epidemiologic data suggest that the prevalence of childhood-onset IBD is increasing, with the greatest percentage increases observed in the youngest children.
- Advances in diagnostic clinical genomics are becoming the integrated standard of care for this complex group with extreme phenotypes.
- Identifying monogenic causal variants using sequencing techniques and understanding the pathways involved allows pathway-specific therapy, with the aim of providing a personalized medicine approach to IBD care.

INTRODUCTION

Inflammatory bowel disease (IBD) is a chronic relapsing inflammatory condition of the gastrointestinal tract that often begins in childhood. Traditionally, it is characterized by 2 major phenotypes: Crohn disease (CD) and ulcerative colitis (UC).

[a] Cell Biology Program, Division of Gastroenterology, Hepatology and Nutrition, Inflammatory Bowel Disease Center, The Hospital for Sick Children, 555 University Avenue, Toronto, ON M5G 1X8, Canada; [b] School of Medicine, Conway Institute, University College Dublin, Belfield, Dublin 4, Ireland; [c] Department of Pediatric Gastroenterology, Hepatology and Nutrition, SickKids, 555 University Avenue, Toronto, Ontario M5G 1X8, Canada; [d] Department of Biochemistry, Institute of Medical Science, University of Toronto, 1 King's College Circle, Toronto, ON M5S 1A8, Canada; [e] Department of Pediatrics, Institute of Medical Science, University of Toronto, 1 King's College Circle, Toronto, ON M5S 1A8, Canada; [f] Division of Gastroenterology, Hepatology and Nutrition, Cell Biology Program, Research Institute, The Hospital for Sick Children, University of Toronto, SickKids, Inflammatory Bowel Disease Centre, 555 University Avenue, Toronto, Ontario M5G 1X8, Canada
* Corresponding author. Division of Gastroenterology, Hepatology and Nutrition, Cell Biology Program, Research Institute, The Hospital for Sick Children, University of Toronto, SickKids, Inflammatory Bowel Disease Centre, 555 University Avenue, Toronto, Ontario M5G 1X8, Canada.
E-mail address: aleixo.muise@sickkids.ca

Gastroenterol Clin N Am 47 (2018) 755–772
https://doi.org/10.1016/j.gtc.2018.07.004
0889-8553/18/© 2018 Elsevier Inc. All rights reserved.
gastro.theclinics.com

Abbreviations	
CD	Crohn disease
CVID	Common variable immunodeficiency
GWAS	Genome-wide association studies
HSCT	Hematopoietic stem cell transplantation
IBD	Inflammatory bowel disease
IPEX	Immune dysregulation, polyendocrinopathy, enteropathy X-linked syndrome
SNP	Single-nucleotide polymorphisms
UC	Ulcerative colitis
WAS	Wiskott Aldrich syndrome
WES	Whole-exome sequencing
WGS	Whole-genome sequencing
XIAP	X-linked inhibitor of apoptosis protein gene

CD can affect any part of the digestive tract and manifests as transmural inflammation, leading to serious complications, such as intestinal stricture formation, fistulization, and development of abscesses.[1] The inflammatory process in UC is confined to the superficial mucosa of the colon only and occurs in a continuous fashion proximally, from the anus.[2] IBD has become a global disease with accelerating incidence in newly industrialized countries.[3] It has been estimated, that 20% to 30% of new cases of IBD present before the age of 20 years.[4] Interestingly, the increasing incidence is most notable in younger children.[5] As per the Paris classification, children diagnosed at age of onset of younger than 10 years are categorized as "A1a," with those diagnosed below this value termed VEO-IBD.[6] However, this age cutoff has been debated in the literature (**Table 1**). These younger children often present with a distinct form of disease, which is phenotypically and genetically different from older-onset IBD. This unique subgroup accounts for 4% to 15% of pediatric IBD.[7–9] Despite recent advances, the etiology of IBD remains largely unknown. It is proposed that an interplay of genetic factors, environment, microbiota, and immune responses are all involved in the pathogenesis of the disease[10] (**Fig. 1**). However, advances in the understanding of the genetic contribution, which appears to be much more significant in younger children, gives us a useful insight into the pathogenesis and potential future therapeutic targets in IBD.

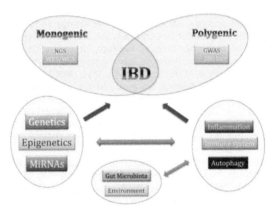

Fig. 1. Proposed etiology of pediatric IBD. miRNA, microRNA; NGS, next-generation sequencing. (*From* Loddo I, Romano C. Inflammatory bowel disease: genetics, epigenetics, and pathogenesis. Front Immunol 2015;6:551; with permission.)

EPIDEMIOLOGY

An epidemiologic shift has been recently reported in adult-onset IBD where societies have become more westernized. Although it is widely accepted that rates of pediatric IBD are increasing worldwide, accurate estimates are lacking.[11] Published international incidence rates for IBD in children range from 0.47 per 100,000 in Saudi Arabia to 15.9 per 100,000 in the South Asian population in British Columbia, Canada.[12,13] The EPIMAD registry, which obtained data from a cohort enrolled in a prospective French population-based registry from 1988 to 2011, suggested a stable rate of VEO-IBD, but an increasing incidence of early-onset IBD (EO-IBD, diagnosis from 6 to 16 years), by 116%.[8] More recently, in a Canadian study, it has been established that the age group with the most rapidly increasing incidence is those aged younger than 5 years (**Fig. 2**).[5] Evidence also suggests that although immigrants to the western world have a lower incidence of IBD than that of nonimmigrants, children of individuals immigrating from some low-prevalence regions in Asia have a similarly high incidence of IBD compared with the children of nonimmigrants.[14,15] This increasing global burden of IBD will pose significant challenges to health care systems around the world. Genetic risk most likely remains static, leading to a postulation that it is an environmental modifier or shift in microbiota or immune response that is driving the increase in incidence in this younger age group, making this a critical cohort of patients that deserve close study to further investigate the etiology of IBD.

CLINICAL PRESENTATION OF VERY EARLY ONSET INFLAMMATORY BOWEL DISEASE

There is a distinct difference to be noted in the presentation of early-onset versus later-onset IBD. In contrast to adult-onset disease, children with UC often present with pancolitis, whereas children with CD often present with ileocolonic disease and only rarely present with ileal disease in isolation.[16–18] Of note, CD in children diagnosed when younger than 8 years is often isolated colonic inflammation (L2), which may lead to a misclassification of UC or indeterminate colitis during the initial evaluation.[8,19] At presentation, there does not appear to be a difference regarding the rates of complicated forms of CD, stricturing (B2), or penetrating (B3) disease.[8] Of the infantile age group (<2 years), for those who present with IBD, there does not appear to be a difference in disease location in the group younger than 2 years old versus those who present in the 3-year to 6-year age group.[8] The exact time point at which age of diagnosis of CD changes from colonic to a more ileal presentation has yet to be determined. The subclassifications of pediatric patients attempted to address this issue. Children diagnosed with disease at younger than 17 years were categorized as a single group in the Montreal Classification for IBD.[6,20] Subsequently, the Paris Modification divided pediatric-onset IBD into 2 groups: A1a, children diagnosed when younger than 10 years of age, and A1b, children diagnosed between 10 to 17 years of age. This age classification addresses the fact that from the age of 7 years, there is a substantial rise in the frequency of patients with a diagnosis of conventional polygenic IBD, particularly CD.[21,22] Serologic patterns have also been noted to differ in those diagnosed with CD <8 years; CBir1 positivity with otherwise negative serology and a low rate of anti–*Saccharomyces cerevisiae* antibodies.[23,24]

Children who present with IBD at age younger than 6 years are often phenotypically and genotypically distinct from older children. A further subgroup, those younger than 2 years, have limited published evidence on their phenotype. From case series, evidence suggests that they often have more severe presentations

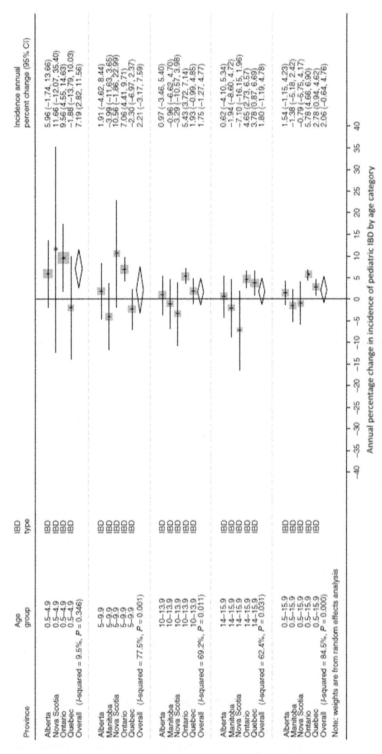

Fig. 2. Increasing incidence of IBD in children younger than 5 years. CI, confidence interval. (*Reprinted by permission from Springer Nature: Benchimol EI, Bernstein CN, Bitton A, et al. Trends in Epidemiology of Pediatric Inflammatory Bowel Disease in Canada: Distributed Network Analysis of Multiple Population-Based Provincial Health Administrative Databases. Am J Gastroenterol. 2017;112(7):1128.*)

and serious infections may complicate their disease course, raising the concerns of immunodeficiency.[25] Those younger than 6 years are also believed to have a more aggressive disease course; however, recent evidence appears to refute this. This group still presents as a heterogeneous population, with some children having very mild disease.[9] Of concern in those presenting at an earlier age are the effects of chronic inflammation on growth and global development.[26] From the EPIMAD registry, rectal bleeding and mucous stools were more frequent at diagnosis in the VEO-IBD group, reflecting a colonic location, whereas weight loss and abdominal pain were the most frequent clinical symptoms in the EO-IBD group.[8,27] There does not appear to be a difference in the frequency of diarrhea or number of extraintestinal manifestations between those who present earlier in childhood as opposed to later.[8] However, morbidity does appear to be higher in the VEO-IBD population, given that they may not respond to conventional therapies, and may have more severe degrees of inflammation, resulting in profound effects on growth and a greater duration of disease.[26,28] Overall, however, Benchimol and colleagues[9] established that children in the VEO-IBD age group had lower emergency department visits and hospitalizations.

DIAGNOSIS OF VERY EARLY ONSET INFLAMMATORY BOWEL DISEASE

Guidelines do not exist for the diagnostic approach to VEO-IBD. Initial steps are the same as in older children: assessment of intestinal and extraintestinal disease phenotypes by clinical, laboratory, radiologic, and endoscopic evaluation. Interestingly, more cases appear to be diagnosed as inpatients, perhaps owing to the younger ages of the children.[8] However, important features to note in the patient's clinical history that can direct further investigative tests include age of symptom onset, history of consanguinity, family history of inflammatory or autoimmune conditions, history of disease in male family members (X-linked disease), or a history of severe or recurrent infections, skin disease, or autoimmunity. These features may suggest a monogenic defect. For those with a high suspicion for monogenic disease, immunology support should be sought to allow for vaccine titers, immunoglobulin profiles, analyses of B-cell and T-cell function, analysis of oxidative burst by neutrophils (using the nitro blue tetrazolium test or a dihydrorhodamine flow cytometry assay), and if necessary, more targeted profiling of the systemic and mucosal immune system. Liaison with pathology colleagues also may be useful to look for apoptosis, thought to be associated with monogenic disease or more specifically villous atrophy or epithelial cell shedding (*NEMO*), severe apoptosis (*TTC7A*), or hypoplastic crypts (*ADAM17*), on biopsy specimens and further staining to investigate features of monogenic disease. Ultimately, the child, especially those with extreme phenotypes, will require whole-exome sequencing (WES) with variant confirmation by Sanger sequencing, complementary DNA sequencing, or polymerase chain reaction methods. Functional validation, if a genetic variant is identified, is important to confirm the variant before taking clinical action. WES has a role in both explanatory and predictive clinical genomics in the VEO-IBD group. Advances in diagnostic clinical genomics are becoming integrated standard of care for this complex group. Mendelian disorder–associated IBD is enriched in infantile and VEO-IBD, but does not exclusively present in this age group.[29] This challenges the clinician to consider the role of genomic medicine beyond the VEO-IBD age group.

Consideration should be given to gene-specific differences in the age of onset. The reported time of onset of IBD-like immunopathology in subgroups, for example,

Table 1
Clinical classifications of pediatric IBD

Group	Classification	Age Range, y	Disease Distribution	Disease Classification	Positive Family History, %	Genetic Contribution
Pediatric-onset IBD	Montreal A1 Paris A1a or A1b	<17	Ileocolonic	CD > UC/IBD-U	10–20	Polygenic inheritance
Early-onset IBD (EO-IBD)	Paris A1a	<10	Predominantly colonic	UC/IBD-U > CD	30–40	Increased contribution of monogenic disease
Very early onset IBD (VEO-IBD)		<6	Colonic, ileal involvement <20%		20	
Infantile (and toddler) onset		<2	Colonic			
Neonatal IBD		<28 d of life	Colonic			

Abbreviations: CD, Crohn disease; IBD, inflammatory bowel disease; IBD-U, IBD-unclassified; UC, ulcerative colitis.

Data from Uhlig HH, Schwerd T, Koletzko S, et al. The diagnostic approach to monogenic very early onset inflammatory bowel disease. Gastroenterology 2014;147(5):990–1007.e3; and Bequet E, Sarter H, Fumery M, et al. Incidence and phenotype at diagnosis of very-early-onset compared with later-onset paediatric inflammatory bowel disease: a population-based study [1988-2011]. J Crohns Colitis 2017;11(5):519–26.

interleukin *(IL)-10* signaling defects, Wiskott Aldrich Syndrome (WAS) or immune dysregulation, polyendocrinopathy, enteropathy X-linked syndrome (IPEX), is infancy and early childhood. However, atypical late onset of IBD has been reported in patients with *WAS* and *IPEX*.[30,31] Age of onset is variable in neutrophil defects and *XIAP* deficiency. Common variable immunodeficiency (CVID) may manifest for the first time in early childhood or as late as the eighth decade of life.[32] Other disorders, such as *GUCY2C* deficiency, typically develop during adulthood. Monogenic phenotypes may change over time, gastrointestinal symptoms can present as an initial or a later finding.[7]

Clinical judgment is required to select which children should undergo WES. The checklist provided in **Box 1** gives some guidance on who should be considered. WES analysis is strengthened when not only the proband (patient) is sequenced, but also direct family members of the proband. This allows investigators to perform family linkage analysis, enabling better information to be drawn from the results. WES analysis is also improved when clear phenotypes can be provided to the investigator; this will allow genotypic phenotypic analysis to be performed, which concentrates the investigator's interest to certain areas of the genome. However, resources have to be made available to those families who engage in genomic medicine, including multidisciplinary team assessment, and pre-sequencing and post-sequencing counseling. With the increased complexity and interplay of genetics, immunology, and gastroenterology, an interdisciplinary approach is vital to provide the best diagnostic and therapeutic supports for patients and their families (**Box 1, Fig. 3**).

GENETICS

The initial suggestion supporting a genetic causation for IBD is highlighted by the high concordance rates for CD in monozygotic twins and the increased risk of familial inheritance of children with parents who have a diagnosis of IBD.[33–36] Genetic factors now are estimated to contribute 20% to 25% of disease heritability.[37] Host genetics are recognized to play a more predominant role in children with a diagnosis of VEO-IBD.[38,39] Evidence suggests that in some cases, VEO-IBD can be considered a monogenic disease, or multigenic enriched with rare variants, often involving genes associated with primary immunodeficiencies.[28,38]

Initially via genetic linkage analysis studies, genetic risk was found in major histocompatibility complex Class II molecules with both UC (*DR2, DR9*, and *DRB1*0103*)

Box 1
Checklist for those who may benefit from investigative clinical genomic testing

- Extreme severe phenotype
- Early age of onset, all younger than 2 years, consider at younger than 6 years
- Severe perianal disease
- Recurrent or atypical infections
- Family history or consanguinity
- Failure of conventional medical treatment
- Early progression to surgery
- Atypical findings on histology; that is, apoptosis
- Hemophagocytic lymphohistiocytosis or early development of tumors

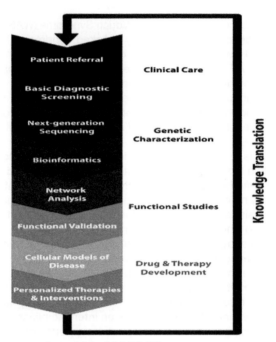

Fig. 3. Diagnostic approach to child with VEO-IBD.

and CD (*DR7, DR3*0103,* and *DQ4*).[40–42] CD risk loci of *IBD1* and *IBD5* were identified from linkage studies with large pedigrees enrolled.[43,44] *NOD2* was one of the key discoveries, which explained the pivotal role of the cross link between intestinal microbiota and the innate immune system in IBD pathogenesis.[45,46]

Genome-wide association studies (GWASs) have rapidly expanded our knowledge of the role of common genetic variants in complex genetic disease pathogenesis (**Table 2**). Currently, more than 230 risk loci have been associated with IBD.[47–49] Initial GWASs focused on adult-onset cohorts, which is often a more polygenic, complex disease. These studies identified specific clinical phenotypic presentations that are associated with NOD2 single-nucleotide polymorphism (SNP) carriers: ileal involvement and surgical resection.[50,51] More recently, genetic association studies have identified variants that are associated with IBD disease severity, such as progression to surgery.[52] These initial GWASs prompted investigators to explore the genetic phenotypic variation of pediatric-onset IBD.

Monogenic defects alter intestinal immune homeostasis via several mechanisms. GWASs identified SNPs associated with IBD risk that are in loci of genes involved in, for example, autophagy, adaptive immunity, maintenance of epithelial integrity, and endoplasmic reticular stress.[47,53,54] GWASs failed to detect large differences between adult-onset and pediatric-onset disease,[55,56] but children often included in these initial studies were older children and adolescents. However, many adult-onset CD SNPs (including *IL23R, NOD2,* and *LRRK2*) play a role in pediatric-onset CD. GWASs that included pediatric-onset–only IBD replicated associations with 8 of 17 UC SNPs (including *IL-10*). Interestingly, pediatric IBD GWASs identified novel SNPs not seen in earlier adult-onset IBD studies (*IL-27*, TNFRSF6B).[55,56] Furthermore, SNPs may have different effects in different age groups; *ZMIZ1* SNP (*rs 1250550*) had a protective effect in pediatric CD, whereas this SNP and others within the region were found to confer increased risk for adult-onset CD.[55,57]

Table 2
Quick reference guide to the more common genetic variants associated with VEO-IBD with some salient clinical features

Gene	Associated Syndrome	Phenotypic Features
Variants influencing intestinal barrier function		
ADAM17	ADAM17 deficiency[67]	Neonatal diarrhea: watery, progresses to bloody
COL7A1	Dystrophic epidermolysis bullosa[68]	Bloody diarrhea
EPCAM	Tufting enteropathy[69]	Neonatal diarrhea
FERMT1	Kindler syndrome[70]	Skin trauma–induced blistering, esophageal and anal stenosis, hemorrhagic colitis
GUCY2	Familial diarrhea[39,71]	Neonatal onset of watery diarrhea
IKBKG (NEMO)	X-linked ectodermal dysplasia and immunodeficiency[72]	Diarrhea, failure to thrive, susceptibility to infection
TTC7A	Familial diarrhea[66]	Enterocolitis, immunodeficiency, recurrent intestinal atresia
Variants impairing development of adaptive immune system		
ARPC1B	WAS-like phenotype and intestinal inflammation[73]	Micro-thrombocytopenia, defects in platelet function, invasive infections, IBD, vasculitis, eosinophilia
DOCK8	Hyper IgM, Hyper IgE syndrome[39]	Susceptibility to infection (staphylococcal) and intestinal inflammation
LRBA	Defects in immune cell populations[65]	Hypogammaglobinemia and intestinal inflammation.
PTEN	PTEN syndrome[74]	Inflammatory polyps, multiple tumors, immune dysregulation, autoimmunity.[75]
RAG1 or RAG 2	Omenn syndrome[76]	Diffuse erythroderma, hepatosplenomegaly, lymphadenopathy, and intestinal disease.
RAG1, RAG2, JAK3, CD45, CD3G, ZAP70, ADA, DCLRE1C	Combined variable immunodeficiency (CVID)[7,77]	
WASP	WAS[78]	Thrombocytopenia, eczema, immune deficiencies and intestinal inflammation
Variants impairing regulatory T cells		
FOXP3 (also IL-2, IL2RA/CD25,MALT1STAT3, STAT 5B, ITCH, STAT1, CTLA4)	IPEX syndrome[76,79] IPEX-like	Colonic disease and enteropathy ± neonatal diarrhea, failure to thrive, infection, skin rash, diabetes, thyroiditis, cytopenias, autoimmunity

(continued on next page)

Gene	Associated Syndrome	Phenotypic Features
Table 2 *(continued)*		
Gene	**Associated Syndrome**	**Phenotypic Features**
Variants in the IL-10/IL-10R pathway		
IL10, IL10RA, IL10RB	Neonatal or infantile VEO-IBD[80]	Severe enterocolitis and perianal disease (+/− arthritis, folliculitis, lymphoma)
IL10RA	Neonatal Crohn disease[81]	Enterocolitis
Variants influencing bacterial recognition and clearance		
CYBB, CYBA, NCF1, NCF2, NCF4	Chronic granulomatous disease (CGD)[82]	Intestinal inflammation and autoimmune disease
ITGB2	IBD phenotype[83]	Bacterial infections, laboratory studies notable for peripheral granulocytes
NCF2	Neonatal colitis[84]	Colitis, severe fistulizing perianal disease, stricturing
Variants affecting innate defense		
XIAP	X-linked lymphoproliferative syndrome (XLP1/2)[61,63]	Severe colonic and perianal fistulizing disease, EBV can result in fatal HLH
TRIM22	IBD phenotype[85]	Granulomatous colitis and perianal disease

Abbreviations: CD, Crohn disease; EBV, Epstein-Barr virus; HLH, Hemophagocytic lymphohistiocytosis; IBD, inflammatory bowel disease; Ig, immunoglobulin; IL, interleukin; IPEX, immune dysregulation, polyendocrinopathy, enteropathy X-linked syndrome; VEO-IBD, very early onset IBD; WAS, Wiskott Aldrich syndrome.

Next-generation sequencing techniques, such as WES, are now one of the accepted approaches used to investigate children with VEO-IBD. The exome includes all coding regions that comprise approximately 1% to 2% of the human genome.[58] This technique enables identification of de novo causative mutations in genes, which may be highly penetrant. One of the first single-gene defects identified were of *IL-10* and *IL-10* receptor in infantile VEO-IBD, which result in the phenotype of severe perianal disease and colitis.[28,59] WES led to the discovery of a hemizygous mutation in X-linked inhibitor of apoptosis protein gene (*XIAP*) in an infant with aggressive colitis.[60] Patients with *XIAP* deficiency develop an X-linked lymphoproliferative type syndrome and Epstein-Barr virus can trigger life-threatening hemophagocytic lymphohistiocytosis.[61] Patients with *XIAP* deficiency can present with pediatric CD[62,63]; however, the penetrance of IBD-like intestinal inflammation in patients with *XIAP* deficiency is approximately 30% to 40%, ranging from neonatal to adult-onset IBD.[61,64] Further studies led to a discovery of a homozygous mutation in LRBA in a patient with common variable immunodeficiency and *TTC7A* in a patient with recurrent intestinal atresia, combined immunodeficiency, and enterocolitis.[65,66] The seminal VEO-IBD paper by Uhlig and colleagues[7] in 2014 lists 50 genetic disorders identified and associated with IBD-like immunopathology.

A more complete method is to perform whole-genome sequencing (WGS), which allows complete investigation of every locus throughout the human genome. The most challenging aspect of WGS is the extensive data load that results, which makes interpretation difficult.

MANAGEMENT OF VERY EARLY ONSET INFLAMMATORY BOWEL DISEASE

It has been well described that children who present early may have a more severe disease course. Children with IBD are more likely to receive corticosteroids, commence immunomodulators, and require surgery in the first year after diagnosis than adults with IBD.[86,87] Kammermeier and colleagues[88] examined a cohort of infantile-onset IBD, in whom 40% required parenteral nutrition, 31% extensive immunosuppression, 29% hematopoietic stem cell transplantation (HSCT), and 19% surgery. However, VEO-IBD represents a cohort, albeit the minority, who may be completely cured of their disease via HSCT. Our growing understanding of the immunopathogenesis of this disease has opened new avenues for developing targeted therapies. Novel tools investigators are using include enteroids as a conduit to further understand the etiology of the disease, along with using them for high-throughput drug screening to target enterocyte defects.[89] Recent advances have challenged investigators to address "actionable" genetic information (**Table 3**). This is the identification of pathogenic genetic variants in patients with IBD that offers individualized treatment pathways, including the appropriate use of HSCT, pathway-specific biologic therapies, and informed use of elective surgery. Importantly, it informs of treatment strategies that may not be appropriate and that may even cause harm. For example, there is evidence that patients with epithelial barrier defects should not be

---

Table 3
Potential "actionable": gene defects recognized in VEO-IBD

Gene Defect	Potential Therapeutic Approach	Contraindications to Therapy
IL10 and IL 10 receptor	HSCT likely curative[80,91]	
FOXP3, IL2RA, CTLA4, MALT1	HSCT likely curative[92]	
XIAP	HSCT likely curative[60]	
SH2D1A	HSCT likely curative[93]	
DCLRE1C	HSCT likely curative[94]	
ZAP70	HSCT likely curative[95]	
WAS	HSCT likely curative[96]	
CGD *CYBB, CYBA, NCF1, NCF2, NCF4*	HSCT likely curative[97] Leukine antibiotics, IL-1 receptor antagonist (Anakinra), possible use to bridge to HSCT or if HSCT not available[98,99]	Anti-TNF contraindicated: increase risk of severe infections, may be fatal[100]
EPCAM		HSCT not helpful[101]
TTC7A		HSCT not helpful[102]
Mevalonate kinase deficiency, *NLRC4* gene defects, IL-10 R deficiency	IL-1 targets[29]	
NLRC4	IL-18, ILR inhibition[103]	
LRBA deficiency	CTLA4 fusion protein: Abatacept (possible use to bridge to HSCT)[104]	
STAT1	HSCT *or* Janus kinase inhibitor Ruxolitinib[105]	

Abbreviations: HSCT, hematopoietic stem cell transplantation; IL, interleukin; TNF, tumor necrosis factor; VEO-IBD, very early onset inflammatory bowel disease.

considered for HSCT, because this does not correct the defect that causes the disease (*NEMO* deficiency or *TTC7A* deficiency).[90] Furthermore, engaging in genomic medicine should provoke referral for family counseling and screening for tumors and infections.[29]

SUMMARY

VEO-IBD is a unique subgroup of potentially phenotypically and genetically different patients from those who present in older age groups. As our understanding evolves, the different components of the immune system, including innate and adaptive responses involved in VEO-IBD are coming to light. As we continue to investigate the pathways involved in VEO-IBD, we gain further insight into the pathophysiology of this complex disease. This knowledge can be directly translated into potential therapeutic targets that will not only influence the care of these young children, but may be applicable to patients who present later. Advances in diagnostic clinical genomics, along with translational studies exploring the functions of these genes, allow for an exciting mechanistic insight into the role of immune dysregulation in intestinal inflammation highlighting the exceptional potential for personalized precision medicine to children with VEO-IBD.

In conclusion, awareness of physicians to extreme phenotypes due to monogenic forms of IBD will accelerate discovery in this field. The further pursuit of phenotypic genotypic relationships in VEO-IBD will give us insight into the complexity of this monogenic disease. Careful study of the pathways involved allows us to gain further understanding of the immune dysregulation in intestinal inflammation. Aiming to provide personalization of IBD care through targeted therapies will be the future goal of IBD therapy.

REFERENCES

1. Baumgart DC, Sandborn WJ. Crohn's disease. Lancet 2012;380(9853): 1590–605.
2. Ordas I, Eckmann L, Talamini M, et al. Ulcerative colitis. Lancet 2012;380(9853): 1606–19.
3. Ng SC, Shi HY, Hamidi N, et al. Worldwide incidence and prevalence of inflammatory bowel disease in the 21st century: a systematic review of population-based studies. Lancet 2017;390(10114):2769–78.
4. Loftus EV Jr. Clinical epidemiology of inflammatory bowel disease: incidence, prevalence, and environmental influences. Gastroenterology 2004;126(6):1504–17.
5. Benchimol EI, Bernstein CN, Bitton A, et al. Trends in epidemiology of pediatric inflammatory bowel disease in Canada: distributed network analysis of multiple population-based provincial health administrative databases. Am J Gastroenterol 2017;112(7):1120–34.
6. Levine A, Griffiths A, Markowitz J, et al. Pediatric modification of the Montreal classification for inflammatory bowel disease: the Paris classification. Inflamm Bowel Dis 2011;17(6):1314–21.
7. Uhlig HH, Schwerd T, Koletzko S, et al. The diagnostic approach to monogenic very early onset inflammatory bowel disease. Gastroenterology 2014;147(5): 990–1007.e3.
8. Bequet E, Sarter H, Fumery M, et al. Incidence and phenotype at diagnosis of very-early-onset compared with later-onset paediatric inflammatory bowel disease: a population-based study [1988-2011]. J Crohns Colitis 2017;11(5):519–26.

9. Benchimol EI, Mack DR, Nguyen GC, et al. Incidence, outcomes, and health services burden of very early onset inflammatory bowel disease. Gastroenterology 2014;147(4):803–13.e7 [quiz: e14–5].

10. Loddo I, Romano C. Inflammatory bowel disease: genetics, epigenetics, and pathogenesis. Front Immunol 2015;6:551.

11. Benchimol EI, Fortinsky KJ, Gozdyra P, et al. Epidemiology of pediatric inflammatory bowel disease: a systematic review of international trends. Inflamm Bowel Dis 2011;17(1):423–39.

12. El Mouzan MI, Saadah O, Al-Saleem K, et al. Incidence of pediatric inflammatory bowel disease in Saudi Arabia: a multicenter national study. Inflamm Bowel Dis 2014;20(6):1085–90.

13. Pinsk V, Lemberg DA, Grewal K, et al. Inflammatory bowel disease in the South Asian pediatric population of British Columbia. Am J Gastroenterol 2007;102(5): 1077–83.

14. Benchimol EI, Mack DR, Guttmann A, et al. Inflammatory bowel disease in immigrants to Canada and their children: a population-based cohort study. Am J Gastroenterol 2015;110(4):553–63.

15. Benchimol EI, Manuel DG, To T, et al. Asthma, type 1 and type 2 diabetes mellitus, and inflammatory bowel disease amongst South Asian immigrants to Canada and their children: a population-based cohort study. PLoS One 2015;10(4): e0123599.

16. Sawczenko A, Sandhu BK, Logan RF, et al. Prospective survey of childhood inflammatory bowel disease in the British Isles. Lancet 2001;357(9262):1093–4.

17. Henriksen M, Jahnsen J, Lygren I, et al. Ulcerative colitis and clinical course: results of a 5-year population-based follow-up study (the IBSEN study). Inflamm Bowel Dis 2006;12(7):543–50.

18. Van Limbergen J, Russell RK, Drummond HE, et al. Definition of phenotypic characteristics of childhood-onset inflammatory bowel disease. Gastroenterology 2008;135(4):1114–22.

19. Abraham BP, Mehta S, El-Serag HB. Natural history of pediatric-onset inflammatory bowel disease: a systematic review. J Clin Gastroenterol 2012;46(7):581–9.

20. Silverberg MS, Satsangi J, Ahmad T, et al. Toward an integrated clinical, molecular and serological classification of inflammatory bowel disease: report of a Working Party of the 2005 Montreal World Congress of Gastroenterology. Can J Gastroenterol 2005;19(Suppl A):5A–36A.

21. Lopez-Granados E, Keenan JE, Kinney MC, et al. A novel mutation in NFKBIA/IKBA results in a degradation-resistant N-truncated protein and is associated with ectodermal dysplasia with immunodeficiency. Hum Mutat 2008;29(6):861–8.

22. Fujii K, Miyashita T, Omata T, et al. Gorlin syndrome with ulcerative colitis in a Japanese girl. Am J Med Genet A 2003;121A(1):65–8.

23. Markowitz J, Kugathasan S, Dubinsky M, et al. Age of diagnosis influences serologic responses in children with Crohn's disease: a possible clue to etiology? Inflamm Bowel Dis 2009;15(5):714–9.

24. Steven LC, Driver CP. Niemann-pick disease type C and Crohn's disease. Scott Med J 2005;50(2):80–1.

25. Ruemmele FM, El Khoury MG, Talbotec C, et al. Characteristics of inflammatory bowel disease with onset during the first year of life. J Pediatr Gastroenterol Nutr 2006;43(5):603–9.

26. Moeeni V, Day AS. Impact of inflammatory bowel disease upon growth in children and adolescents. ISRN Pediatr 2011;2011:365712.

27. Gupta N, Bostrom AG, Kirschner BS, et al. Presentation and disease course in early- compared to later-onset pediatric Crohn's disease. Am J Gastroenterol 2008;103(8):2092–8.

28. Glocker EO, Frede N, Perro M, et al. Infant colitis—it's in the genes. Lancet 2010; 376(9748):1272.

29. Uhlig HH, Muise AM. Clinical genomics in inflammatory bowel disease. Trends Genet 2017;33(9):629–41.

30. Baud O, Goulet O, Canioni D, et al. Treatment of the immune dysregulation, polyendocrinopathy, enteropathy, X-linked syndrome (IPEX) by allogeneic bone marrow transplantation. N Engl J Med 2001;344(23):1758–62.

31. Okou DT, Mondal K, Faubion WA, et al. Exome sequencing identifies a novel FOXP3 mutation in a 2-generation family with inflammatory bowel disease. J Pediatr Gastroenterol Nutr 2014;58(5):561–8.

32. Ameratunga R, Lehnert K, Woon ST, et al. Review: diagnosing common variable immunodeficiency disorder in the era of genome sequencing. Clin Rev Allergy Immunol 2018;54(2):261–8.

33. Tysk C, Lindberg E, Jarnerot G, et al. Ulcerative colitis and Crohn's disease in an unselected population of monozygotic and dizygotic twins. A study of heritability and the influence of smoking. Gut 1988;29(7):990–6.

34. Orholm M, Munkholm P, Langholz E, et al. Familial occurrence of inflammatory bowel disease. N Engl J Med 1991;324(2):84–8.

35. Orholm M, Binder V, Sorensen TI, et al. Concordance of inflammatory bowel disease among Danish twins. Results of a nationwide study. Scand J Gastroenterol 2000;35(10):1075–81.

36. Colombel JF, Grandbastien B, Gower-Rousseau C, et al. Clinical characteristics of Crohn's disease in 72 families. Gastroenterology 1996;111(3):604–7.

37. Park JH, Wacholder S, Gail MH, et al. Estimation of effect size distribution from genome-wide association studies and implications for future discoveries. Nat Genet 2010;42(7):570–5.

38. de Ridder L, Weersma RK, Dijkstra G, et al. Genetic susceptibility has a more important role in pediatric-onset Crohn's disease than in adult-onset Crohn's disease. Inflamm Bowel Dis 2007;13(9):1083–92.

39. Uhlig HH. Monogenic diseases associated with intestinal inflammation: implications for the understanding of inflammatory bowel disease. Gut 2013;62(12): 1795–805.

40. Stokkers PC, Reitsma PH, Tytgat GN, et al. HLA-DR and -DQ phenotypes in inflammatory bowel disease: a meta-analysis. Gut 1999;45(3):395–401.

41. Forcione DG, Sands B, Isselbacher KJ, et al. An increased risk of Crohn's disease in individuals who inherit the HLA class II DRB3*0301 allele. Proc Natl Acad Sci U S A 1996;93(10):5094–8.

42. Toyoda H, Wang SJ, Yang HY, et al. Distinct associations of HLA class II genes with inflammatory bowel disease. Gastroenterology 1993;104(3):741–8.

43. Rioux JD, Silverberg MS, Daly MJ, et al. Genomewide search in Canadian families with inflammatory bowel disease reveals two novel susceptibility loci. Am J Hum Genet 2000;66(6):1863–70.

44. Hugot JP, Laurent-Puig P, Gower-Rousseau C, et al. Mapping of a susceptibility locus for Crohn's disease on chromosome 16. Nature 1996;379(6568):821–3.

45. Hugot JP, Chamaillard M, Zouali H, et al. Association of NOD2 leucine-rich repeat variants with susceptibility to Crohn's disease. Nature 2001;411(6837): 599–603.

46. Ogura Y, Bonen DK, Inohara N, et al. A frameshift mutation in NOD2 associated with susceptibility to Crohn's disease. Nature 2001;411(6837):603–6.
47. Jostins L, Ripke S, Weersma RK, et al. Host-microbe interactions have shaped the genetic architecture of inflammatory bowel disease. Nature 2012;491(7422): 119–24.
48. Liu JZ, van Sommeren S, Huang H, et al. Association analyses identify 38 susceptibility loci for inflammatory bowel disease and highlight shared genetic risk across populations. Nat Genet 2015;47(9):979–86.
49. de Lange KM, Moutsianas L, Lee JC, et al. Genome-wide association study implicates immune activation of multiple integrin genes in inflammatory bowel disease. Nat Genet 2017;49(2):256–61.
50. Cuthbert AP, Fisher SA, Mirza MM, et al. The contribution of NOD2 gene mutations to the risk and site of disease in inflammatory bowel disease. Gastroenterology 2002;122(4):867–74.
51. Li E, Hamm CM, Gulati AS, et al. Inflammatory bowel diseases phenotype, *C. difficile* and NOD2 genotype are associated with shifts in human ileum associated microbial composition. PLoS One 2012;7(6):e26284.
52. Lee JC, Biasci D, Roberts R, et al. Genome-wide association study identifies distinct genetic contributions to prognosis and susceptibility in Crohn's disease. Nat Genet 2017;49(2):262–8.
53. Anderson CA, Boucher G, Lees CW, et al. Meta-analysis identifies 29 additional ulcerative colitis risk loci, increasing the number of confirmed associations to 47. Nat Genet 2011;43(3):246–52.
54. Parkes M, Barrett JC, Prescott NJ, et al. Sequence variants in the autophagy gene IRGM and multiple other replicating loci contribute to Crohn's disease susceptibility. Nat Genet 2007;39(7):830–2.
55. Imielinski M, Baldassano RN, Griffiths A, et al. Common variants at five new loci associated with early-onset inflammatory bowel disease. Nat Genet 2009; 41(12):1335–40.
56. Kugathasan S, Baldassano RN, Bradfield JP, et al. Loci on 20q13 and 21q22 are associated with pediatric-onset inflammatory bowel disease. Nat Genet 2008; 40(10):1211–5.
57. Franke A, McGovern DP, Barrett JC, et al. Genome-wide meta-analysis increases to 71 the number of confirmed Crohn's disease susceptibility loci. Nat Genet 2010;42(12):1118–25.
58. Bick D, Dimmock D. Whole exome and whole genome sequencing. Curr Opin Pediatr 2011;23(6):594–600.
59. Moran CJ, Walters TD, Guo CH, et al. IL-10R polymorphisms are associated with very-early-onset ulcerative colitis. Inflamm Bowel Dis 2013;19(1):115–23.
60. Worthey EA, Mayer AN, Syverson GD, et al. Making a definitive diagnosis: successful clinical application of whole exome sequencing in a child with intractable inflammatory bowel disease. Genet Med 2011;13(3):255–62.
61. Rigaud S, Fondaneche MC, Lambert N, et al. XIAP deficiency in humans causes an X-linked lymphoproliferative syndrome. Nature 2006;444(7115):110–4.
62. Speckmann C, Lehmberg K, Albert MH, et al. X-linked inhibitor of apoptosis (XIAP) deficiency: the spectrum of presenting manifestations beyond hemophagocytic lymphohistiocytosis. Clin Immunol 2013;149(1):133–41.
63. Zeissig Y, Petersen BS, Milutinovic S, et al. XIAP variants in male Crohn's disease. Gut 2015;64(1):66–76.
64. Yang X, Kanegane H, Nishida N, et al. Clinical and genetic characteristics of XIAP deficiency in Japan. J Clin Immunol 2012;32(3):411–20.

65. Alangari A, Alsultan A, Adly N, et al. LPS-responsive beige-like anchor (LRBA) gene mutation in a family with inflammatory bowel disease and combined immunodeficiency. J Allergy Clin Immunol 2012;130(2):481–8.e2.

66. Avitzur Y, Guo C, Mastropaolo LA, et al. Mutations in tetratricopeptide repeat domain 7A result in a severe form of very early onset inflammatory bowel disease. Gastroenterology 2014;146(4):1028–39.

67. Blaydon DC, Biancheri P, Di WL, et al. Inflammatory skin and bowel disease linked to ADAM17 deletion. N Engl J Med 2011;365(16):1502–8.

68. Zimmer KP, Schumann H, Mecklenbeck S, et al. Esophageal stenosis in childhood: dystrophic epidermolysis bullosa without skin blistering due to collagen VII mutations. Gastroenterology 2002;122(1):220–5.

69. Vetrano S, Rescigno M, Cera MR, et al. Unique role of junctional adhesion molecule-a in maintaining mucosal homeostasis in inflammatory bowel disease. Gastroenterology 2008;135(1):173–84.

70. Ussar S, Moser M, Widmaier M, et al. Loss of Kindlin-1 causes skin atrophy and lethal neonatal intestinal epithelial dysfunction. PLoS Genet 2008;4(12):e1000289.

71. Fiskerstrand T, Arshad N, Haukanes BI, et al. Familial diarrhea syndrome caused by an activating GUCY2C mutation. N Engl J Med 2012;366(17):1586–95.

72. Karamchandani-Patel G, Hanson EP, Saltzman R, et al. Congenital alterations of NEMO glutamic acid 223 result in hypohidrotic ectodermal dysplasia and immunodeficiency with normal serum IgG levels. Ann Allergy Asthma Immunol 2011;107(1):50–6.

73. Kahr WH, Pluthero FG, Elkadri A, et al. Loss of the Arp2/3 complex component ARPC1B causes platelet abnormalities and predisposes to inflammatory disease. Nat Commun 2017;8:14816.

74. Driessen GJ, IJspeert H, Wentink M, et al. Increased PI3K/Akt activity and deregulated humoral immune response in human PTEN deficiency. J Allergy Clin Immunol 2016;138(6):1744–7.e5.

75. Heindl M, Handel N, Ngeow J, et al. Autoimmunity, intestinal lymphoid hyperplasia, and defects in mucosal B-cell homeostasis in patients with PTEN hamartoma tumor syndrome. Gastroenterology 2012;142(5):1093–6.e6.

76. Shearer WT, Dunn E, Notarangelo LD, et al. Establishing diagnostic criteria for severe combined immunodeficiency disease (SCID), leaky SCID, and Omenn syndrome: the Primary Immune Deficiency Treatment Consortium experience. J Allergy Clin Immunol 2014;133(4):1092–8.

77. Agarwal S, Smereka P, Harpaz N, et al. Characterization of immunologic defects in patients with common variable immunodeficiency (CVID) with intestinal disease. Inflamm Bowel Dis 2011;17(1):251–9.

78. Derry JM, Ochs HD, Francke U. Isolation of a novel gene mutated in Wiskott-Aldrich syndrome. Cell 1994;79(5). following 922.

79. Barzaghi F, Passerini L, Bacchetta R. Immune dysregulation, polyendocrinopathy, enteropathy, x-linked syndrome: a paradigm of immunodeficiency with autoimmunity. Front Immunol 2012;3:211.

80. Engelhardt KR, Shah N, Faizura-Yeop I, et al. Clinical outcome in IL-10- and IL-10 receptor-deficient patients with or without hematopoietic stem cell transplantation. J Allergy Clin Immunol 2013;131(3):825–30.

81. Shim JO, Hwang S, Yang HR, et al. Interleukin-10 receptor mutations in children with neonatal-onset Crohn's disease and intractable ulcerating enterocolitis. Eur J Gastroenterol Hepatol 2013;25(10):1235–40.

82. Marks DJ, Miyagi K, Rahman FZ, et al. Inflammatory bowel disease in CGD reproduces the clinicopathological features of Crohn's disease. Am J Gastroenterol 2009;104(1):117–24.
83. Ventham NT, Kennedy NA, Adams AT, et al. Integrative epigenome-wide analysis demonstrates that DNA methylation may mediate genetic risk in inflammatory bowel disease. Nat Commun 2016;7:13507.
84. Muise AM, Xu W, Guo CH, et al. NADPH oxidase complex and IBD candidate gene studies: identification of a rare variant in NCF2 that results in reduced binding to RAC2. Gut 2012;61(7):1028–35.
85. Li Q, Lee CH, Peters LA, et al. Variants in TRIM22 that affect NOD2 signaling are associated with very-early-onset inflammatory bowel disease. Gastroenterology 2016;150(5):1196–207.
86. Hyams J, Markowitz J, Lerer T, et al. The natural history of corticosteroid therapy for ulcerative colitis in children. Clin Gastroenterol Hepatol 2006;4(9): 1118–23.
87. Jakobsen C, Bartek J Jr, Wewer V, et al. Differences in phenotype and disease course in adult and paediatric inflammatory bowel disease—a population-based study. Aliment Pharmacol Ther 2011;34(10):1217–24.
88. Kammermeier J, Dziubak R, Pescarin M, et al. Phenotypic and genotypic characterisation of inflammatory bowel disease presenting before the age of 2 years. J Crohns Colitis 2017;11(1):60–9.
89. Sato T, Clevers H. Growing self-organizing mini-guts from a single intestinal stem cell: mechanism and applications. Science 2013;340(6137):1190–4.
90. Chen R, Giliani S, Lanzi G, et al. Whole-exome sequencing identifies tetratricopeptide repeat domain 7A (TTC7A) mutations for combined immunodeficiency with intestinal atresias. J Allergy Clin Immunol 2013;132(3):656–64.e7.
91. Murugan D, Albert MH, Langemeier J, et al. Very early onset inflammatory bowel disease associated with aberrant trafficking of IL-10R1 and cure by T cell replete haploidentical bone marrow transplantation. J Clin Immunol 2014;34(3):331–9.
92. Charbit-Henrion F, Jeverica AK, Begue B, et al. Deficiency in mucosa-associated lymphoid tissue lymphoma translocation 1: a novel cause of IPEX-like syndrome. J Pediatr Gastroenterol Nutr 2017;64(3):378–84.
93. Booth C, Gilmour KC, Veys P, et al. X-linked lymphoproliferative disease due to SAP/SH2D1A deficiency: a multicenter study on the manifestations, management and outcome of the disease. Blood 2011;117(1):53–62.
94. Rohr J, Pannicke U, Doring M, et al. Chronic inflammatory bowel disease as key manifestation of atypical ARTEMIS deficiency. J Clin Immunol 2010;30(2): 314–20.
95. Cuvelier GD, Rubin TS, Wall DA, et al. Long-term outcomes of hematopoietic stem cell transplantation for ZAP70 deficiency. J Clin Immunol 2016;36(7): 713–24.
96. Ngwube A, Hanson IC, Orange J, et al. Outcomes after allogeneic transplant in patients with Wiskott-Aldrich syndrome. Biol Blood Marrow Transplant 2018; 24(3):537–41.
97. Chiriaco M, Salfa I, Di Matteo G, et al. Chronic granulomatous disease: clinical, molecular, and therapeutic aspects. Pediatr Allergy Immunol 2016;27(3): 242–53.
98. Kato K, Kojima Y, Kobayashi C, et al. Successful allogeneic hematopoietic stem cell transplantation for chronic granulomatous disease with inflammatory complications and severe infection. Int J Hematol 2011;94(5):479–82.

99. Freudenberg F, Wintergerst U, Roesen-Wolff A, et al. Therapeutic strategy in p47-phox deficient chronic granulomatous disease presenting as inflammatory bowel disease. J Allergy Clin Immunol 2010;125(4):943–6.e1.

100. Uzel G, Orange JS, Poliak N, et al. Complications of tumor necrosis factor-alpha blockade in chronic granulomatous disease-related colitis. Clin Infect Dis 2010; 51(12):1429–34.

101. Kammermeier J, Drury S, James CT, et al. Targeted gene panel sequencing in children with very early onset inflammatory bowel disease—evaluation and prospective analysis. J Med Genet 2014;51(11):748–55.

102. Kammermeier J, Lucchini G, Pai SY, et al. Stem cell transplantation for tetratricopeptide repeat domain 7A deficiency: long-term follow-up. Blood 2016; 128(9):1306–8.

103. Canna SW, Girard C, Malle L, et al. Life-threatening NLRC4-associated hyperinflammation successfully treated with IL-18 inhibition. J Allergy Clin Immunol 2017;139(5):1698–701.

104. Lo B, Zhang K, Lu W, et al. Autoimmune disease. Patients with LRBA deficiency show CTLA4 loss and immune dysregulation responsive to abatacept therapy. Science 2015;349(6246):436–40.

105. Weinacht KG, Charbonnier LM, Alroqi F, et al. Ruxolitinib reverses dysregulated T helper cell responses and controls autoimmunity caused by a novel signal transducer and activator of transcription 1 (STAT1) gain-of-function mutation. J Allergy Clin Immunol 2017;139(5):1629–40.e2.

Gastrointestinal Development

Implications for Management of Preterm and Term Infants

Mary W. Lenfestey, MD[a], Josef Neu, MD[b],*

KEYWORDS

- Neonatal nutrition • Gastroesophageal reflux • Gastrointestinal motility
- Inflammation • Microbiome

KEY POINTS

- The gastrointestinal tract is a complex organ system that provides neural, endocrine, exocrine, and immunologic functions, in addition to managing the digestion and absorption of nutrients.
- Parenteral nutrition is used in infants unable to meet nutritional needs with enteral feeds. The composition of parenteral nutrition is being explored to evaluate the effect of different nutrient sources on health and morbidity.
- Gastroesophageal reflux is a common diagnosis for both term and preterm infants; preterm infants are also predisposed to gastrointestinal dysmotility caused by immature gastrointestinal development.
- The gastrointestinal tract is a source of antigen exposure for the immune system; inflammation within the gastrointestinal tract can result in systemic responses and has been correlated to several different diseases.
- The gastrointestinal microbiome is an area of interest for a variety of infant conditions, including necrotizing enterocolitis and colic.

INTRODUCTION

The gastrointestinal (GI) tract is composed of a multitude of luminal structures: the oropharynx, esophagus, stomach, duodenum, jejunum, ileum, cecum, and colon perform functions critical to many facets of health. There have been many advances in

Disclosures: None (M.W. Lenfestey). Funding from Infant Bacterial Therapeutics (not relevant to this topic) (J. Neu).
[a] Department of Pediatrics, University of Florida, PO Box 100296, Gainesville, FL 32610, USA;
[b] Department of Pediatrics, University of Florida, 6516 Southwest 93rd Avenue, Gainesville, FL 32610, USA
* Corresponding author.
E-mail address: neuj@peds.ufl.edu

Gastroenterol Clin N Am 47 (2018) 773–791
https://doi.org/10.1016/j.gtc.2018.07.005
0889-8553/18/© 2018 Elsevier Inc. All rights reserved.

gastro.theclinics.com

the understanding of normal GI development. Although traditionally thought to be primarily an organ system for absorption of nutrients and excretion of waste, data obtained from both human and animal studies over the past several decades have shown that the GI tract contributes to overall health in a much broader manner.[1] It provides neural, endocrine, exocrine, and immunologic functions in addition to the digestion and absorption of nutrients[2] (**Fig. 1**). There are likely correlations between abnormal GI tract function and a variety of pediatric diseases, including obesity, allergy and atopic disease, autoimmune diseases, and neurodevelopmental outcomes. This article explores the normal development of the GI tract and clinical conditions pertinent to the preterm and term infant population that correlate with pathologic development, with a focus on anatomy, absorption and nutrition, motility, and immunologic interplay with the microbiome.

ANATOMIC AND HISTOLOGIC NORMS

One of the most incredible features of intestinal development is the dramatic rate at which this tissue grows throughout prenatal and postnatal periods. There is an

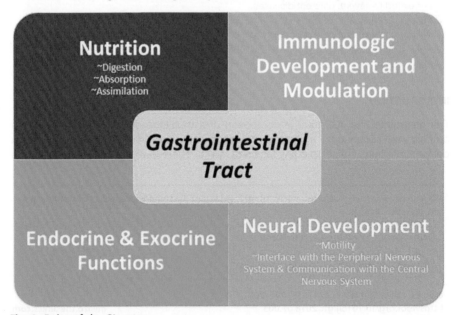

Fig. 1. Roles of the GI system.

estimated 1000-fold increase in size from week 5 through week 40 of gestation.[3] Autopsy data have been useful in determining average small intestinal length for prenatal age: 125 cm by 20 weeks, 200 cm by 30 weeks, and 275 cm at term. This growth continues, ultimately reaching a length of approximately 575 cm by 20 years of life.[4] When considering the impressive surface area produced by the development of villi, finger-like projections critical to the absorption of nutrients, adults have an estimated 200 m^2 of mucosa in contact with external antigens, including food particles, medications, and microbes.[5] The large intestine is approximately 60 cm in a full-term infant, which increases up to 150 cm by adulthood.[6]

The GI tract initially begins as a simple tubular structure that forms in the fourth week of gestation and quickly polarizes along the anterior-posterior axis. Continued cellular division results in the formation of the endoderm, mesoderm, and ectoderm layers, from which the primary components of the GI tract arise. Endoderm gives rise to the epithelial cells, which further differentiate to encompass all of the cell types necessary for digestion and absorption. The mesoderm gives rise to the cells of the muscularis layers and the lamina propria, and include smooth muscle, vascular, and lymphatic contributions. The ectoderm gives rise to migrating neural crest cells, from which the enteric nervous system derives (**Fig. 2**).

There are 3 sections of the embryologic GI structure: the foregut, midgut, and hindgut. The esophagus, stomach, duodenum, pancreas, and hepatobiliary system develop from the foregut. The remainder of the small bowel, the jejunum and ileum, as well as the cecum, ascending colon, and the proximal two-thirds of the transverse colon develop from the midgut. The hindgut is the precursor for the remaining transverse colon, the descending and sigmoid colon, rectum, and the anal canal (**Fig. 3**). This ontogeny is clinically relevant, because each derivative component shares common sources of blood supply, innervation, and lymphatic drainage with those derived from the same precursor. The exception to this is the anal canal, which receives innervation, blood supply, and lymphatics from both hindgut derivatives and pelvic sources.[5]

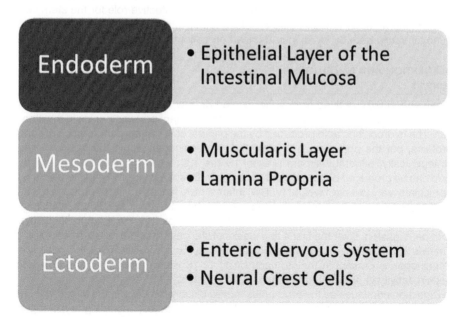

Fig. 2. Derivatives of the GI tract.

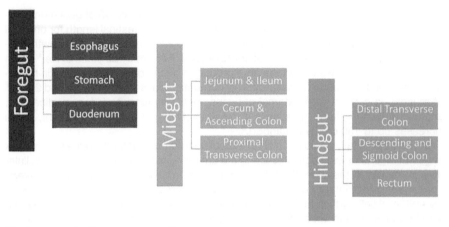

Fig. 3. Embryologic precursors of GI anatomy.

The GI epithelial histology is diverse, with variations in cell types and function between anatomic regions. Gastric mucosa includes acid-producing parietal cells, chief cells, and neuroendocrine cells. The intestinal epithelium acts a barrier to antigens and microbes through interenterocyte tight junctions. Failure to maintain the integrity of tight junctions has been correlated with several diseases, including inflammatory bowel disease, celiac disease, and type I diabetes. Enterocytes are responsible for absorbing nutrients. There are also several types of secretory cells, including Paneth cells (which secrete antimicrobial factors), goblet cells (which secrete protective mucin), and the enteroendocrine cells (which modulate an array of GI functions through their secretion of hormones).[2] Cells are produced via mitosis within the crypt of the intestine, after which most cell types migrate upwards toward the tip of the villus. Paneth cells remain in the crypt area, serving a protective role for the stem cells found in this area.[7] Eventually, cells are sloughed off into the lumen; the rate of cellular turnover varies both by location and based on patient factors.

ABSORPTION AND NUTRITION
Proteins

Whey and casein, derived from either human or cow's milk, are the primary protein sources for term and preterm infants. Digestion of dietary proteins begins in the stomach. The hydrochloric acid produced by the parietal cells begins denaturation of some proteins, but the primary role is activation of pepsinogen within the gastric lumen. Ontogenically, parietal cells are present by the 13th week of gestation and gastric acid can be produced by the second trimester.[8,9] Despite this activity, preterm infants, particularly very low birth weight (VLBW) infants, have limited ability to produce gastric acid compared with their term counterparts. Gastric pH is typically 5.5 to 7 within the first 24 to 48 hours after birth, and has been found to be fairly resistant to stimulation with pentagastrin. Over the first 4 to 8 weeks of life, gastric acid production doubles.[10] There is also evidence of the capability for proteolysis as early as 16 weeks' gestation. Pepsinogen is present in the stomach by 17 to 18 weeks' gestation, and postnatal pepsin activity is proportionate to the infant's maturity.[11]

Digestion continues as the food bolus moves distally throughout the intestines. The pancreas produces several important digestive enzymes, including trypsinogen, chymotrypsinogen, and carboxypeptidase. The presence of food in the proximal small intestine initiates production and release of enterokinase from the epithelial cells, which cleaves the pancreatic zymogens into their active forms. Enterokinase activity occurs by 24 weeks' gestation but only at 25% of the level found in older children.[12] There has been speculation that this may limit preterm infants' ability to digest and absorb proteins adequately. In normal digestion, larger protein molecules are cleaved into smaller oligopeptides, dipeptides, and single amino acid units. These units are absorbed by a variety of mechanisms, including cotransport with hydrogen ions and sodium-dependent transporters.

Given that there are several mechanisms that seem to have suboptimal function in preterm infants compared with term infants, the clinical question arises as to how this practically affects the ability of preterm infants to adequately digest protein nutrition. As mentioned earlier, gastric acid is necessary both for intraluminal denaturation of proteins and to cleave pepsinogen into active pepsin. Because preterm infants are known to have a reduced capability to produce gastric acid, it is reasonable to suggest they may be less apt to initiate gastric protein digestion. A recent study that supports this theory, by Demers-Mathieu and colleagues,[13] compared the gastric digestion capacity in preterm infants with that in term infants. Several preterm infants (24–32 weeks' gestation) and term infants (38–40 weeks' gestation) were given human milk controlled to a pH of 4.5. Gastric content evaluation 2 hours postfeed indicated less evidence of gastric protein digestion in the preterm group. Milk protease levels were not different between the term and preterm mothers' milk.

With regard to enteral nutrition choices, there are many studies to support that human milk is the best option for most preterm infants. Feeds of human milk have been associated with better neurodevelopmental outcomes and lower rates of infections and necrotizing enterocolitis compared with formula; factors including secretory immunoglobulin A (IgA), lactoferrin, growth factors, and cytokines present in human milk have been hypothesized to contribute to these findings.[14] Cow's milk formula is often used in preterm infants if mother's milk is not available and the infant has aged past the criteria to use donor breast milk. Cow's milk protein–derived fortifiers are also used commonly to fortify human milk to meet preterm infant nutritional needs. Another clinical question that has arisen based on an understanding that preterm infants have decreased activity of enterokinase and other peptidases is whether hydrolyzed protein formulas would be better tolerated and possibly provide better nutrition for this population. A study by Mihatsch and colleagues[15] evaluated the time to full feeds in preterm infants receiving either a hydrolyzed protein preterm formula or a standard preterm formula; the group receiving hydrolyzed protein formula had better tolerance of feeds and a shorter overall time to achieving full feeds compared with infants receiving standard formula. Because human milk was not reliably available, human milk feeds were not included in the study. However, despite this interesting result, there is no consensus as to whether or not hydrolyzed formula provides a benefit compared with standard preterm formulas, and this area merits further investigation.

Carbohydrates

Salivary and pancreatic amylases hydrolyze complex carbohydrates into oligosaccharides, which are further hydrolyzed at the epithelial brush border to monosaccharides ready for absorption. The intestinal epithelial absorptive enzymes include lactase, sucrase, maltase, isomaltase, and glucoamylase; these hydrolases are fully active in term infants. Preterm infants have sucrase, maltase, and isomaltase that are close to full activity but often have poor lactase activity. Lactase activity increases significantly between 24 and 40 weeks' gestation.[12]

Amylase is the primary enzyme responsible for hydrolyzing complex carbohydrates and starches into oligosaccharides. Salivary amylase may begin digestion of oral feeds by hydrolyzing up to 18 to 29 glucose units.[16] However, pancreatic amylase is responsible for most of the initial carbohydrate hydrolysis. Although pancreatic amylase production begins as early as week 14 to 16 of gestation, secretion of this enzyme is still limited and does not reach adult levels until 2 years of age.[17,18] The limited contribution of salivary amylase is not able to overcome this deficiency; in addition, many preterm infants are fed via feeding tubes that bypass the oral cavity, further reducing the efficacy of salivary amylase. As such, there are higher amounts of undigested starches that pass into the colon. Microbes within the large intestine ultimately digest starches with production of hydrogen gas and short-chain fatty acids (SCFAs), which can be absorbed and used as a fat-based energy source. There are data to suggest that SCFAs, particularly butyrate, may alter proliferation, differentiation, and turnover of colon epithelium.[19] It also serves as a fuel source to these cells, and may affect immune modulation within the intestine.[20] Many preterm formulas use partially hydrolyzed starches, such as corn syrup solids; however, increasingly hydrolyzed starch base correlates with increasing osmolarity of the formula.

Lactose is the primary carbohydrate source in mammalian milk. Despite a relative lactase deficiency in the preterm population, it is unusual to have clinical symptoms of lactose intolerance. With gradual enteral feed advancement, preterm infants generally do not receive large quantities of lactose abruptly. Especially while enteral nutrition only accounts for less than 40% to 50% of total nutrition, the amount of lactose present is unlikely to overwhelm the lactase capacity. Also, as described earlier, excess lactose that goes undigested by the lactase in the brush border is used effectively in the colon by conversion into beneficial SCFAs. Small intestine lactase activity can be modulated by feeding route and the feeding substrate. Preterm infants who received enteral feeds at 4 days of life had 100% and 60% more lactase activity at days 10 and 28 of life, respectively, compared with preterm infants who had feeds initiated after day of life 15. Lactase activity was higher in human milk–fed infants than those receiving formula at 10 days of life.[21] The location of lactase on the villus structure makes this enzyme vulnerable to intestinal damage. Lactase is located in midvillus to upper villus, whereas sucrase, maltase, and glucoamylase are located in the midvillus.[22] In clinical scenarios that result in mucosal damage, such as ischemia or infection, the distal villi are first to be affected and last to be fully regenerated. As such, there may be transient deficiency in lactase within this period; it is unclear how often this translates to clinical symptoms of lactose intolerance.

Lipids

Triglycerides are the most common source of dietary lipids and contribute approximately half of the nonprotein energy content in human milk and formula.[3] Digestion of lipids begins with the breakdown of large collections of triglycerides via micellar emulsification by bile acids. This process results in the formation of many smaller droplets of triglycerides, which increases the surface area available for interaction with lipase. Lipase serves to hydrolyze the lipids into monoglycerides and free fatty acids, which can be absorbed into the enterocytes. Long-chain fatty acids and monoglycerides are absorbed into the enterocyte, and through a reesterification process within the cell are converted into chylomicrons, which exit the cell and are transported via the lymphatic system; they ultimately enter the blood circulation via the thoracic duct. Medium-chain triglycerides (MCTs) do not require bile acids for digestion, and, once absorbed into the enterocyte, pass directly into the portal venous system (**Fig. 4**). Because of these differences in digestion and absorption, MCT is the

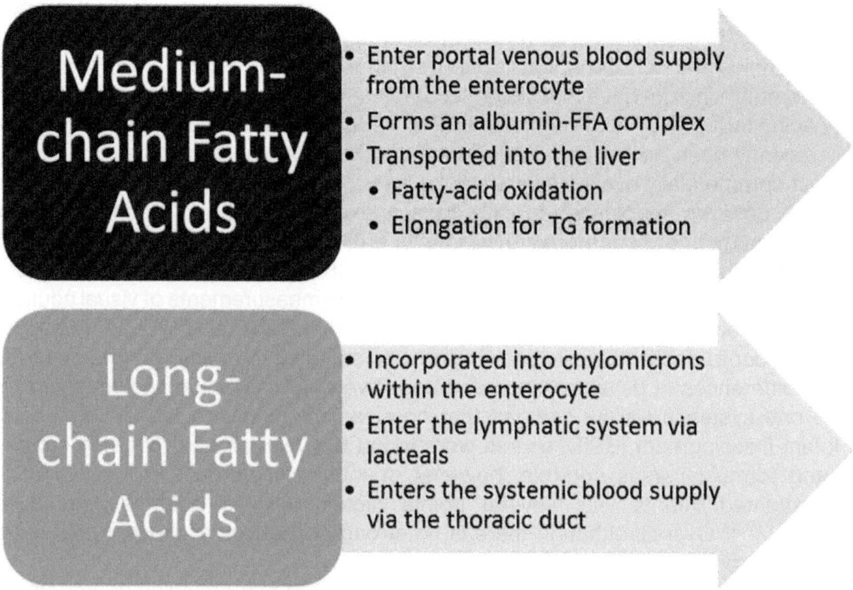

Medium-chain Fatty Acids	• Enter portal venous blood supply from the enterocyte
	• Forms an albumin-FFA complex
	• Transported into the liver
	  • Fatty-acid oxidation
	  • Elongation for TG formation

Long-chain Fatty Acids	• Incorporated into chylomicrons within the enterocyte • Enter the lymphatic system via lacteals • Enters the systemic blood supply via the thoracic duct

Fig. 4. Differences in long-chain and medium-chain fatty acid metabolism. TG, triglyceride.

recommended lipid source in the setting of lymphatic obstructions. There has also been a question as to whether providing primarily MCT-based lipids, as opposed to long-chain triglycerides, would promote better absorption and nutrition for preterm infants. However, a Cochrane Review found that there are no data to support this; no difference in the rate of necrotizing enterocolitis, growth, or other morbidities was identified in a comparison of MCT-based with long-chain triglyceride–based feeds.[23]

There are many forms of lipase: lingual, gastric, pancreatic, and epithelial cell lipase. Human milk has lipase present in colostrum and both term and preterm mothers' milk; this substance is absent in cow's milk and formulas. Human milk lipase has been termed a bile-salt–stimulated lipase because it is activated in the small intestine in the presence of bile acids. This enzyme may help to facilitate long-chain triglyceride digestion for infants fed with breast milk.[24] Lipase has been identified as present in the stomach of fetuses early in gestation; however, progression of the functional capacity of the enzyme is not fully understood.[25] Lingual lipase, secreted from glands at the base of the tongue, has been identified in gastric aspirates as early as gestational age 6 months. Activity of this lipase is lower at birth in infants at 26 weeks' gestation, peaks around week 30 to 32, and gradually declines to lower levels near term.[26] There are 2 primary forms of pancreatic lipase: pancreatic lipase, which is more active against insoluble substrates, and pancreatic carboxylase esterase, which is more active against soluble substrates. Both term and preterm infants have a relative pancreatic insufficiency compared with older children, with lower levels of pancreatic lipases noted at birth; these levels increase to near-adult levels by 6 months of life.[27] As mentioned earlier, bile acids are also critical to normal fat digestion and absorption. They are synthesized and excreted from the liver via the biliary system. VLBW preterm infants have lower concentration of these bile acids in the duodenum than their term counterparts because of both lower synthesis by the immature hepatocytes and less ileal resorption of bile.[28,29]

In order to prevent an essential fatty acid deficiency, adequate dietary intake of linoleic and linolenic fatty acids is required. Under normal circumstances, the body converts these 18-carbon fatty acids into long-chain polyunsaturated fatty acids (LCPUFAs) with greater than 20 carbons. These LCPUFAs are required for formation of eicosanoids and central nervous system structures.[30] There is debate as to whether or not preterm infants have the ability to complete this conversion of dietary essential fatty acids into LCPUFAs. Preformed LCPUFAs are present in human milk and have only recently been added into premature infant formulas; however, they are lacking in most commercially available intravenous lipid formulations. Most premature infant formulas now are supplemented with docosahexaenoic acid and arachidonic acid. Because many of the micropremature infants are very ill after birth, limited intake of enteral nutrition may result in deficient intake of LCPUFAs during this time.[31] Several studies support improved behavioral and physiologic measurements of visual acuity in patients receiving formulas supplemented with docosahexaenoic acid (omega-3 LCPUFA) compared with those receiving unsupplemented formulas.[32,33] Studies evaluating differences in developmental and cognitive outcomes have shown mixed results: one systemic review deemed that no clear differences in the Bayley Scales of Infant Development (BSID) scores were found between groups receiving supplemented formula versus controls; however, mental development in the LCPUFA-supplemented infants was several points higher than in controls with BSID version II.[30,34] Overall, although there is no strong consensus at present, this nutritional topic merits further study.

With regard to lipid absorption, it has been suggested that providing homogenized pasteurized human milk (donor breast milk) may improve preterm infant growth. A randomized controlled trial by De Oliveira and colleagues[35] compared a small number of tube fed preterm infants provided either standard Holder-pasteurized human milk with pasteurized milk that was homogenized with ultrasonication. Gastric aspirate samples indicated an increased gastric lipolysis level and reduced gastric emptying rate in the group receiving homogenized milk; with improved lipolysis, this may suggest a means by which to improve lipid digestion and absorption in this population.

Parenteral lipids are typically derived from a vegetable source that is rich in omega-6 instead of omega-3 LCPUFAs; this provides most of the essential fatty acids in the form of linoleic acid. Omega-3 fatty acids have less of a systemic inflammatory effect,[36] and adult data support omega-3 fatty acids reducing inflammation and several diseases, such as rheumatoid arthritis and coronary artery disease. Although there are no data available for the preterm infant population, neonatal rat studies have shown decreased rates of necrotizing enterocolitis with omega-3 supplementation.[37] New intravenous lipid preparations are available, with fish oil as a component, which provides a source of omega-3 fatty acids. There are studies that indicate that lipid emulsions using formulations of soybean oil, olive oil, MCT, and fish oil are safe and well tolerated[38,39] as well as a growing body of data that indicate this lessens the degree of parenteral nutrition–associated liver disease.[40]

Given the potential antiinflammatory influence of omega-3 fatty acids, this is an area that merits further investigation to better evaluate whether modifying preterm infants' diets could modify the course of diseases associated with systemic inflammation, such as neurodevelopmental outcomes or chronic lung disease. There are some data to support the correlation of lower docosahexaenoic acid levels and the development of chronic lung disease.[41]

MOTILITY AND MECHANICAL GASTROINTESTINAL FUNCTIONS

To meet nutritional requirements for growth and development by solely enteral means, infants must have adequate GI motor functions. This process is complex and includes the ability to take in a food source orally and coordinate a suck-swallow-breathe process safely. Once the food bolus is within the stomach, abnormal motility patterns can result in clinical issues such as gastroesophageal reflux and feeding intolerance related to gastric emptying delay. Because of GI immaturity, preterm infants face several barriers in taking oral feeds.

Oral Feeding Skills

In utero, suck and swallow are present by 17 to 18 weeks' gestation. However, it is common to have suck-swallow incoordination in preterm infants, particularly those born at less than 32 to 34 weeks; this is caused by a constellation of factors. Preterm infants have inadequately developed orofacial musculature, which results in difficulties latching adequately onto nipples and an inefficient suck and transfer of milk.[42] Under normal circumstances, respiration is inhibited by the act of swallowing as a protective mechanism against aspiration. However, preterm infants have cardiorespiratory immaturity and have an increased incidence of swallows that occur with inspiration compared with term infants; this behavior increases their risk of feed-related apnea, bradycardia, oxygen desaturations, and aspiration.[2,3] To circumvent the suck-swallow-breathe incoordination, feeds are provided via enteral tubes (nasogastric [NG] or orogastric [OG]), generally through a corrected age of 33 to 34 weeks, at which age most infants have developed oral coordination comparable with full-term infants. However, the use of NG/OG tubes has risks. Some studies suggest an increased risk of gastroesophageal reflux and aspiration pneumonia with the use of NG tubes; continually propping open the lower esophageal sphincter may more readily allow the reflux of gastric contents into the esophagus.[43] The continuous presence of a negative sensory stimulus may also contribute to the development of oral aversions in this at-risk group. Early feeding therapy and oral skill development is very important in preterm infants.

Gastroesophageal Reflux

Gastroesophageal reflux (GER) describes the movement of gastric contents into the esophagus and is a normal physiologic process that occurs in humans several times per day. GER disease (GERD) occurs when reflux is associated with distressing symptoms or complications. The true incidence of GERD is difficult to quantify, because symptoms are nonspecific. Clinically, infants suspected of having GERD are empirically managed with feed modifications and/or antireflux medications. If this fails, then further studies may be conducted. It is important to consider limitations in methods of evaluation; pH probes can be helpful in identifying acid reflux, but impedance studies provide more accurate information for the presence of both acid and nonacid reflux.

Transient relaxation of the lower esophageal sphincter is the most significant mechanism for causing GER in both preterm and term infants; this is normal reflux mediated by the vagal nerve triggered by a distention of the proximal stomach that activates intramural inhibitory neurons, which release nitric oxide to relax the lower esophageal sphincter. Infants with delayed gastric emptying or otherwise impaired motility have more of the transient relaxations, correlating with increased GER. With regard to esophageal maturity, preterm infants have slower propagation velocities and a longer contraction phase than older children. The lower esophageal sphincter resting pressure is only 4 mm Hg at 28 weeks' gestation, compared with 18 mm Hg in full-term infants (which is equivalent to adult pressures).[44] Because of these factors, there can be a dramatic increase in reflux episodes with fluctuations in abdominal pressure.[45]

GER is commonly blamed for apneas and bradycardia in preterm infants based on mostly anecdotal or circumstantial correlations. There have been studies that show apnea associated with conditions that mimic reflux. One study by Davies and colleagues[46] induced apnea with instillation of small amounts of liquid into the pharynx of preterm infants. However, another study by Page and Jeffery[47] instead observed that apnea and bradycardia occurred with laryngeal infusion of normal saline or water during sleep, but pharyngeal administration only correlated with increased swallowing. Regardless, studies have not been able to document a true causal relationship between GER and apnea.[43,45] Other studies have not found significant differences in preterm infants in terms of body weight or weekly weight gains but did find that preterm infants with GERD had longer hospital stays than infants without GERD.[48]

GER symptoms are typically treated initially, and often empirically, with acid-suppression medications such as H_2 antagonists (ranitidine, famotidine, nizatidine) and proton pump inhibitors (PPIs; omeprazole, lansoprazole, esomeprazole). However, the use of these medications has risks. An increasing body of data correlates H_2 antagonists and PPIs with necrotizing enterocolitis. Animal studies show increased bacterial translocation in newborn rats treated with H_2 antagonists.[49] Retrospective studies note an increased incidence of gram-negative bacteremia and necrotizing enterocolitis in preterm infants receiving PPIs and H_2 antagonists.[50,51] A case-controlled cross-sectional study by Gupta and colleagues[52] showed decreased fecal microbial diversity, increased Proteobacteria and decreased Firmicutes in preterm infants receiving H_2 antagonist therapy (**Fig. 5**). This finding supports that decreased ability to produce gastric acid results in pathogenic changes in the GI microbiome, which clinically predisposes this vulnerable population to necrotizing enterocolitis.

Term infants are also commonly treated for possible reflux; as with preterm infants, this is often a clinical diagnosis based on regurgitation and/or fussiness and crying. With large numbers of pediatric patients on acid-suppression therapy, there has been increasing interest in the safety of these therapies in the last decade, particularly regarding long-term PPI use. There is a solid body of adult data that correlates long-term PPI therapy and alterations in the GI flora, increased rate of respiratory infections (community-acquired pneumonia), increased rate of enteric infections (*Clostridium difficile*), vitamin B_{12} deficiency, hypomagnesemia, and calcium deficiency and osteoporosis.[53] There are fewer data available for children at this time. One pediatric review by Tolia and Boyer[54] identified an increased incidence of diarrhea and constipation, as well as increased gastrin level, but did not identify vitamin B_{12} deficiency. Because acid suppression continues to be administered commonly to both preterm and term infants, this is an area that requires further investigation; in the meantime, it is prudent to note that these medications have risks, and administration warrants careful consideration.[54,55]

Abnormal Gastric and Intestinal Motility

The motility patterns of the stomach and intestines are closely related, and normal function depends on feedback provided from within the GI tract. Gastric emptying delay is more common in preterm infants than term infants,[56,57] and, as described earlier, greater gastric residual volumes can worsen reflux. Gastroantral transit varies from 8 to 96 hours in preterm infants to 4 to 12 hours in adults. In adults and older children, duodenal receptors sensing lipids, carbohydrates, acid, and increasing osmolality all signal to decrease gastric emptying. However, it is unknown whether these mechanisms contribute in the same manner in infants born at less than 32 weeks' gestation, because there are few data available. Small bowel motility patterns are also abnormal in preterm infants and are incompletely developed in infants before

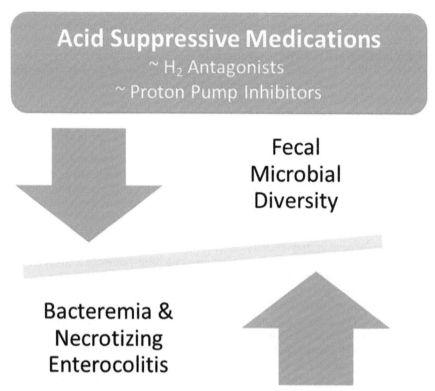

Fig. 5. Use of H_2 antagonists and PPIs in preterm infants has been associated with increased incidence of necrotizing enterocolitis (NEC) and gram-negative rod bacteremia, and correlates with changes in fecal microbial diversity. (*Data from* Refs.[50–52])

28 weeks' gestation. Motilin receptors and cyclic motilin release are not present until 32 weeks' gestation, with migrating myoelectric complexes first noted at 33 to 34 weeks' gestation.[58]

Caloric density of feeds is inversely related to gastric emptying speed in infants born between 32 and 39 weeks' gestation.[59] During the last trimester in utero, fetuses swallow approximately 450 mL of low-caloric-density amniotic fluid per day.[60] Preterm infants often have difficulty tolerating high-caloric-density feeds; a proposed solution is to provide formula lower in fat and carbohydrate, which physiologically promotes faster gastric emptying. However, this approach is impractical, because preterm infants have increased nutritional and metabolic demands that such formulas would likely not meet. Transpyloric feeds are often used, especially for infants with apnea or aspiration. However, there is no evidence that this practice has an effect on mortality or morbidity in this population.[3] Promotility agents, such as erythromycin and metoclopramide, are used in both term and preterm infants to help promote gastric emptying. Erythromycin binds to neural motilin receptors and stimulates antral migrating motor complexes. There are data that support efficacy in improving feeding tolerance without significant side effects in preterm infants; however, other studies found mixed results.[61] Of note, there have been correlations between erythromycin and arrhythmias and pyloric stenosis. Metoclopramide is primarily a dopamine D_2 antagonist but also has some agonistic effect on serotonin (5-HT$_4$) receptors and weak inhibition of 5-HT$_3$ receptors; it has a promotility effect by enhancing antral contractions and decreasing postprandial fundus relaxation. Metoclopramide has clear efficacy in improving gastric emptying times in both term and preterm infants[62]; however, the medication has known side effects of extrapyramidal movements or tardive dyskinesia, which are difficult to monitor in infants. Cisapride has been used commonly in the past but has been removed from the market in the United States because of reports of cardiac arrhythmias.

IMMUNE FUNCTION, GASTROINTESTINAL INFLAMMATION, AND THE MICROBIOME

Significant transitions occur within the neonatal GI tract. The neonatal period is an active time for development of both innate and adaptive immune function; this corresponds with major shifts in the GI microbiome. Although the in utero environment was once thought to be sterile, recent studies identified microbes in the amniotic fluid, placenta, and infant meconium, indicating prenatal microbe exposure.[63–65] These microbes likely contribute to intestinal development, with beginnings of colonization before birth. Expansion and diversification of the microbiome continues from birth through the second year of life and beyond; changes often correlate with dietary advancements and alterations.[66]

Commensal bacteria develop a symbiotic relationship with the GI epithelium and gut-associated lymphoid tissue. Bacteria and their associated metabolic by-products can penetrate the submucosa and interact with the gut-associated lymphoid tissue, which affects immune tolerance; this is important to allow coexistence with GI microbes without developing inappropriate inflammatory responses or reducing the immune response to pathogens. Toll-like receptors (TLRs) are one mechanism involved in immune homeostasis. TLRs are involved with cell signaling in response to bacterial products such as lipopolysaccharides; these receptors enhance the ability of epithelial cells to withstand inflammatory damage. There are several differences in both TLR subtype activity and function in preterm infants compared with full-term infants. Preterm infants have higher activity of TLR4, which correlates with reduced ability to recover from cell injury and mucosal barrier dysfunction; this is a proposed mechanism for the increased risk of necrotizing enterocolitis in preterm infants.[67,68] Dysregulation of the GI microbiome has been associated with a variety of diseases, including obesity, inflammatory bowel disease, atopic disease, celiac disease, and necrotizing enterocolitis.[69–72]

As described earlier, the GI tract of premature infants is immature and less capable of defense against enteral pathogens. Epithelial mucosal barriers are less functional, and there are both qualitative and quantitative deficiencies in GI immune cells. Abnormal motility patterns and decreased production of gastric acid, proteolytic enzymes, secretory IgA, and antimicrobial peptides (primarily from Paneth cells) all contribute to the increased risk of dysbiosis and bacterial overgrowth.[73] Clinically, this translates to an increase risk of bacterial translocation, necrotizing enterocolitis, and a systemic inflammatory response.[74]

Several patient factors influence the GI flora of infants, including mode of delivery, diet, gestational age, and antibiotic exposure[75] **(Fig. 6)**. Preterm infants tend to have higher exposure to pathogenic bacteria given prolonged hospital courses in neonatal intensive care units than do term infants. Although many factors are capable of elucidating changes in the microbiome, the following select factors are discussed further in this article: the effects of antibiotic exposure, use of parenteral nutrition, and feeding patterns.

Antibiotics are the most commonly used class of medications in the neonatal intensive care unit.[76] Preterm infants, especially VLBW, commonly show a variety of

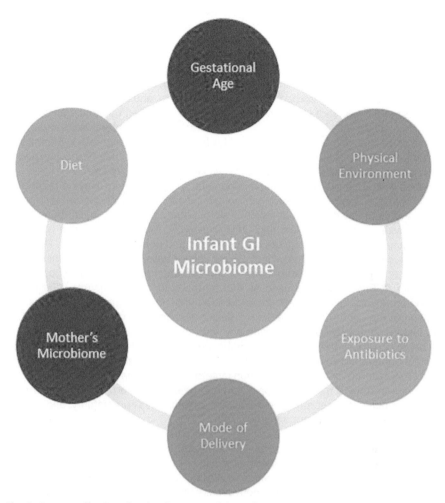

Fig. 6. Factors affecting the development of the infant GI microbiome.

nonspecific behaviors that may be related to infection or simply caused by prematurity. Because symptoms are ambiguous, and morbidity and mortality of sepsis are high, preterm infants are routinely given prolonged empiric courses of antibiotics. However, culture-proven bacteremia and sepsis are only present in 1% to 2% of VLBW infants. In the past decade, there is an increasing body of data to correlate early and prolonged antibiotic exposure with necrotizing enterocolitis, sepsis, and death.[77,78] Clearly, given the significant risks of sepsis, the authors are not suggesting that clinicians forgo antibiotics in this critically ill population; however, consideration regarding the clinical suspicion for infection must be weighed against the risk of prolonged antibiotic therapy given the available data.

Because of GI immaturity, VLBW infants often require at least partial parenteral nutrition. These infants are critically ill after birth and delaying enteral feeds has been a common practice in the past. However, administering only parenteral feeds without enteral stimulation alters GI physiology in a negative manner. Many neuroendocrine factors, such as gastrin, cholecystokinin, motilin, and vasoactive intestinal peptide, are stimulated by the presence of enteral nutrition and help to regulate GI functions with trophic mucosal effects. Lack of enteral nutrition results in an imbalance in the neuroendocrine hormones and can contribute to GI dysfunction.[79] Exclusively using parenteral nutrition has also been correlated with decreased production of secretory IgA and increased mucosal atrophy with resultant increase in bacterial translocation, systemic inflammatory response, and sepsis.[80] Animal studies have shown a reversal of total parenteral nutrition–associated bacterial translocation and inflammation with enteral feeds.[81] Rapid advancement of enteral feeds in preterm infants correlates with faster attainment of full feeds without an increase in necrotizing enterocolitis.[82] Early enteral nutrition is protective, helps to improve GI motility, and in most clinical scenarios should be initiated within the first days of life.[3]

Breast milk supports healthy GI development in a multitude of ways. Breast milk contains epithelial growth factor, erythropoietin, insulinlike growth factor, and antiinflammatory interleukin 10, all of which likely provide protective benefits by encouraging tissue growth and limiting inflammation.[83] Human milk also contains oligosaccharides, which contribute both prebiotic and postbiotic functions. Prebiotic roles include promoting the growth of certain taxa of beneficial bacteria within the infant GI tract.[2] Postbiotic effect occurs with fermentation of the residual oligosaccharides into SCFAs, which are used as fuel by the colonocyte. Butyrate, one of the SCFAs produced, has also been found to strengthen intercellular tight junctions.[3] In addition to the contributions mentioned earlier, human milk contains immunoglobulins, lactoferrin, lysozyme, and white blood cells that are likely protective for infants. Antibodies in breast milk are reflective of the mother's GI and respiratory flora; infants in close contact have similar flora to their mothers, with maternal antibodies in the breast milk tailored for optimal protection (enteromammary immune system).[3] Human milk feeds (mother's milk or donor milk) have been correlated with improved outcomes, including less necrotizing enterocolitis, retinopathy of prematurity, and sepsis, and improved neurodevelopmental outcomes.[83–86]

The GI tract is a dynamic organ system that can drive a systemic inflammatory response. With initial damage to the GI epithelium, a local response with cytokines and toxic mediators develops. These cytokines and chemokines are capable of creating a systemic response that often serves to promote increased intestinal permeability with further local GI immune activation, which creates a cyclic feedback process. There are several mechanisms and theories suggested as to how this occurs, but this is outside of the scope of this article.[87]

Given the known correlation of microbiota shifts before necrotizing enterocolitis, probiotic use as a preventive therapy has been studied in preterm infants as a possible means to modify the microbiome. Probiotics are currently classified as a supplement or food product, not as a drug, thus are not subject to the same stringent regulations as other medications. At present, the use of probiotics for necrotizing enterocolitis is controversial.[88] Some studies have shown benefit in prevention of necrotizing enterocolitis. Two studies found that preterm infants receiving daily feeds supplemented with a probiotic mixture (*Bifidobacterium infantis*, *Streptococcus thermophilus*, and *Bifidobacteria bifidus* in one study, and *Lactobacillus acidophilus* and *Bifidobacterium infantis* in the other) had decreased necrotizing enterocolitis, late-onset sepsis, and death.[89,90] However, other studies have not found statistically significant benefits,[91] and more worrisome findings of sepsis related to probiotic use in immunocompromised infants have been reported.[92–97] Further studies are needed to investigate probiotic strain and dose efficacy and safety before widespread, routine use in the preterm population is appropriate.

SUMMARY

The GI tract is an important organ system that performs a myriad of functions for preterm and term infants. This article explores several areas of normal development, including anatomic and histologic norms; anomalies in these processes can correlate clinically with a host of congenital diseases. Preterm infants have special challenges related to the immature, underdeveloped GI tract that manifest as inefficient digestion and absorption of nutrients and abnormal motility, which can present as reflux and feeding intolerance. Sources of nutrition and methods of feeding advancement for preterm infants are currently important topics of interest and study. The immunologic role of the GI tract has become well recognized, as has its role in systemic inflammation. Overall, it is important to recognize that the GI system has significant effects on systemic health for preterm and term infants.

REFERENCES

1. Montgomery RK, Mulberg AE, Grand RJ. Development of the human gastrointestinal tract: twenty years of progress. Gastroenterology 1999;116:702–31.
2. Neu J. Digestive-absorption functions in fetuses, infants and children and the developing microbiome of the fetus and newborn. In: Poli RA, Abman SH, Rowtich DH, et al, editors. Fetal and neonatal physiology, vol. 1, 5th edition. Philadelphia, PA: Elsevier; 2017. p. 897–908.
3. Neu J, Douglas-Escobar M, Fucile S. Gastrointestinal development: implications for infant feeding. In: Duggan C, Watkins JB, Koletzko B, et al, editors. Nutrition in pediatrics, vol. 1, 5th edition. Shelton, CT: People's Medical Publishing House; 2016. p. 387–98.
4. Weaver LT, Austin S, Cole TJ. Small intestinal length: a factor essential for gut adaptation. Gut 1991;32:1321–3.
5. Mezoff EA, Shroyer NF. Anatomy and physiology of the small and large intestines. In: Wyllie R, Hyams JS, Kay M, editors. Pediatric gastrointestinal and liver disease. 5th edition. Philadelphia, PA: Elsevier; 2016. p. 2–21.
6. Gray H, Warwick R, Williams PL. Gray's anatomy. 36th edition. Philadelphia: Saunders; 1980. p. xvii, 1578.
7. Clevers HC, Bevins CL. Paneth cells: maestros of the small intestinal crypts. Annu Rev Physiol 2013;75:289–311.
8. Kelly EJ, Brownlee KG, Newell SG. Gastric secretory function in the developing human stomach. Early Hum Dev 1992;31:163–6.
9. Kelly EJ, Lagopoulos M, Primrose JN. Immunocytochemical localisation of parietal cells and G cells in the developing human stomach. Gut 1993;34:1057–9.
10. Hyman PE, Clarke DD, Everett SL, et al. Gastric acid secretory function in preterm infants. J Pediatr 1985;106(3):467–71.
11. Werner B. Peptic and tryptic capacity of the digestive glands in newborns: a comparison between premature and full-term infants. Acta Paediatr Jpn 1948; 35n(Suppl 5):1.
12. Antonowicz I, Lebenthal E. Developmental pattern of small intestinal enterokinase and disaccharidase activities in the human fetus. Gastroenterology 1977;72(6): 1299–303.
13. Demers-Mathieu V, Underwood MA, Borghese R, et al. Premature infants have lower gastric digestion capacity for human milk proteins than term infants. J Pediatr Gastroenterol Nutr 2018;66(5):816–21. Post Acceptance: November 10, 2017.

14. Schanler RJ. The use of human milk for premature infants. Pediatr Clin North Am 2001;48(1):207–19.

15. Mihatsch WA, Franz AR, Hogel J, et al. Hydrolyzed protein accelerates feeding advancement in very low birthweight infants. Pediatrics 2002;110(6):1199–203.

16. Murray RD, Kerzner B, Sloan HR, et al. The contribution of salivary amylase to glucose polymer hydrolysis in premature infants. Pediatr Res 1986;20(2):211–28.

17. Davis MM, Hodes ME, Munsick RA, et al. Pancreatic amylase expression in human pancreatic development. Hybridoma 1986;5:137–45.

18. McClean P, Weaver LT. Ontogeny of human pancreatic exocrine function. Arch Dis Child 1993;68:62–5.

19. Leonel AJ, Alvarez-Leite JI. Butyrate: implications for intestinal function. Curr Opin Clin Nutr Metab Care 2012;15:474–9.

20. Arpaia N, Campbell C, Fan X, et al. Metabolites produced by commensal bacteria promote peripheral regulatory T-cell generation. Nature 2013;504:451–5.

21. Schulman RJ, Schanler RJ, Lau C, et al. Early feeding, feeding tolerance, and lactase activity in preterm infants. J Pediatr 1998;133(5):645–9.

22. Boyle JT, Celano P, Koldovsky O. Demonstration of a difference in expression of maximal lactase and sucrase activity along the villus in the adult rat jejunum. Gastroenterology 1980;79(3):503–7.

23. Klenoff-Brumberg HL, Genen LH. High versus low medium chain triglyceride content of formula for promoting short term growth of preterm neonates. Cochrane Database Syst Rev 2003;(1):CD002777.

24. Freed LM, York CM, Homosh P, et al. Bile salt-stimulated lipase of human milk: characteristics of the enzyme in the milk of mothers of premature and full-term infants. J Pediatr Gastroenterol Nutr 1987;6:598–604.

25. Ménard D, Monfils S, Tremblay E. Ontogeny of human gastric lipase and pepsin activities. Gastroenterology 1995;108:1650–6.

26. Hamosh M, Scanlon JW, Ganot D, et al. Fat digestion in the newborn. Characterization of lipase in gastric aspirates of premature and term infants. J Clin Invest 1981;67:838–46.

27. Zoppi G, Andreotti G, Pajno-Ferrara F, et al. Exocrine pancreas function in premature and full term neonates. Pediatr Res 1972;6:880–6.

28. Balistreri WF. Immaturity of hepatic excretory function and the ontogeny of bile acid metabolism. J Pediatr Gastroenterol Nutr 1983;2(Suppl 1):S207–2014.

29. Boehm G, Braun W, Moro G, et al. Bile acid concentrations in serum and duodenal aspirates of healthy preterm infants: effects of gestational and postnatal age. Biol Neonate 1997;71(4):207–14.

30. Georgieff MK, Innis SM. Controversial nutrients that potentially affect preterm neurodevelopment: essential fatty acids and iron. Pediatr Res 2005;57(5 Ptx2):99R–103R.

31. Lapillonne A, Jensen CL. Reevaluation of the DHA requirement for the premature infant. Prostaglandins Leukot Essent Fatty Acids 2009;81:143–50.

32. SanGiovanni JP, Parra-Cabrera S, Colditz GA, et al. Meta-analysis of dietary essential fatty acids and long-chain polyunsaturated fatty acids as they relate to visual resolution acuity in healthy preterm infants. Pediatrics 2000;105(6):1292–8.

33. Morale SE, Hoffman DR, Castaneda YS, et al. Duration of long-chain polyunsaturated fatty acids availability in the diet and visual acuity. Early Hum Dev 2005;81(2):197–203.

34. Smithers LG, Gibson RA, McPhee A, et al. Effect of long-chain polyunsaturated fatty acid supplementation of preterm infants on disease risk and

neurodevelopment: a systematic review of randomized controlled trials. Am J Clin Nutr 2008;87(4):912–20.

35. De Oliveira SC, Bellanger A, Menard O, et al. A impact of homogenization of pasteurized human milk on gastric digestion in the preterm infant: a randomized controlled trial. Clin Nutr ESPEN 2017;20:1–11.

36. Calder PC. Can n-3 polyunsaturated fatty acids be used as immunomodulatory agents? Biochem Soc Trans 1996;24(1):211–20.

37. Caplan MS, Russell T, Xiao Y, et al. Effect of polyunsaturated fatty acid (PUFA) supplementation on intestinal inflammation and necrotizing enterocolitis (NEC) in a neonatal rat model. Pediatr Res 2001;49(5):647–52.

38. Rayyan M, Devlieger H, Jochum F, et al. Short-term use of parenteral nutrition with a lipid emulsion containing a mixture of soybean oil, olive oil, medium chain tri-glycerides and fish oil. A randomized double blind study in preterm infants. JPEN J Parenter Enteral Nutr 2012;36(1_suppl):81S–94S.

39. Le HD, de Meijer VE, Robinson EM, et al. Parenteral fish-oil-based lipid emulsion improves fatty acid profiles and lipids in parenteral nutrition-dependent children. Am J Clin Nutr 2011;94:749–58.

40. Angsten G, Finkel Y, Lucas S, et al. Improved outcome in neonatal short bowel syndrome using parenteral fish oil in combination with omega-6/9 lipid emulsions. JPEN J Parenter Enteral Nutr 2012;36(5):587–95.

41. Martin CR, Dasilva DA, Cluette-Brown JE, et al. Decreased postnatal docosahex-aenoic and arachidonic acid blood levels in premature infants are associated with neonatal morbidities. J Pediatr 2011;159:743–9.e1-2.

42. Lau C, Smith EO, Schanler RJ. Coordination of suck-swallow and swallow respiration in preterm infants. Acta Paediatr Jpn 2003;92(6):721–7.

43. Poets CF. Gastroesophageal reflux: a critical review of its role in preterm infants. Pediatrics 2004;113(2):e128–32.

44. Jadcherla SR. Gastroesophageal reflux in the neonate. Clin Perinatol 2002;29(1):135–58.

45. Newell SJ, Booth IW, Morgan ME, et al. Gastro-oesophageal reflux in preterm infants. Arch Dis Child 1989;64(6):780–6.

46. Davies AM, Koenig JS, Thach BT. Upper airway chemoreflex responses to saline and water in preterm infants. J Appl Physiol (1985) 1988;64:1412–20.

47. Page M, Jeffery HE. Airway protection in sleeping infants in response to pharyngeal fluid stimulation in the supine position. Pediatr Res 1998;44:691–8.

48. Frakaloss G, Burke G, Sanders MR. Impact of gastroesophageal reflux on growth and hospital stay in premature infants. J Pediatr Gastroenterol Nutr 1998;26:146–50.

49. Basaran UN, Celayir S, Eray N, et al. The effect of an H2-receptor antagonist on small-bowel colonization and bacterial translocation in newborn rats. Pediatr Surg Int 1998;13(2–3):118–20.

50. Graham PL 3rd, Begg MD, Larson E, et al. Risk factors for late onset gram-negative sepsis in low birth weight infants hospitalized in the neonatal intensive care unit. Pediatr Infect Dis J 2006;25(2):113–7.

51. Guillet R, Stoll BJ, Cotten CM, et al. Association of H2-blocker therapy and higher incidence of necrotizing enterocolitis in very low birth weight infants. Pediatrics 2006;117(2):e137–42.

52. Gupta RW, Tran L, Norori J, et al. Histamine-2 receptor blockers alter the fecal microbiota in premature infants. J Pediatr Gastroenterol Nutr 2013;56:397–400.

53. Chen IL, Gao WY, Johnson AP, et al. Proton pump inhibitor use in infants: FDA reviewer experience. J Pediatr Gastroenterol Nutr 2012;54(1):8–14.

54. Tolia V, Boyer K. Long-term proton pump inhibitor use in children: a retrospective review of safety. Dig Dis Sci 2008;53(2):385–93.

55. Ward RM, Kearns GL. Proton pump inhibitors in pediatrics. Paediatr Drugs 2013; 15(2):119–31.

56. Cavell B. Gastric emptying in infants fed human milk or infant formula. Acta Paediatr Scand 1981;70(5):639–41.

57. Cavell B. Reservoir and emptying function of the stomach of the premature infant. Acta Paediatr Scand Suppl 1982;296:60–1.

58. Berseth CL. Gastrointestinal motility in the neonate. Clin Perinatol 1996;23(2): 179–90.

59. Lebenthal E, Siegel M. Understanding gastric emptying: implications for feeding the healthy and compromised infant. J Pediatr Gastroenterol Nutr 1985;4(1):1–3.

60. Pritchard JA. Fetal swallowing and amniotic fluid volume. Obstet Gynecol 1966; 28(5):606–10.

61. Patole S, Rao S, Doherty D. Erythromycin as a prokinetic agent in preterm neonates: a systematic review. Arch Dis Child Fetal Neonatal Ed 2005;90(4):F301–6.

62. Hyman PE, Abrams C, Dubois A. Effect of metoclopramide and bethanechol on gastric emptying in infants. Pediatr Res 1985;19(10):1029–32.

63. Aagaard K, Ma J, Antony KM, et al. The placenta harbors a unique microbiome. Sci Transl Med 2014;6:237ra265.

64. DiGiulio DB. Diversity of microbes in amniotic fluid. Semin Fetal Neonatal Med 2012;17:2–11.

65. Moles L, Gómez M, Heilig H, et al. Bacterial diversity in meconium of preterm neonates and evolution of their fecal microbiota during the first month of life. PLoS One 2013;8:e66986.

66. Langhendries JP. Early bacterial colonisation of the intestine: why it matters? Arch Pediatr 2006;13:1526–34.

67. Leaphart CL, Cavallo J, Gribar SC, et al. A critical role for TLR4 in the pathogenesis of necrotizing enterocolitis by modulating intestinal injury and repair. J Immunol 2007;179:4808–20.

68. Neu J, Walker WA. Necrotizing enterocolitis. N Engl J Med 2011;364:255–64.

69. Dicksved J, Halfvarson J, Rosenquist M, et al. Molecular analysis of the gut microbiota of identical twins with Crohn's disease. ISME J 2008;2:716–27.

70. Daniel H, Moghaddas Gholami A, Berry D, et al. High-fat diet alters gut microbiota physiology in mice. ISME J 2014;8:295–308.

71. Wang Y, Hoenig JD, Malin KJ, et al. 16S rRNA gene-based analysis of fecal microbiota from preterm infants with and without necrotizing enterocolitis. ISME J 2009;3:944–54.

72. Penders J, Thijs C, van den Brandt PA, et al. Gut microbiota composition and development of atopic manifestations in infancy: the KOALA birth cohort study. Gut 2007;56:661–7.

73. Claud EC. Neonatal necrotizing enterocolitis-inflammation and intestinal immaturity. Antiinflamm Antiallergy Agents Med Chem 2009;8:248–59.

74. Martin CR, Walker WA. Intestinal immune defenses and the inflammatory response in necrotizing enterocolitis. Semin Fetal Neonatal Med 2006;11:369–77.

75. Bjorkstrom MV, Hall L, Sodelund S, et al. Intestinal flora in very low-birth weight infants. Acta Paediatr 2009;98:1762–7.

76. Clark RH, Bloom BT, Spitzer AR, et al. Reported medication use in the neonatal intensive care unit: data from a large national data set. Pediatrics 2006;117: 1979–87.

77. Cotten CM, Taylor S, Stoll B, et al. Prolonged duration of initial empirical antibiotic treatment is associated with increased rates of necrotizing enterocolitis and death for extremely low birth weight infants. Pediatrics 2009;123:58–66.
78. Kuppala VS, Meinzen-Derr J, Morrow AL, et al. Prolonged initial empirical antibiotic treatment is associated with adverse outcomes in premature infants. J Pediatr 2011;159:720–5.
79. Johnson LR. The trophic action of gastrointestinal hormones. Gastroenterology 1976;70:278–88.
80. Hermsen JL, San Y, Kudsk KA. Food fight! Parenteral nutrition, enteral stimulation and gut-derived mucosal immunity. Langenbecks Arch Surg 2009;394:17–30.
81. Wildhaber BE, Yang H, Spencer AU, et al. Lack of enteral nutrition-effects on the intestinal immune system. J Surg Res 2005;123(1):8–16.
82. Karagol BS, Zencirogly A, Okumus N, et al. Randomized controlled trial of slow vs. rapid enteral feeding advancements on the clinical outcomes of preterm infants with birth weight 750-1250g. JPEN J Parenter Enteral Nutr 2013;37(2):223–8.
83. Meizen-Derr J, Poindexter B, Wrage L, et al. Role of human milk in extremely low birth weight infants' risk of necrotizing enterocolitis or death. J Perinatol 2009; 29(1):57–62.
84. Howie PW, Forsyth JS, Ogston SA, et al. Protective effect of breast feeding against infection. BMJ 1990;300:11–6.
85. Heller CD, O'Shea M, Yao Q, et al. Human milk intake and retinopathy of prematurity in extremely low birth weight infants. Pediatrics 2007;120:1–9.
86. Isaacs EB, Fischl BR, Quinn BT, et al. Impact of breast milk on IQ, brain size, and white matter development. Pediatr Res 2010;67:357–62.
87. Clark JA, Coopersmith CM. Intestinal crosstalk: a new paradigm for understanding the gut as the "motor" of critical illness. Shock 2007;28(4):384–93.
88. Neu J. Gastrointestinal development and meeting the nutritional needs of premature infants. Am J Clin Nutr 2007;85(2):629S–34S.
89. Lin HC, Su BH, Chen AC, et al. Oral probiotics reduce the incidence and severity of necrotizing enterocolitis in very low birth weight infants. Pediatrics 2005;115: 1–4.
90. Bin-Nun A, Bromiker R, Wilschanski M, et al. Oral probiotics prevent necrotizing enterocolitis in very low birth weight neonates. J Pediatr 2005;147:192–6.
91. Dani C, Biadaioli R, Bertini G, et al. Probiotics feeding in prevention of urinary tract infection, bacterial sepsis and necrotizing enterocolitis in preterm infants. A prospective double-blind study. Biol Neonate 2002;82:103–8.
92. Berger RE. *Lactobacillus* sepsis associated with probiotic therapy. J Urol 2005; 174:1843.
93. De Groote MA, Frank DN, Dowell E, et al. *Lactobacillus rhamnosus* GG bacteremia associated with probiotic use in a child with short gut syndrome. Pediatr Infect Dis J 2005;24:278–80.
94. Jones PM, Gupta SK. Colic and gastrointestinal gas. In: Wyllie R, Hyams JS, Kay M, editors. Pediatric gastrointestinal and liver disease. 5th edition. Philadelphia, PA: Elsevier; 2016. p. 115–23.
95. Koonce T, Mounsey A, Rowland K. Colicky baby? Here's a surprising remedy. J Fam Pract 2011;60(1):34–6.
96. Mugambi MN, Musekiwa A, Lombard M, et al. Synbiotics, probiotics, or prebiotics in infant formula for full term infants: a systematic review. Nutr J 2012;11: 81, p1–32.
97. Anabrees J, Indrio F, Paes B, et al. Probiotics for infantile colic: a systematic review. BMC Pediatr 2013;13:186.

Multiplex Nucleic Acid Amplification Testing to Diagnose Gut Infections
Challenges, Opportunities, and Result Interpretation

Neil W. Anderson, MD[a], Phillip I. Tarr, MD[b],*

KEYWORDS

• Children • Diagnosis • Diarrhea • Gastroenteritis • Multiplex PCR

KEY POINTS

• Classical microbiologic testing of stool for the diagnosis of enteric infections is labor intensive, slow, and often incomplete.
• Multiplex nucleic acid testing is a sensitive culture-independent technology that is fast and detects viruses, bacteria, and parasites.
• Multiplex nucleic acid testing has drawbacks, including cost, detection of pathogens that are of uncertain clinical significance in North American children, and the inability to produce bacteria for DNA fingerprinting by disease control authorities.

THE CHALLENGES OF DIAGNOSTIC ENTERIC MICROBIOLOGY

Establishing an infectious etiology for an episode of gastroenteritis, and especially an episode in which diarrhea predominates, has appeal. However, current (classical) tests rely on bacterial growth and colony characterization, agglutination, antigen testing, and microscopy, which are technologies dating to the late 1800s. These techniques are applied to highly diverse pathogens (bacteria, viruses, and parasites), and often do not produce timely and helpful diagnoses. In this article, we review current (classical) enteric infection diagnostic technology, survey newly available

Disclosure Statement: Dr. Tarr was supported by P30DK052574 (Administrative Core).
[a] Division of Laboratory and Genomic Medicine, Barnes Jewish Hospital, Washington University in St. Louis School of Medicine, 660 South Euclid Avenue, CB 8118, St Louis, MO 63110, USA;
[b] Division of Gastroenterology, Hepatology and Nutrition, Department of Pediatrics, Washington University in St. Louis School of Medicine, 660 South Euclid Avenue, CB 8208, St Louis, MO 63110, USA
* Corresponding author.
E-mail address: tarr@wustl.edu

Gastroenterol Clin N Am 47 (2018) 793–812
https://doi.org/10.1016/j.gtc.2018.07.006
0889-8553/18/© 2018 Elsevier Inc. All rights reserved.

gastro.theclinics.com

Abbreviations	
EAggEC	Enteroaggregative *Escherichia coli*
EPEC	Enteropathogenic *Escherichia coli*
ETEC	Enterotoxigenic *Escherichia coli*
FDA	Food and Drug Administration
PCR	Polymerase chain reaction
STEC	Shiga toxin-producing *Escherichia coli*

multiplex nucleic acid amplification tests that are now being introduced for enteric pathogen detection, discuss the challenges and opportunities of this new technology, and offer a set of frequently asked questions about test results that are generated. Our perspective is based largely on the North American and European literature and focuses on infections in childhood. We do not offer specific treatment regimens and urge consultation to obtain the most up-to-date recommendations regarding appropriate therapy.

Enteric Pathogen Overview

The diagnostic microbiologist seeking pathogens in the stool of a child with diarrhea has a daunting task. First, there are many different pathogens to seek. Bona fide and candidate causes of gastroenteritis include bacteria (*Aeromonas* spp., *Campylobacter* spp., *Clostridioides* [formerly *Clostridium*] *difficile*, Shiga toxin-producing *Escherichia coli* [STEC] O157, non-O157 STEC, enteropathogenic *E coli* [EPEC], enteroaggregative *E coli* [EAggEC], and enterotoxigenic *E coli* [ETEC], *Plesiomonas shigelloides*, *Salmonella* spp., *Shigella* spp., and *Yersinia entercolitica*), and *Vibrio* spp., viruses (adenoviruses 40 and 41, astroviruses, noroviruses, rotaviruses, sapoviruses, and human bocaviruses), and protozoa (*Cryptosporidium*, *Cyclospora cayatenensis*, *Giardia lamblia*, *Blastocystis hominis*, *Dientamoeba fragilis*, and *Entamoeba histolytica*). Patients whose immune systems are compromised are prone to gastroenteritis caused by these organisms, and also by *Cystoisospora* (formerly *Isospora*) *belli* and *Microsporidium* spp. However, classical microbiology testing in North America and Europe seeks only a subset of these agents.

The requesting physician, too, faces challenges when the laboratory reports a positive result. Children without diarrhea excrete *Aeromonas*,[1] adenoviruses,[2] and *Cryptosporidium*[3] at frequencies similar to, and sometimes greater than, children with diarrhea. The etiologic role of *C difficile* in childhood diarrhea is difficult to establish until children are about 3 years old.[3] Even after that age, many children will excrete *C difficile* without symptoms of *C difficile* infection. All STEC belonging to serotype O157:H7 are pathogens and usually cause severe disease. In contrast, most non-O157:H7 STEC cause milder infections, and have minimal risk of precipitating the hemolytic uremic syndrome, unless they contain a gene encoding Shiga toxin 2. However, culture reports rarely include Shiga toxin genotype.

Current (Classical) Enteric Diagnostic Technology

Approximately 30% of stool weight consists of bacteria belonging to diverse species, making stool an exceedingly complex specimen type from which to isolate a bacterial pathogen.[4] Culture strategies enrich for bacterial pathogens and help the technologist to identify specific agents among a population of commensal bacteria. For example, Hektoen enteric and xylose, lysine, deoxycholate agars contain high concentrations of bile salts, which suppress background bacteria and select for *Salmonella* and *Shigella* spp. They also contain pH indicators and specific substrates to differentiate colonies that represent the agents of interest.

However, despite enrichment, selection, and differentiating culture strategies, nonpathogenic bacteria can overgrow pathogenic bacteria in inoculated stool. Even after detecting a suspicious colony, final identification requires biochemical and antigen testing or mass spectrometry. To cover the breadth of possible bacterial pathogens, microbiologists use multiple plates of selective and/or differentiating agar. Omitting even a single agar or enrichment technique could eliminate the possibility of finding a pathogen that is best (or even exclusively) detected on that medium. These enrichment and confirmatory steps obligate at least 24 hours to perform, limiting their value in the real-time management of patients. Different kinds of techniques (microscopy, special stains of stool smears, antigen testing) are used to find pathogenic viruses, protozoa, and C difficile. **Table 1** summarizes the nonmolecular tests that microbiologists currently use to find pathogens in children in high-income countries. Although individual reagents are inexpensive, the diverse technologies to detect these diverse pathogens (**Fig. 1**), and the costs of trained laboratory personnel to staff these tests, are not.

Current enteric testing technology has additional problems related to specimen type and transport. The Infectious Diseases Society of America recommends that stool samples (not swabs) be sent for microbiologic evaluation.[12] However, patients with diarrhea often do not produce stool while they are on site,[13,14] causing logistic issues in getting specimens to the laboratory. Recent publications suggest that swab specimens are almost as worthwhile as bulk stool specimens for microbiologic diagnosis, but of overall greater yield when considering the pragmatic value of obtaining diagnostic material at the visit.[15–19] C difficile and virus antigen testing require bulk stools, as does microscopy for parasites. When stools are sent to distant referral laboratories, time is lost in transit. Also, if testing does not commence immediately on receipt in the laboratory, diagnosis is further delayed.

For all of these reasons, it is understandably frustrating for practitioners or systems to develop logical testing protocols with existing technology, especially because few such episodes are caused by agents that can be treated, or are reportable to public health authorities. This is particularly true for viral gastroenteritis, which often resolves spontaneously, and the detection of a virus does not preclude parallel testing to confirm that a more actionable bacterial or protozoal pathogen is not also present. Clearly, the field is ready for new approaches to enteric diagnosis that are rapid, use small volumes of specimen, and provide results relevant to multiple different pathogens.

Overview of Multiplex Nucleic Acid Amplification Tests

Multiplex nucleic acid amplification tests can identify, in a single assay on a single specimen, nucleic acids of bacterial, viral, and protozoal origin, thereby obviating piecemeal testing to find an enteric pathogen. Many of the newly available multiplex nucleic acid tests do not require special expertise to perform, so results can be offered around the clock, near the point of care. The cost of current instruments preclude deployment outside laboratories at the point of care, but this might change in the future.

Multiplex nucleic acid amplification tests share similar design characteristics, and all sequentially apply nucleic acid extraction, primer binding and nucleic acid amplification, detection of the amplification products, and generation of a report. Although early multiplex nucleic acid tests required multiple instruments to perform these steps, there is a general trend toward consolidating these steps to make the assays quicker and more user friendly. A common example of this assay format is the use of a single cartridge into which stool or extracted nucleic acid is loaded. The cartridge contains the

Table 1
Examples of "classical" (i.e., non-molecular) techniques to identify common enteric pathogens in stool in high-income countries. Some pathogens are detected by multiple different technologies

Technology	Agents Detected
Bacteria[a]	
Blood agar plate	Aeromonas spp., P. shigelloides, Vibrio spp.
Campylobacter selective agar, incubation at 42°C	Campylobacter spp.
C. difficile toxin antigen detection in stool	C. difficile
Cytotoxicity with neutralization of C. difficile toxin	C. difficile
Toxigenic culture	C. difficile
Chromogenic agar plates	STEC O157:H7,[b] non-O157:H7 STEC[b]
Shiga toxin antigen detection on broth enrichment culture	STEC O157:H7,[c] non-O157:H7 STEC[c]
Hektoen enteric agar	Salmonella spp., Shigella spp.
Selenite F broth	Salmonella spp.
Shigella selective agar	Shigella spp.
Thiosulfate bile salt agar	Vibrio spp.
Yersinia selective agar	Y. enterocolitica
Viruses	
Enzyme immunoassay[d]	Adenovirus 40 and 41, norovirus,[e] rotavirus
Parasites	
Enzyme immunoassay[f]	Cryptosporidium, Giardia
Microscopy – wet mount, concentration, and trichrome staining	B. hominis, Cryptosporidium, D. fragilis, E. histolytica, Giardia
Microscopy - Wet mounts, autofluorescence, and acid-fast staining	Cryptosporidium, Cyclospora, Cystoisospora
Microscopy	Cryptosporidium, Cyclospora

[a] Some laboratories report *Edwardsiella tarda* and *Staphylococcus aureus* in stool cultures based on local custom or special requests. Institutional expertise should guide the response, depending on the clinical context.
[b] Some chromogenic agars identify only STEC O157:H7 (including sorbitol MacConkey agar with or without tellurite and cefixime), and some identify non-O157 STEC.
[c] After a broth culture is positive for Shiga toxin, further analysis is needed to determine if the toxin is produced by an STEC O157:H7 or a non-O157 STEC. 10-15% of STEC O157:H7 are not detected by Shiga toxin assays but are detected on sorbitol MacConkey agar culture of stool,[3,5–10] so the CDC recommends against using the toxin assay as an exclusive screen for STEC O157:H7.[11]
[d] These enzyme immunoassays detect only single viruses, so it is necessary to specify the agent(s) of interest.
[e] Norovirus EIA is FDA cleared for outbreak investigation but not for routine diagnosis.
[f] Some enzyme immunoassays detect *Cryptosporidium* and *Giardia*, and others detect only one of these agents. Because the symptoms of these infections overlap, it is best to test for both.

reagents (buffers, primers, enzymes) needed to generate an amplicon and all reactions occur in the cartridge. An instrument accepts the loaded cartridge and drives the fluidics to move materials within the cartridge. The instrument also heats and cools the cartridge to perform the amplification reaction, the optics to detect the amplified targets, and the software to interpret the signals and to generate a report.

Regardless of the assay format, the first step in all multiplex nucleic acid tests is the extraction of nucleic acids from bacteria, viruses, and protozoa from the stool. Nuclease inhibitors are present in this step to preserve the integrity of the extracted RNA and DNA. Depending on assay format, this step is accomplished in a cartridge or using a standalone extraction instrument.

In the second step, oligonucleotide probes that bind to loci in pathogens of interest are mixed with the extracted DNA in a chamber that also contains optimized buffers for polymerase chain reaction (PCR). The ideal primer pair binds to loci that are found only or predominantly in organisms of interest (ie, are specific), and that are always or almost always present in all organisms of interest (ie, are conserved). The definitions of specificity and conservation vary according to pathogen. In some situations, a single primer pair provides specificity and sensitivity, whereas in other situations, primer pairs that bind to a combination of loci are needed to increase specificity.

In the third step, after primer binding, nucleic acids are amplified through PCR in the presence of enzymes, nucleotides, and buffers. This step may occur in a standalone thermocycler or within a test cartridge, depending on the assay.

The final step of all multiplex nucleic acid tests is the detection of amplified products. This step is accomplished in various ways, ranging from target specific fluorescent probes to sorting of products using oligonucleotide probes and flow cytometry. Each method generates signals that report presence of an organism of interest. As noted, the software might require that more than 1 locus be present before a positive report is generated.

The Earliest Multiplex Nucleic Acid Test Technology

The feasibility, accuracy, and speed of laboratory-developed PCR detection were first demonstrated for bacterial enteric pathogens,[20–23] but these assays were confined to laboratories with the expertise and infrastructure to build in-house tests compliant with CLIA requirements. Early commercial multiplex nucleic acid test kits sought a limited set of bacterial enteric pathogens. The EntericBio RealTime Gastro Panel 1 (EntericBio, Limerick, Ireland) tested stool for the presence of *Campylobacter* spp., *Salmonella* spp., *Shigella* spp., and STEC.[24] The RIDA GENE-gastrointestinal kits (R-Biopharm, Darmstadt, Germany) and the Seeplex Diarrhea ACE detection systems (SeeGene, Seoul, Korea) offered similarly focused panels, although one could achieve added breadth by running multiple different panels simultaneously.[25,26] Each assay was simple to use, and as sensitive as, and more rapid than, culture-based diagnostics. However, these assays were not cleared by the US Food and Drug Administration (FDA).

Current Multiplex Nucleic Acid Test Systems

The FDA has recently cleared several multiplex nucleic acid tests to detect a spectrum of enteric pathogens. These tests require between approximately 1 and 5 hours to generate results. The ProGastro SSCS assay (Hologic, Marlborough, MA), Gen-Probe Prodesse (Hologic), the Verigene enteric pathogens test (Luminex, Austin, TX), and the BD MAX Extended Enteric Bacterial Panel (Becton, Dickinson and Company, Franklin Lakes, NJ) seek a limited number of highly actionable bacterial pathogens, and one, the BD MAX Enteric Parasite panel, is limited to detecting diarrheagenic parasites. Other tests detect a broader range of targets. **Table 2** describes characteristics of each of the currently available FDA-cleared multiplex nucleic acid tests as described on their websites on January 28, 2018, and the pathogens that they identify. It is possible that future iterations of these test systems will encompass different (expanded) target panels, with increased specificity.

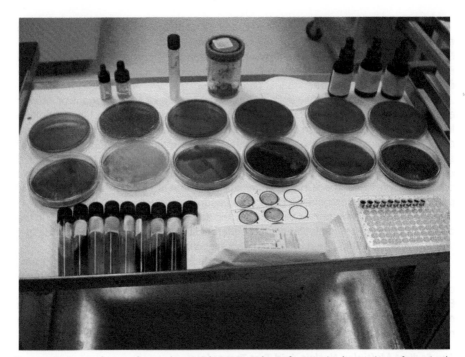

Fig. 1. Media used to perform a bacterial enteric culture from a single specimen for a single patient, ca. 2005, to detect *Aeromonas, Campylobacter,* O157:H7, and non-O157 Shiga toxin-producing *Escherichia coli, Plesiomonas, Salmonella, Shigella,* and *Yersinia.* Viruses and parasites are not detected by these reagents. (*Courtesy of* Patricia Sellenriek, St Louis, Missouri.)

Overall, these assays have very good analytical performance characteristics. When compared with standard methods, the BioFire FilmArray Gastrointestinal Panel is 100% sensitive for 12 of 22 targets and greater than 94.5% sensitive for 7 of 22 targets in 1556 prospectively collected diarrheal stools from patients being evaluated for infectious gastroenteritis.[27] As expected, stools from patients with bloody diarrhea have greater yields of bacterial pathogens than do diarrheal stools without visible blood.[28] This test performed equivalently to the Luminex xTAG Gastrointestinal Panel, except for *Aeromonas* spp.[29] The Luminex xTAG Gastrointestinal Panel was greater than 90% sensitive for each pathogen[30] in 254 clinical stools specimens. A 4-site, 901 specimen trial, demonstrated similar sensitivity.[31] Interestingly, 65% of detections were of targets not requested by physicians. The test performed similarly in adults and children,[22] with a mixed pathogen detection rate of 7%. This test performed equivalently to the BioFire FilmArray Gastrointestinal Panel, except for *Yersinia enterocolitica.*[29] The Verigene enteric pathogens test performance was equivalent to the Luminex xTAG Gastrointestinal Panel and BioFire FilmArray Gastrointestinal Panel.[32] The BD MAX Extended Enteric Bacterial Panel had greater than 97.6% positive agreement and 99.7% negative agreement (for *Vibrio* spp., ETEC, *P shigelloides,* and *Y enterocolitica*) in 2410 unformed stool specimens, when compared with a combination of culture and PCR.[34] The ProGastro SSCS assay Gen-Probe Prodesse was more sensitive than culture of 1153 unique specimens.[35]

Multiplex Nucleic Acid Amplification Tests Opportunities and Challenges

Multiplex nucleic acid amplification tests have 3 major attributes: the breadth of targets detected, rapid turnaround, and the ability to bring highly accurate microbial detection capacity to settings where microbiologic expertise and resources are difficult to maintain. The expanded target range offers etiologies that current classical testing overlooks, because a comprehensive evaluation obligates separate requests for bacterial, viral, and parasitic pathogens. The frequent finding of viral pathogens is not surprising in view of recent data that demonstrate that norovirus is responsible for approximately one-third of undiagnosed cases of diarrhea.[3,36] The rapid turnaround of results for actionable pathogens enables decisions about treatment and hospitalization and provide etiology-based prognoses, even while patients are still on site. This finding was illustrated in a multisite 2018 study showing that patients tested by a multiplex nucleic acid test (n = 1887; all age groups included) received results rapidly (median of 18 hours vs 47 hours for culture) and were more likely to receive targeted antibiotic therapy.[37] Interestingly, this study also demonstrated that the number of patients placed on antibiotic therapy increased after test implementation.

Despite these attributes, multiplex nucleic acid tests are costly, detect organisms that have variable (if any) clinical significance, and often find nucleic acid evidence of multiple different agents within a single specimen. Some data suggest that this technology can reduce overall expenditures in the evaluation of children and adults with diarrhea,[38,39] but formal cost assessments are difficult to perform because there are no acceptable independent reference standards.[38,40] Public health authorities use genetic analyses of pathogens to confirm or refute common origin, and typing requires a pure isolate, which multiplex nucleic acid tests do not produce. Hence, multiplex nucleic acid tests could have major, and adverse, effects on efforts to control outbreaks. The Centers for Disease Control and Prevention report that, although culture-independent diagnostic technologies, including multiplex nucleic acid tests, increase the detection rates of reportable bacterial enteric pathogens, the number of isolates available for typing is diminishing.[41] Also, in a small subset of infections, antibiotics are warranted to treat the infection and, without a bacterial isolate, susceptibilities cannot be determined. Finally, clinicians must make treatment decisions based on multiplex nucleic acid amplification test results, but their knowledge is based on decades of data built on classical microbiologic diagnostic technology. It is not known if culture-derived data apply to the agents reported on multiplex nucleic acid amplification tests, which is generally more sensitive than cultures.

An additional challenge relates to specimen type accepted by multiplex nucleic acid amplification tests. Multiplex nucleic acid amplification tests are cleared for testing on stool, but stool can be difficult to produce (and/or collect) on command, particularly in children. Waiting to obtain a specimen can delay patient care. As such, investigators have explored the possibility of using rectal swabs to detect stool pathogens. Swab specimens were used to compare the BD MAX Enteric Bacterial Panel and stool cultures in 272 subjects and swabs were quite acceptable for gastrointestinal pathogen molecular testing.[42] This finding was substantiated in a large, multisite, outpatient cohort study of children with diarrhea,[43] which reported a 57% pathogen yield for stool and a 67% pathogen yield for rectal swabs, taking into account the pragmatic value of obtaining rectal swabs on site. However, none of the currently FDA-cleared multiplex nucleic acid amplification tests permit the use of rectal swab specimens. Nonetheless, these studies support the value of rectal swabs, suggesting that manufacturers should include them in future assay design and laboratories should consider validating them as acceptable specimen types.

Multiplex Nucleic Acid Amplification Testing and Clinical Considerations

Clinical context is important in selecting any test and interpreting the results. Multiplex nucleic acid amplification tests pose particular challenges, because clinicians

Table 2
Current (January 2018) multiplex nucleic acid tests for enteric pathogen detection

Agents Detected	BioFire FilmArray Gastrointestinal[a,27–29]	Luminex xTAG Gastrointestinal Pathogen Panel[b,22,29–31]	Verigene Enteric Pathogens Test[c,32]	BD MAX Enteric Bacterial Panel[d,33]	BD MAX Extended Enteric Bacterial Panel[e,34]	BD MAX Enteric Parasite Panel[f]	The ProGastro SSCS Assay Gen-Probe Prodesse[g,35]
Campylobacter	Yes	Yes	Yes	Yes	Yes	No	Yes
Toxigenic *Clostridioides difficile*	Yes	Yes	No	No	No	No	No
Escherichia coli O157:H7	Yes	Yes	No	No	No	No	No
Non-O157:H7 STEC	Yes	Yes	Yes	Yes	Yes	No	Yes
EAggEC	No	No	No	No	No	No	No
EPEC	Yes	No	No	No	No	No	No
ETEC	Yes	No	No	No	No	No	No
Salmonella	Yes	Yes	Yes	Yes	Yes	No	Yes
Shigella spp./EIEC[h]	Yes	Yes	Yes	Yes	Yes	No	Yes
Plesiomonas spp.	Yes	No	No	No	Yes	No	No
Vibrio spp.	Yes	Yes	Yes	No	Yes	No	No
Yersinia enterocolitica	Yes	Yes[i]	Yes	No	Yes	No	No
Adenovirus 40/41	Yes	Yes	No	No	No	No	No

Astrovirus	Yes	No	No	No	No	No
Norovirus	Yes	Yes	Yes	No	No	No
Rotavirus	Yes	Yes	Yes	No	No	No
Sapovirus (I, II, IV, V)	Yes	No	No	No	No	No
Cryptosporidium	Yes	Yes	No	No	Yes	No
Cyclospora	Yes	No	No	No	No	No
Entamoeba histolytica	Yes	Yes	No	No	Yes	No
Giardia lamblia	Yes	Yes	No	No	Yes	No

Targeted microbes are as listed on company website on January 28, 2018. Specific URLs are provided for each product.

Abbreviation: STEC, Shiga toxin-producing Escherichia coli.

a http://www.biofiredx.com/wp-content/uploads/2016/03/IS-MRKT-PRT-0234-07-FilmArray-Gastrointestinal-Panel-Information-Sheet.pdf.
b https://www.luminexcorp.com/clinical/infectious-disease/gastrointestinal-pathogen-panel/.
c https://www.luminexcorp.com/clinical/infectious-disease/gastrointestinal-disease/enteric-pathogens-test/.
d http://moleculardiagnostics.bd.com/wp-content/uploads/2017/08/Enteric-Bacterial-Panel-Info-Sheet.pdf.
e http://moleculardiagnostics.bd.com/wp-content/uploads/2017/08/Extended-Enteric-Bacterial-Panel-Info-Sheet.pdf.
f http://moleculardiagnostics.bd.com/wp-content/uploads/2017/08/Enteric-Parasite-Panel-Info-Sheet.pdf.
g http://www.hologic.com/sites/default/files/package%20inserts/11192-EN-IFU-PI.pdf.
h Shigella and enteroinvasive E coli are reported jointly because the target locus (ipaH) detects both agents. In reality, most signals of ipaH are from Shigella.
i Detected by test kits used outside of the United States.

traditionally apply some selectivity when ordering stool microbiology tests, but panels return results that may not have been requested and/or anticipated. Moreover, the ability to generate organism-specific signals greatly exceeds our ability to interpret the findings. To the extent possible, we encourage using panels appropriate to the condition. For acute diarrhea in the community setting, we recommend panels that seek *Campylobacter*, *Salmonella*, and *Shigella* spp., STEC, and *Y enterocolitica*, and, for chronic diarrhea, we recommend a panel that includes parasites and, depending on the age of the child, *C difficile* (**Table 3**).

In reality, however, the laboratory will decide the technology to offer and individual providers will probably have little opportunity to select the panel. Because the provider might not be able to choose wisely the tests to be performed, it is important to interpret wisely the results that the laboratory returns. **Table 4** offers our opinions regarding positive signals that might obligate treatment using data available in early 2018. Generally, we believe that an organism is a pathogen if it has caused outbreaks of infections or shows repeated association with cases in case-control studies. This table does not include bona fide or candidate viral diarrheal pathogens. Also, we wish to note that technology and test menu options are likely to change in this fast moving diagnostic field.

Multiplex nucleic acid amplification test laboratory reports might be ambiguous; for example, the primers for *Campylobacter* detect *Campylobacter jejuni* as well as other *Campylobacter* species, so the report might state, "*Campylobacter* species detected." Similarly, primers for *Cryptosporidium* detect but do not differentiate between *C parvum* and *C hominis*, and primers for *Vibrio* detect non-cholera species as well as *V cholerae*, although the BioFire FilmArray Gastrointestinal Panel (BioMérieux, Marcy-l'Étoile, France) will additionally specify *V cholerae*. Based on our current understanding of diarrhea epidemiology and etiology in North America, it is reasonable to assume that a report that *Campylobacter* not otherwise specified is detected means that *C jejuni* is in the stool (although occasionally this might represent a non-*jejuni* species), and that *Cryptosporidium* reflects presence of either *C parvum* or *C hominis* (which would each be managed similarly). *Vibrio* not otherwise specified almost certainly represents a non-cholera species (eg, *V parahaemolyticus* or *V vulnificus*) if the infection is domestically acquired.

Ambiguous or nonreport of the STEC genotype is much more problematic. If the report does not specify which Shiga toxin genes are present, it is critical to request more information from the laboratory, because the multiplex nucleic acid amplification test might have provided the genotype, depending on the particular system. This information is important because a child infected with an STEC that contains the gene encoding Shiga toxin 2 is at much greater risk of developing hemolytic uremic syndrome than if the infecting STEC does not encode Shiga toxin 2. Alternatively, if the laboratory reports the presence of *E coli* O157:H7, the clinician can assume that the patient is infected with a pathogen that contains the gene encoding Shiga toxin 2. Ideally, microbiology laboratories, which are responsible for the report content presented to the provider, will release results that offer clarity regarding the genotype of the toxin detected (see **Table 4**).

Diarrheagenic *E coli* other than STEC warrant comment. Classical microbiology tests will not detect EPEC, ETEC, or EAggEC, but some multiplex nucleic acid amplification tests will now inform physicians of the presence or absence of these agents in stools submitted for evaluation. EAggEC are associated with domestically acquired diarrhea in North American children based on case-control studies from New Haven, Baltimore, Cincinnati, and Seattle.[1,3,49] However, many control children in these studies excreted EAggEC, and antibiotics are of unproven benefit in these infections, so it is not clear how actionable the finding of an EAggEC in stool would be. Some data suggest that atypical EPEC cause diarrhea in North American children,[1] but ETEC and EPEC do not seem to be major causes of pediatric gastroenteritis[3,49] on this continent. Traveler's diarrhea in adults and older students can be caused by ETEC and EAggEC,[50] but the etiology of diarrhea in the returning child traveler is not well-studied. We wish to note that future data might demonstrate that some EPEC, ETEC, and EAggEC cause pediatric gastroenteritis in North America, especially because these bacteria are phylogenetically quite diverse and that within these classes, some agents might be more virulent than others. However, we strongly urge against empirically treating EPEC, ETEC, and EAggEC infections with antibiotics without sufficient clinical or epidemiologic justification.

Providers should consider multiplex nucleic acid amplification test results in the context of the presentation. For example, finding evidence of an STEC in the stool of a patient who has had several weeks of nonbloody diarrhea would rarely be actionable, especially if the readout states that the gene encoding Shiga toxin 1 is present and that the gene encoding Shiga toxin 2 is absent. Conversely, the presence of *E coli* O157:H7, or any STEC for that matter, in a child with acute painful bloody diarrhea, would probably be best treated by admission to hospital, intravenous volume expansion,[45] and avoidance of antibiotics.[44,46–48]

Even if a multiplex nucleic acid amplification test suggests the presence of a pathogen, it is important to consider noninfectious causes for diarrhea, especially if the diarrhea is prolonged. For example, it might be reasonable to administer a brief course of antibiotics to treat *Aeromonas* spp., but if the patient does not improve, or also has lost weight loss and/or is anemic, the illness could be noninfectious in origin. In North America and Europe, the incidence of childhood and adolescent-onset inflammatory bowel disease is high, and attributing causality to a questionably credible pathogen could delay appropriate treatment for Crohn's disease or ulcerative colitis.

The simple presence or absence of specific agents might not be as helpful a readout as would be calculation of pathogen burden in the stool.[51,52] Specifically, when pathogen density in stool is considered, it becomes easier to differentiate the symptomatic from the asymptomatic state. It is likely that future iterations of nucleic acid testing of stool will include density of target as an independent variable, rather than simple

Table 3 Context-informed diagnostic strategies		
Characteristics of illness	Diarrhea duration <10 d, visible blood in stool, painful diarrhea, or >5 bowel movements in prior 24 h, or fever[a]	Diarrhea duration >1 wk All ages, nonbloody diarrhea[d]
Pathogens on panel	Bacterial enteric pathogen panel[b]	Parasites, *Clostridioides difficile*[c] Viruses

[a] Many patients with bacterial enteric infections, and especially those caused by Shiga toxin-producing *Escherichia coli* (STEC), do not have fevers on presentation. Hence, the absence of a fever is not a good reason to decide not to perform a stool culture.
[b] *Campylobacter*, *Salmonella*, and *Shigella* spp., O157:H7 and non-O157 STEC and *Yersinia enterocolitica*.[c]
[c] We would not seek *C difficile* in a child under 3 years of age. Healthy children without diarrhea might excrete *Cryptosporidium*, so a positive result should be interpreted cautiously, although if the symptoms are appropriate we would treat.
[d] Viruses detected in multiplex nucleic acid amplification tests are helpful if they enable the provider to offer guidance about the self-limited nature of the illness.

Table 4
Agents detected by multiplex nucleic acid amplification tests, and possible courses of action

Courses of Action	Agent
Agents that are frequently and appropriately treated with antimicrobials at all ages	*Campylobacter* spp., *Cryptosporidium, Giardia, Entamoeba histolytica, Aeromonas,*[a] *Plesiomonas, Vibrio* spp., *Shigella* spp., *Yersinia*
Agents that might be appropriately treated with antibiotics depending on the circumstance	ETEC in a returned traveler with watery diarrhea *Salmonella* spp. if there is suspicion of extraintestinal dissemination, patient is immunocompromised, or organism is *Salmonella typhi* (which requires further testing to identify) *Clostridioides difficile* in children over age 3, but this organism is often excreted by children in the absence of diarrhea.[3]
Agents that would best be treated with intravenous volume expansion, and avoidance of antibiotics.[44-48]	*Escherichia coli* O157:H7, and any STEC that contains a gene encoding Shiga toxin 2. If the laboratory cannot tell you this information, you should assume that the pathogen contains the Shiga toxin 2 gene, pending further analysis. You should also assume that all *E coli* O157:H7 contain the gene encoding Shiga toxin 2.
Agents sought and reported on multiplex nucleic acid amplification tests that are probably pathogens[1,3,49] in some circumstances, but healthy North American children can excrete these bacteria, and it is not known if antibiotics shorten diarrhea duration	EAggEC, EPEC, ETEC[b] (except in returned travelers)

These recommendations reflect the personal opinions of the authors.

Abbreviations: EAggEC, enteroaggregative *Escherichia coli*; EPEC, enteropathogenic *Escherichia coli*; ETEC, enterotoxigenic *Escherichia coli*; STEC, Shiga toxin-producing *Escherichia coli*.

[a] Aeromonas is not currently sought on multiplex nucleic acid amplification tests, but we include it in this table because it is reported by classic microbiologic testing.

[b] In a teenage returned traveler, we might consider antibiotic treatment of an EAggEC or and ETEC infection, but the adult literature supports treatment only of ETEC-related traveler's diarrhea.

presence or absence. Along these lines, nucleic acid amplification technology is usually amenable to target quantification, thereby enabling pathogen density to be calculated.

Multiplex nucleic acid amplification tests demonstrate the presence of multiple bona fide or candidate pathogens in diarrheal stools, largely because they can detect viruses and bacteria in a single specimen.[22,36] Unfortunately, the literature does not offer sufficient guidance regarding the prognostic, therapeutic, or pathogenic significance of multiple candidate or bona fide pathogens in stools of patients with diarrhea.

Multiplex nucleic acid amplification tests also compel us to examine the laboratory–physician interface, because this technology detects organisms that will be unfamiliar to many clinicians. We, therefore, believe that it is incumbent upon the diagnostic laboratory to put the signals that multiplex nucleic acid amplification tests generate in context. For example, the evidence that EAggEC, ETEC, or EPEC cause diarrhea in North American children is weak, but their detection might prompt treatment. A thoughtfully annotated report, reflecting the strong possibility that these agents are not the cause of the symptoms and the probable lack of value of antibiotics, could avert unnecessary use of antibiotics in response to these findings. Another example in which data conveyance is important relates to Shiga toxin genotype. If the multiplex nucleic acid amplification test identifies the specific Shiga toxin gene(s) present in the stool, the report should be explicit, and not merely state that the specimen is positive for Shiga toxin 1 and/or 2. The report should inform the recipient that *E coli* that produce Shiga toxin 2 (with or without Shiga toxin 1) have profoundly greater associations with the hemolytic uremic syndrome than those that produce only Shiga toxin 1. Such annotations should be generated by experienced local stakeholders, including infectious diseases, gastroenterology, and hospital infection control experts, and public health authorities.

Finally, attention should be paid to nonanalytical considerations relevant to multiplex nucleic acid amplification tests. The first consideration is that, as the time required to analyze the specimen diminishes, pretesting and posttesting logistics occupy increasing proportions of the turnaround time, defined as the interval between the specimen leaving the patient and the time that the doctor receives the results. If the specimen is sent to a distant testing site or analysis does not commence immediately after the laboratory receives the stool, then the advantage of rapid time to result diagnostic technology is diminished accordingly. We encourage all clinicians who submit stool specimens to know the lag time before testing begins, the rapidity with which results can be expected to return, and the mode of reporting. The urgency of finding or excluding the presence of some bacterial enteric pathogens (especially STEC) rivals the urgency of a positive blood culture. Hence, it is important to convey such findings as soon as they are generated. The results should be actively transmitted, that is, via telephone, and not deposited into an electronic database awaiting their discovery by a clinician. The second consideration is the high unit cost of current multiplex nucleic acid amplification tests. In acute bloody diarrhea, the value of rapid and accurate diagnosis is immense. However, most episodes of childhood nonbloody diarrhea are caused by viruses, and the reassuring value of identifying a causative agent must be weighed against the cost of performing the test.

We are increasingly approached by providers who receive the results of multiplex nucleic acid amplification tests. Most questions revolve around which organisms reported are actionable, either when detected as single findings or in combination with other agents, how to interpret results that note the presence of genes encoding Shiga toxins, and whether or not the incidental finding of *C difficile* toxin genes in a stool relates to the illness. In Appendix 1, we provide a list of frequently asked questions by providers, and our current responses.

SUMMARY

Rapid, accurate, and easy-to-use technology, close to or at points of care, will revolutionize our ability to diagnose and treat enteric infections. The abandonment of disparate technologies for finding pathogens in stool, the minimization of bulk stool transport requirements, and the short time to results will improve our ability to care for patients with gastrointestinal infections. However, these nonculture diagnostics are currently quite problematic for public health authorities who need isolates to type. As data and improved technology emerge, it will be important for providers to remain up to date with recommendations regarding the pathogenicity of the agents that the multiplex nucleic acid amplification tests detect, and the appropriate action(s) to take in response.[54]

ACKNOWLEDGMENTS

The authors thank Ms Maida Redzic for skillful assistance in article preparation, Drs Carey-Ann Burnham, Peter Putnam, Linda Chui, Otto Vanderkooi, David Sonderman,

Rob Shulman, and the faculty of the Washington University School of Medicine Divisions of Pediatric Gastroenterology, Hepatology, and Nutrition, and Infectious Diseases, for helpful comments on the text.

REFERENCES

1. Cohen MB, Nataro JP, Bernstein DI, et al. Prevalence of diarrheagenic Escherichia coli in acute childhood enteritis: a prospective controlled study. J Pediatr 2005;146(1):54–61.
2. Melamed R, Storch GA, Holtz LR, et al. Case-control assessment of the roles of noroviruses, human bocaviruses 2, 3, and 4, and novel polyomaviruses and astroviruses in acute childhood diarrhea. J Pediatric Infect Dis Soc 2017;6(3): e49–54.
3. Denno DM, Shaikh N, Stapp JR, et al. Diarrhea etiology in a pediatric emergency department: a case control study. Clin Infect Dis 2012;55(7):897–904.
4. Stephen AM, Cummings JH. The microbial contribution to human faecal mass. J Med Microbiol 1980;13(1):45–56.
5. Schindler EI, Sellenriek P, Storch GA, et al. Shiga toxin-producing Escherichia coli: a single-center, 11-year pediatric experience. J Clin Microbiol 2014;52(10): 3647–53.
6. Carroll KC, Adamson K, Korgenski K, et al. Comparison of a commercial reversed passive latex agglutination assay to an enzyme immunoassay for the detection of Shiga toxin-producing Escherichia coli. Eur J Clin Microbiol Infect Dis 2003; 22(11):689–92.
7. Church DL, Emshey D, Semeniuk H, et al. Evaluation of BBL CHROMagar O157 versus sorbitol-MacConkey medium for routine detection of Escherichia coli O157 in a centralized regional clinical microbiology laboratory. J Clin Microbiol 2007;45(9):3098–100.
8. Fey PD, Wickert RS, Rupp ME, et al. Prevalence of non-O157:H7 Shiga toxin-producing Escherichia coli in diarrheal stool samples from Nebraska. Emerg Infect Dis 2000;6(5):530–3.
9. Klein EJ, Stapp JR, Clausen CR, et al. Shiga toxin-producing Escherichia coli in children with diarrhea: a prospective point-of-care study. J Pediatr 2002;141(2): 172–7.
10. Lockary VM, Hudson RF, Ball CL. Shiga toxin-producing Escherichia coli, Idaho. Emerg Infect Dis 2007;13(8):1262–4.
11. Gould LH, Bopp C, Strockbine N, et al. Recommendations for diagnosis of Shiga toxin–producing Escherichia coli infections by clinical laboratories. MMWR Recomm Rep 2009;58(RR-12):1–14.
12. Baron EJ, Miller JM, Weinstein MP, et al. A guide to utilization of the microbiology laboratory for diagnosis of infectious diseases: 2013 recommendations by the Infectious Diseases Society of America (IDSA) and the American Society for Microbiology (ASM)(a). Clin Infect Dis 2013;57(4):e22–121.
13. Freedman SB, Eltorki M, Chui L, et al. Province-wide review of pediatric Shiga toxin-producing Escherichia coli case management. J Pediatr 2017;180: 184–90.e1.
14. Klein EJ, Boster DR, Stapp JR, et al. Diarrhea etiology in a Children's Hospital Emergency Department: a prospective cohort study. Clin Infect Dis 2006;43(7): 807–13.
15. Goldfarb DM, Steenhoff AP, Pernica JM, et al. Evaluation of anatomically designed flocked rectal swabs for molecular detection of enteric pathogens in

children admitted to hospital with severe gastroenteritis in Botswana. J Clin Microbiol 2014;52(11):3922–7.

16. Arvelo W, Hall AJ, Estevez A, et al. Diagnostic performance of rectal swab versus bulk stool specimens for the detection of rotavirus and norovirus: implications for outbreak investigations. J Clin Virol 2013;58(4):678–82.

17. Gustavsson L, Westin J, Andersson LM, et al. Rectal swabs can be used for diagnosis of viral gastroenteritis with a multiple real-time PCR assay. J Clin Virol 2011; 51(4):279–82.

18. Kabayiza JC, Andersson ME, Welinder-Olsson C, et al. Comparison of rectal swabs and faeces for real-time PCR detection of enteric agents in Rwandan children with gastroenteritis. BMC Infect Dis 2013;13:447.

19. Rodrigues A, de Carvalho M, Monteiro S, et al. Hospital surveillance of rotavirus infection and nosocomial transmission of rotavirus disease among children in Guinea-Bissau. Pediatr Infect Dis J 2007;26(3):233–7.

20. Cunningham SA, Sloan LM, Nyre LM, et al. Three-hour molecular detection of Campylobacter, Salmonella, Yersinia, and Shigella species in feces with accuracy as high as that of culture. J Clin Microbiol 2010;48(8):2929–33.

21. Guion CE, Ochoa TJ, Walker CM, et al. Detection of diarrheagenic Escherichia coli by use of melting-curve analysis and real-time multiplex PCR. J Clin Microbiol 2008;46(5):1752–7.

22. Mengelle C, Mansuy JM, Prere MF, et al. Simultaneous detection of gastrointestinal pathogens with a multiplex Luminex-based molecular assay in stool samples from diarrhoeic patients. Clin Microbiol Infect 2013;19(10):E458–65.

23. de Boer RF, Ott A, Kesztyus B, et al. Improved detection of five major gastrointestinal pathogens by use of a molecular screening approach. J Clin Microbiol 2010; 48(11):4140–6.

24. Koziel M, Kiely R, Blake L, et al. Improved detection of bacterial pathogens in patients presenting with gastroenteritis by use of the EntericBio real-time Gastro Panel I assay. J Clin Microbiol 2013;51(8):2679–85.

25. Higgins RR, Beniprashad M, Cardona M, et al. Evaluation and verification of the Seeplex Diarrhea-V ACE assay for simultaneous detection of adenovirus, rotavirus, and norovirus genogroups I and II in clinical stool specimens. J Clin Microbiol 2011;49(9):3154–62.

26. Reddington K, Tuite N, Minogue E, et al. A current overview of commercially available nucleic acid diagnostics approaches to detect and identify human gastroenteritis pathogens. Biomol Detect Quantif 2014;1(1):3–7.

27. Buss SN, Leber A, Chapin K, et al. Multicenter evaluation of the BioFire FilmArray gastrointestinal panel for etiologic diagnosis of infectious gastroenteritis. J Clin Microbiol 2015;53(3):915–25.

28. Piralla A, Lunghi G, Ardissino G, et al. FilmArray GI panel performance for the diagnosis of acute gastroenteritis or hemorrhagic diarrhea. BMC Microbiol 2017;17(1):111.

29. Khare R, Espy MJ, Cebelinski E, et al. Comparative evaluation of two commercial multiplex panels for detection of gastrointestinal pathogens by use of clinical stool specimens. J Clin Microbiol 2014;52(10):3667–73.

30. Navidad JF, Griswold DJ, Gradus MS, et al. Evaluation of Luminex xTAG gastrointestinal pathogen analyte-specific reagents for high-throughput, simultaneous detection of bacteria, viruses, and parasites of clinical and public health importance. J Clin Microbiol 2013;51(9):3018–24.

31. Stark SI, Rosenfeld LE, Kleinman CS, et al. Atrial dissociation: an electrophysiologic finding in a patient with transposition of the great arteries. J Am Coll Cardiol 1986;8(1):236–8.

32. Huang RS, Johnson CL, Pritchard L, et al. Performance of the Verigene(R) enteric pathogens test, Biofire FilmArray gastrointestinal panel and Luminex xTAG(R) gastrointestinal pathogen panel for detection of common enteric pathogens. Diagn Microbiol Infect Dis 2016;86(4):336–9.

33. Anderson NW, Buchan BW, Ledeboer NA. Comparison of the BD MAX enteric bacterial panel to routine culture methods for detection of Campylobacter, enterohemorrhagic Escherichia coli (O157), Salmonella, and Shigella isolates in preserved stool specimens. J Clin Microbiol 2014;52(4):1222–4.

34. Simner PJ, Oethinger M, Stellrecht KA, et al. Multisite evaluation of the BD max extended enteric bacterial panel for detection of Yersinia enterocolitica, enterotoxigenic Escherichia coli, vibrio, and plesiomonas shigelloides from stool specimens. J Clin Microbiol 2017;55(11):3258–66.

35. Buchan BW, Olson WJ, Pezewski M, et al. Clinical evaluation of a real-time PCR assay for identification of Salmonella, Shigella, Campylobacter (Campylobacter jejuni and C. coli), and Shiga toxin-producing Escherichia coli isolates in stool specimens. J Clin Microbiol 2013;51(12):4001–7.

36. Nicholson MR, Van Horn GT, Tang YW, et al. Using multiplex molecular testing to determine the etiology of acute gastroenteritis in children. J Pediatr 2016;176: 50–6.e2.

37. Cybulski RJ Jr, Bateman AC, Bourassa L, et al. Clinical impact of a multiplex gastrointestinal PCR panel in patients with acute gastroenteritis. Clin Infect Dis 2018. [Epub ahead of print].

38. Goldenberg SD, Bacelar M, Brazier P, et al. A cost benefit analysis of the Luminex xTAG Gastrointestinal Pathogen Panel for detection of infectious gastroenteritis in hospitalised patients. J Infect 2015;70(5):504–11.

39. Beal SG, Tremblay EE, Toffel S, et al. A gastrointestinal PCR panel improves clinical management and lowers health care costs. J Clin Microbiol 2018;56(1) [pii: e01457-17].

40. Freeman K, Mistry H, Tsertsvadze A, et al. Multiplex tests to identify gastrointestinal bacteria, viruses and parasites in people with suspected infectious gastroenteritis: a systematic review and economic analysis. Health Technol Assess 2017;21(23):1–188.

41. Marder EP, Cieslak PR, Cronquist AB, et al. Incidence and trends of infections with pathogens transmitted commonly through food and the effect of increasing use of culture-independent diagnostic tests on surveillance - foodborne diseases active surveillance network, 10 U.S. Sites, 2013-2016. MMWR Morb Mortal Wkly Rep 2017;66(15):397–403.

42. DeBurger B, Hanna S, Powell EA, et al. Utilizing BD MAX enteric bacterial panel to detect stool pathogens from rectal swabs. BMC Clin Pathol 2017;17:7.

43. Freedman SB, Xie J, Nettel-Aguirre A, et al. Enteropathogen detection in children with diarrhoea, or vomiting, or both, comparing rectal flocked swabs with stool specimens: an outpatient cohort study. Lancet Gastroenterol Hepatol 2017; 2(9):662–9.

44. Davis TK, McKee R, Schnadower D, et al. Treatment of Shiga toxin-producing Escherichia coli infections. Infect Dis Clin North Am 2013;27(3):577–97.

45. Grisaru S, Xie J, Samuel S, et al. Associations between hydration status, intravenous fluid administration, and outcomes of patients infected with Shiga toxin-

producing Escherichia coli: a systematic review and meta-analysis. JAMA Pediatr 2017;171(1):68–76.

46. Freedman SB, Xie J, Neufeld MS, et al. Shiga toxin-producing Escherichia coli infection, antibiotics, and risk of developing hemolytic uremic syndrome: a meta-analysis. Clin Infect Dis 2016;62(10):1251–8.

47. Davis TK, Van De Kar NC, Tarr PI. Shiga toxin/verocytotoxin-producing Escherichia coli infections: practical clinical perspectives. Microbiol Spectr 2014;2(4). EHEC-0025-2014.

48. Holtz LR, Neill MA, Tarr PI. Acute bloody diarrhea: a medical emergency for patients of all ages. Gastroenterology 2009;136(6):1887–98.

49. Nataro JP, Mai V, Johnson J, et al. Diarrheagenic Escherichia coli infection in Baltimore, Maryland, and New Haven, Connecticut. Clin Infect Dis 2006;43(4):402–7.

50. DuPont HL. Therapy for and prevention of traveler's diarrhea. Clin Infect Dis 2007; 45(Suppl 1):S78–84.

51. Barletta F, Ochoa TJ, Mercado E, et al. Quantitative real-time polymerase chain reaction for enteropathogenic Escherichia coli: a tool for investigation of asymptomatic versus symptomatic infections. Clin Infect Dis 2011;53(12):1223–9.

52. Liu J, Platts-Mills JA, Juma J, et al. Use of quantitative molecular diagnostic methods to identify causes of diarrhoea in children: a reanalysis of the GEMS case-control study. Lancet 2016;388(10051):1291–301.

53. Centers for Disease Control and Prevention. Culture-independent diagnostic tests. 2016. Available at: https://www.cdc.gov/foodsafety/challenges/cidt.html. Accessed March 5, 2018.

54. Imdad A, Retzer F, Thomas LS, et al. Impact of culture-independent diagnostic testing on recovery of enteric bacterial infections. Clin Infect Dis 2018;66(12): 1892–8.

APPENDIX 1: FREQUENTLY ASKED QUESTIONS

Herein we provide responses to questions we have been asked by physicians regarding multiplex nucleic acid amplification test reports. These responses reflect our current approach to these situations, but might change as new data emerge. We also acknowledge that center-specific practice preferences might vary from ours.

The laboratory tells me that my patient's stool contains an enteroaggregative Escherichia coli (EAggEC; or enterotoxigenic E coli [ETEC] or enteropathogenic E coli [EPEC]). What does this mean?

Current data suggest EPEC and ETEC are rarely, if ever, pathogens in children in high-income countries, although in some situations (watery diarrhea in a patient with recent international travel) we might consider an ETEC to be etiologic, especially in an adolescent. EAggEC are probably pathogens, but it is far from clear that antibiotics are helpful. EAggEC are also isolated from stools from patients with a spectrum of illness,[3] including bloody diarrhea (see **Table 4**).

My patient's stool test says that a Shiga toxin-producing E coli (STEC) is present. What should I do?

It is critical to know if the Shiga toxin signal comes from an *E coli* that contains a gene encoding Shiga toxin 2 (all *E coli* O157:H7 contain this gene). Hence, if the report states that the patient is infected with *E coli* O157:H7 and/or an STEC that contains the Shiga toxin 2 gene, we strongly encourage that the patient be hospitalized and receive intravenous volume expansion with isotonic crystalloid.[44,47,48] If your laboratory confirms that the gene encoding Shiga toxin 2 is absent, the patient has a much lower risk of developing hemolytic uremic syndrome. If you cannot obtain assurance that the gene encoding Shiga toxin 2 is absent, you should consider this patient to be at risk of developing hemolytic uremic syndrome and expand the volume accordingly. Also, the positive result might be based on an enzyme immunoassay that does not differentiate between toxin genotypes. We strongly encourage dialogue with your microbiologist, who can help to interpret the findings.

The laboratory tells me that they tested for Shiga toxin with an enzyme immunoassay, and that my patient is infected with a STEC, but they cannot tell me if it is an E coli O157:H7 or if the Shiga toxin is Shiga toxin 2. Might this patient develop hemolytic uremic syndrome?

In some situations, the laboratory will report that a stool specimen contains an organism that produces Shiga toxin, as determined by an enzyme immunoassay and not by multiplex nucleic acid amplification test. This is probably an antigen test on a broth culture. You should treat the patient as if the specimen contains *E coli* O157:H7, pending further microbiologic evaluation.

My patient is infected with Aeromonas (or Plesiomonas). What should I do?

These bacteria are probably pathogens, although children without diarrhea can excrete *Aeromonas*. We generally recommend treatment for these agents, but if the diarrhea persists despite antibiotic treatment, consider an alternative diagnosis, especially inflammatory bowel disease. If a patient has other findings of inflammatory bowel disease (eg, anemia, hypoalbuminemia), we encourage consideration of this diagnosis (and referral), even if you have not completed the treatment for the *Aeromonas*.

My patient's stool was positive for Shigella/enteroinvasive E coli. What does that mean?

The diagnostic target for *Shigella* and enteroinvasive *E coli* is a gene called *ipaH*, but current multiplex nucleic acid amplification tests do not further differentiate between the 2 species. However, enteroinvasive *E coli* are quite rare in the developed world. Hence, your patient is almost certainly infected with *Shigella*, which is generally treated with antibiotics, and not an enteroinvasive *E coli*.

My patient is recovering from an E coli O157:H7 (or Campylobacter, Salmonella, Shigella, or Yersinia) infection. The health department will not let the child return to day care until 2 stool tests are negative. The molecular test continues to be positive. What should I do?

Disease control authorities increasingly recognize the challenge of highly sensitive nonculture diagnostics.[53,54] You should defer to them regarding the number of specimens and testing modality (culture or multiplex nucleic acid amplification test) before a child is cleared to return to daycare. You should also consider cost to the family for such tests, especially because the information received will not be of clinical benefit to the patient and multiplex nucleic acid amplification test charges could be several hundred dollars per test. Classical microbiology charges are probably less and could be considered in this circumstance.

What do multiplexed nucleic acid amplification tests miss?

Current multiplex nucleic acid amplification tests do not detect several species that could be clinically important in the right setting, such as *Blastocystis hominis*, *Dientamoeba fragilis*, *Cystoisospora belli*, *Microsporidium* spp., or helminths. Classical microscopy for these agents is recommended, although dedicated polymerase chain reaction is available and preferred for some targets (ie, *Microsporidium* spp.). Current multiplex nucleic acid amplification tests also do not detect agents that cause diarrhea in immunosuppressed patients, such as *Brachyspira*, cytomegalovirus, herpes simplex virus, and *Mycobacterium* spp. These pathogens are best detected by histology and/or specific polymerase chain reaction.

I did not want the laboratory to test my 18-month-old patient with diarrhea for C difficile, but a positive result came back anyway. Can I ignore it?

We almost never consider *C difficile* to be a pathogen in children less than 3 years old. In fact, we are skeptical that *C difficile* is a pathogen in older children, but we cannot clearly define an age at which we would absolutely prescribe treatment. Again, the credibility of this attribution depends on the context of the illness.

I have an 8-year-old patient with diarrhea and the report states that C difficile is present and so is another pathogen. Which organism is causing the diarrhea? The patient took antibiotics for a sinus infection until 3 weeks ago.

This answer depends on which organism is co-identified with the *C difficile*. If the patient is coinfected with *Salmonella* or an STEC, ignore (ie, do not treat) the *C difficile*. If the patient is coinfected with *Campylobacter*, *Shigella*, or *Yersinia*, treat that pathogen first. If the symptoms worsen or persist, we might then consider treating the *C difficile*. If the patient is infected with an EAggEC, ETEC, EPEC, or a viral pathogen, we would treat the *C difficile*. These recommendations assume that the patient is older than 3 years of age.

I remember hearing that 3 stool examinations are needed before one can be confident a parasite is not present. Does this apply to multiplex nucleic acid amplification tests?

The literature is split on the number of microscopic examinations to definitively exclude the presence of *Giardia* or *Cryptosporidium*. Current antigen tests for these agents are quite sensitive, so it is probably not necessary to examine more than 1 stool before confidently excluding the presence of one of these pathogens. Multiplex nucleic acid amplification tests are probably also quite sensitive. However, multiplex nucleic acid amplification tests are expensive and protozoal gastroenteritis in North American children is rare. Hence, without data to the contrary, we do not recommend performing more than 1 multiplex nucleic acid amplification test to exclude the presence of *Giardia* or *Cryptosporidium*.

How can I help my local health department in the multiplex nucleic acid amplification test era?

Because multiplex nucleic acid amplification tests do not produce viable STEC, *Campylobacter*, *Salmonella*, *Shigella*, or *Yersinia*, public health investigators have no isolates to DNA fingerprint (and, soon, to whole genome sequence). Such linkage between isolates is critical, because health departments need to devote epidemiologic resources to pathogens of apparent common origin, especially if their vehicle could still be in commerce. It would be ideal to attempt to recover such reportable bacterial enteric pathogens as soon as a multiplex nucleic acid amplification test identifies a positive specimen, but to do so requires a skilled laboratory and multiplex nucleic acid amplification tests are likely to supplant enteric diagnostic microbiology expertise in the community. Also, it might be difficult to request that a patient come back to the center to provide a stool for culture after they have returned home and a microbiologic diagnosis is provided. However, if bulk stool was submitted to the laboratory for multiplex nucleic acid amplification test diagnosis, then sufficient material might be leftover to set up a culture. We hope that multiplex nucleic acid amplification tests, because of their probable greater sensitivity than stool cultures, might identify patients infected with reportable bacterial enteric pathogens more frequently than do classical microbiology tests, and thereby target isolation efforts to positive specimens. Ideally, clinical laboratories and manufacturers will develop protocols to seamlessly incorporate bacterial culture to augment multiplex nucleic acid amplification test diagnosis, probably by setting aside stool or transport media before introducing the specimen stool into the multiplex nucleic acid amplification test cartridge. This set aside will be very helpful in the event pathogen isolation is required.

New Insights into the Pathogenesis and Treatment of Malnutrition

Grace E. Thaxton, BS[a], Peter C. Melby, MD[b],
Mark J. Manary, MD[c,d,e], Geoffrey A. Preidis, MD, PhD[f],*

KEYWORDS

- Undernutrition • Therapeutic foods • Prenatal • Perinatal • Epigenetics
- Protein deficiency • Immune deficiency • Intestinal microbiota

KEY POINTS

- Prenatal and perinatal influences can have lifelong and intergenerational effects on nutritional status, primarily via epigenetic modifications.
- Protein deficiency results in hepatic dysfunction driven by loss of peroxisomes and mitochondrial impairment.
- Compromised gut barrier function increases nutrient needs and predisposes to infection and systemic inflammation.
- Malnutrition-associated immune deficiencies are driven by lymphoid atrophy, cell cycle arrest of progenitor cells, and impaired effector function.
- The intestinal microbiota can contribute to malnutrition and represents a promising therapeutic target.

INTRODUCTION

Malnutrition affects 52 million children under age 5 years, contributing to 45% of child mortality. Chronic malnutrition results in stunting (low height for age), present in 155

Disclosure Statement: The authors have no commercial or financial conflicts to disclose.
[a] Department of Microbiology and Immunology, University of Texas Medical Branch, 301 University Boulevard, Galveston, TX 77555-0435, USA; [b] Center for Tropical Diseases, Division of Infectious Diseases, Department of Internal Medicine, University of Texas Medical Branch, 301 University Boulevard, Galveston, TX 77555-0435, USA; [c] Department of Pediatrics, Washington University at St. Louis, One Brookings Drive, St Louis, MO 63110-1093, USA; [d] School of Public Health and Family Medicine, College of Medicine, Private Bag 360. Chichiri, Blantyre 3, Malawi; [e] United States Department of Agriculture/Agricultural Research Service, Children's Nutrition Research Center, 1100 Bates Street, Houston, TX 77030, USA; [f] Section of Gastroenterology, Hepatology, and Nutrition, Department of Pediatrics, Baylor College of Medicine, Texas Children's Hospital, Feigin Tower, 1102 Bates Avenue, Suite 860, Houston, TX 77030, USA
* Corresponding author.
E-mail address: geoffrey.preidis@bcm.edu

Gastroenterol Clin N Am 47 (2018) 813–827
https://doi.org/10.1016/j.gtc.2018.07.007
0889-8553/18/© 2018 Elsevier Inc. All rights reserved.

gastro.theclinics.com

Abbreviations	
GH	Growth hormone
HMO	Human milk oligosaccharides
IUGR	Intrauterine growth restriction
IL	Interleukin
LPS	Lipopolysaccharide
MUAC	Mid-upper arm circumference
PPARα	Peroxisome proliferator-activated receptor alpha
RUTF	Ready-to-use therapeutic food
SAM	Severe acute malnutrition
WHO	World Health Organization
WHZ	Weight-for-height z score

million children—87 million in Asia and 59 million in Africa. The 16.9 million children with severe wasting (low weight for height), including 12.6 million in Asia and 4.1 million in Africa,[1] have a 9.4-fold greater chance of dying compared with healthy-weight children.[2] The World Health Organization (WHO) defines severe acute malnutrition (SAM) as mid-upper arm circumference (MUAC) less than 115 mm or weight-for-height z score (WHZ) less than -3 for ages 6 months to 59 months. Both acute and chronic malnutrition can cause long-term cognitive deficits. Low birthweight, stunting, and wasting correlate with lower scores on intelligence tests, developmental delays, and decreased lifetime earnings, perpetuating the poverty-malnutrition cycle.[3]

The WHO recommends that all children with SAM are treated with therapeutic foods. Children with minimal appetite or medical complications should receive inpatient treatment with therapeutic milk (F-75 and later F-100) and an antibiotic with gram-negative coverage and then be transitioned to community-based treatment with ready-to-use therapeutic food (RUTF). Children should be monitored until recovery, defined as WHZ greater than or equal to -2 or MUAC greater than or equal to 125 mm and greater than or equal to 2 weeks without edema.[4] Despite these guidelines, SAM mortality rates in the hospital setting remain as high as 10% to 40%, and meta-analyses examining long-term outcomes reveal mixed results.[5,6] Among the key barriers to improving care is an incomplete understanding of mechanisms underlying the metabolic and physiologic abnormalities of SAM.

Recent insights into the pathogenesis of malnutrition instill hope that better outcomes might soon be possible. This review highlights new evidence relevant to 5 topics, including early-life determinants of malnutrition, the role of protein deficiency in the development and perpetuation of malnutrition, the drivers of malnutrition-associated immune deficiencies, impaired gut barrier function and resulting inflammation, and potential roles of the intestinal microbiota in the pathogenesis and treatment of malnutrition.

PRENATAL AND PERINATAL FACTORS

Intrauterine growth restriction (IUGR), being small for gestational age, and preterm birth all contribute to child mortality[7] and malnutrition.[8] Maternal micronutrient status is 1 determinant of low birthweight and IUGR. Iron supplementation during pregnancy reduces the risk of low birthweight and child mortality within the first 5 years of life,[9] and multiple micronutrient supplementation during pregnancy increases birthweight and decreases infant mortality.[10] Low vitamin D receptor expression has been observed in placentas of IUGR pregnancies,[11] and single-nucleotide polymorphisms in placental genes governing vitamin D metabolism are associated with low birthweight.[12] IUGR can be driven by many other factors, including low insulin-like growth factor 1 (IGF-1)[13] (discussed later), highlighting the complex, systemic nature of metabolic derangements in malnutrition.

Low birthweight could promote malnutrition via fetal epigenetic alterations.[14] Differential DNA methylation in infants with IUGR was observed in genes involved in lipid metabolism, transcriptional regulation, metabolic disease, and T-cell development.[15] Although a "thrifty phenotype" may be protective during early-life nutrient deprivation, its persistence into adulthood can have detrimental effects. Adult survivors of infant or prenatal famines have increased rates of obesity, diabetes, and cardiovascular diseases.[16] Epigenetic changes caused by episodes of prenatal or childhood malnutrition can persist for generations[17]; however, some changes can be rescued by early nutrient supplementation in preclinical models.[18]

Maternal genotype also influences the risk of child malnutrition. For example, vitamin D status and fetal growth are impacted by maternal variants of vitamin D metabolizing genes.[19] IUGR might be avoided in certain cases by individualizing prenatal supplementation regimens. Similarly, mothers lacking a functional *FUT2* gene secrete lower concentrations of fucosylated human milk oligosaccharides in breast milk and are more likely to have stunted children.[20] When nutritional quality of breast milk is inadequate, complementary feeding might be required to reduce an infant's risk of malnutrition.

THE ROLE OF PROTEIN DEFICIENCY

Significant food insecurity arising seasonally or with political or natural crises increases the incidence of malnutrition and child mortality. SAM incidence is highest in the rainy season, or preharvest hungry period, and declines just after harvest.[21] One recent study in India found that children with SAM had increased odds of relapse if they completed treatment during seasons of moderate or severe food insecurity.[22] Just as important as macronutrient quantity are protein quality and digestibility.[23] Protein inadequacy, which correlates with stunting,[24] is highest in Africa and southern Asia.[25] Up to 70% of protein consumption in these regions is in the form of cereals and roots, which lack many of the essential amino acids found in animal meat and dairy proteins.

Although stunted children have lower circulating levels of all essential amino acids, it is uncertain whether this results from inadequate intake, increased catabolism, or both. Malnourished children are particularly deficient in arginine, glycine, glutamine, asparagine, glutamate, and serine.[26] These amino acids serve in a variety of biological roles, including protein synthesis, enterocyte growth, bile acid conjugation, intestinal barrier function, and neurotransmitter biosynthesis. Serum amino acids are sensed by, and influence the activity of, the mTORC1 pathway, a master regulator of growth.[27] Protein synthesis, proteolysis, and bone growth are inhibited during SAM, because lipolysis and fatty acid oxidation meet a greater proportion of energy needs.[28–30] Decreased circulating polyunsaturated fatty acid levels further suggest compensatory fat catabolism in SAM,[31] whereas elevated cortisol and growth hormone (GH) and decreased leptin and insulin may reflect hormonal regulation of these processes.[28,32] Decreased leptin is a strong independent predictor of mortality in children with SAM.[28,30]

Protein deficiency also results in liver dysfunction (**Fig. 1**). The most dramatic manifestation is steatosis,[33] although mechanisms by which this occurs are poorly understood. A murine model of protein deficiency linked mitochondrial dysfunction and loss of peroxisomes to impaired fatty acid oxidation and steatosis. By activating the nutrient-sensing nuclear receptor peroxisome proliferator-activated receptor alpha

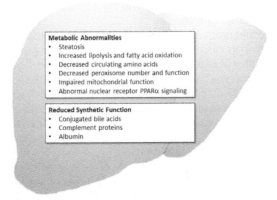

Metabolic Abnormalities
- Steatosis
- Increased lipolysis and fatty acid oxidation
- Decreased circulating amino acids
- Decreased peroxisome number and function
- Impaired mitochondrial function
- Abnormal nuclear receptor PPARα signaling

Reduced Synthetic Function
- Conjugated bile acids
- Complement proteins
- Albumin

Fig. 1. Effects of malnutrition on liver structure and function.

(PPARα), peroxisome numbers and fatty acid oxidation and steatosis were normalized. Peroxisome loss was associated with decreased markers of bile acid synthesis,[34] suggesting that peroxisomal dysfunction may contribute to the altered bile acid profiles observed in SAM. Specifically, children with SAM have increased total bile acids in serum, whereas their intestine contains decreased conjugated and increased secondary bile acids.[35] Secondary bile acids, deoxycholic acid and lithocholic acid, products of metabolism by gut microbes, can be toxic to intestinal epithelial cells, increasing permeability and apoptosis.[36] Thus, although liver dysfunction and microbiome alterations influence bile acid metabolism, the resulting bile acid changes may in turn cause liver and intestinal dysfunction. In a neonatal mouse model of protein deficiency, primary and secondary bile acid content within liver was decreased greater than 80%; mice exhibited evidence of oxidative stress, inflammation, autophagy, and liver dysfunction.[37] Decreased intestinal conjugated bile acids likely also contribute to the impaired fat digestion, fat-soluble vitamin deficiencies, and small bowel bacterial overgrowth that contribute to the clinical picture of SAM.

COMPROMISED GUT BARRIER FUNCTION

Malnutrition affects all organ systems, including the intestinal mucosa (**Fig. 2**). Hallmark histologic changes include mucosal and villous atrophy, crypt branching, and narrowing of the brush border.[38] Malnourished children also have inflammatory cells infiltrating the lamina propria, increased numbers and activity of CD3 cells, increased macrophage number and activity, and reduced interleukin (IL)-10 production.[39] Animal models of protein malnutrition reveal an inverse relationship between dietary protein quantity and the severity of intestinal histopathology.[40,41]

This intestinal damage impairs digestion and absorption of macronutrients and micronutrients, resulting in increased nutritional requirements.[42] In this context, proteins from breast milk and animal sources are more bioavailable than those derived from plants, which could explain why dairy proteins improve growth in children with SAM.[43,44] Compared with other carbohydrates, lactose is often more easily digested by children with SAM.[45]

Animal models of malnutrition exhibit minimal intestinal histopathology unless an infectious insult is provided. Nonetheless, human studies and animal models suggest that malnutrition (with or without infection) impairs intestinal barrier function[41,46] by altering the expression of antimicrobial peptides[41] and tight junction proteins.[47,48]

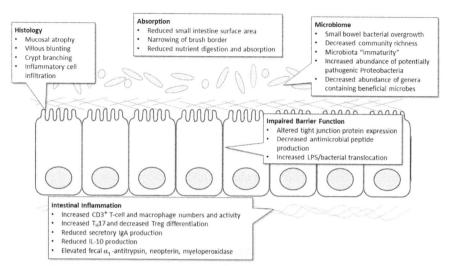

Fig. 2. Effects of malnutrition on intestinal function. Observations predominantly from clinical studies, although some mechanistic data are from preclinical models of malnutrition.

Historically, intestinal absorption and permeability has been assessed with the lactulose:mannitol test, which has high variability in children due to inaccurate carbohydrate dosing, incorrect urine collection, variable rates of gastric emptying or renal excretion, and concurrent diarrhea.[49] Recent studies have sought to identify biomarkers that correlate with intestinal damage, inflammation, and barrier function. Promising candidates include serum endotoxin core antibody; circulating bacterial products, such as lipopolysaccharide (LPS) and flagellin; and fecal markers, including α_1-antitrypsin, myeloperoxidase, and neopterin.[50] Serum LPS and bacterial 16S DNA are elevated in children with SAM, and correlate with decreased expression of mucosal repair peptides and IGF-1, which suggests GH resistance.[47] Thus, decreased barrier function and bacterial translocation may contribute to chronic inflammation and growth failure by modulating the GH/IGF-1 axis.[29,32] Not surprisingly, intestinal and systemic inflammatory markers and elevated GH predict mortality in malnourished children.[32,51]

IMMUNE DEFICIENCIES ATTRIBUTED TO MALNUTRITION

Malnutrition causes deficits in both adaptive and innate immune function, leading to increased childhood mortality from infectious disease.[52] These deficits are multifactorial, driven in part by impaired immune cell production and function. Animal models of protein malnutrition demonstrate bone marrow atrophy and decreased numbers of hematopoietic stem cells and hematopoietic progenitor cells. Cell cycle arrest occurs in the latter due to reduced expression of cell cycle proteins and increased expression of inhibitory proteins.[53] Bone marrow mesenchymal stem cells are more likely to differentiate into adipocytes in protein-malnourished mice, further limiting their ability to produce cytokines.[54] Bone marrow polymorphonuclear cells from protein-malnourished mice also exhibit reduced migration and IL-1β production in response to LPS challenge.[55] Lymphoid organs, including thymus, spleen, and lymph nodes, also show atrophy, reduced cellularity, arrested cell cycle, and impaired cellular function in acute malnutrition.[56]

In addition to the reduced cellularity of hematopoietic and lymphoid tissues, a shortened lifespan from increased apoptosis also contributes to reduced numbers of circulating monocytes, macrophages, dendritic cells, and natural killer cells.[56] Circulating innate immune cells from malnourished mice also exhibit impaired cytokine expression in response to LPS as a result of nuclear factor κB dysregulation.[56] In addition to protein deficiency, multiple micronutrient deficiencies can contribute to immune dysfunction.[56] In preclinical models, natural killer cell and neutrophil functions are restored by reversal of vitamin A deficiency and vitamin C deficiency, respectively.[57,58]

Reduced numbers and function of innate immune cells contribute to deficits in adaptive immunity. Dendritic cells from severely malnourished children have reduced HLA-DR expression and consequently are unable to stimulate T cells.[59] Peripheral blood mononuclear cells from malnourished children underexpress helper T-cell (T_H)1 differentiation cytokines and overexpress T_H2 cytokines, contributing to their inability to clear certain infections.[60,61] CD3[+] T cells from cord blood of children with IUGR revealed hypermethylation of genes that participate in T-cell regulation and activation and metabolic diseases.[62] T cells from malnourished children also overexpress the apoptotic marker CD95.[60] CD8[+] T cells from malnourished mice recover their functional deficits when transferred to a healthy mouse,[63] suggesting that environmental cues contribute to impaired function. T cells require glucose uptake and metabolism—both leptin-dependent processes. Low leptin levels in malnutrition inhibit T-cell activation and skew differentiation of T cells from T_H1 to T_H2.[64,65] Leptin also protects against thymic atrophy, prevents apoptosis of innate immune cells, and improves cytokine production in macrophages and T cells in models of malnutrition.[65,66] Changes to the gut microbiota drive differentiation of T_H17 cells over regulatory T cells, because transcription factors for each cell type are sensitive to different commensal species.[67] Finally, deficits in mucosal immunity in malnourished children can result in poor response to mucosal vaccines.[68] In a mouse model of malnutrition, poor secretory IgA production mediated decreased response to *Salmonella* and cholera vaccines.[69]

Malnutrition also impairs hepatic synthesis of complement proteins, especially in children with edematous malnutrition, among whom low circulating C3 correlates with low serum albumin.[52] Increased consumption of complement, however, measured via elevated circulating levels of the C3 degradation product C3d, might also contribute to the low levels reported in numerous studies of malnourished children.[35]

INTESTINAL MICROBIOTA AS A CAUSE AND THERAPEUTIC TARGET FOR MALNUTRITION

Enteropathogens induce malnutrition, mediating growth impairment by reducing nutrient absorption and increasing nutrient and energy needs.[70] Most malnourished children in low-income countries harbor multiple pathogens.[71] As the number of pathogens isolated from stool increases, weight-for-age z scores and height-for-age z scores decrease.[72] A single episode of diarrhea can have an impact on mortality and linear growth for 2 months to 3 months after infection.[51,71] Even in the absence of diarrhea, however, the malnourished gut microbiota is abnormal.[73–75] Decades ago, culture-dependent studies revealed bacterial overgrowth in the proximal gastrointestinal tract, and microbial DNA sequencing technologies have facilitated a more detailed characterization of this malnutrition-associated dysbiosis[75] (**Box 1**). Numerous factors may drive these microbiome alterations. For example, a monotonous diet containing specific nondigestible dietary carbohydrates[20,76] provides a selective advantage to microbes that metabolize these substrates. Likewise, inflammation can alter the microbiome by triggering an immune response in which

---

Box 1
Summary of features that characterize the gut microbiota from malnourished children

The fecal microbiome derived from malnourished versus healthy children is characterized by

- Increased relative abundance of pathogenic genera within the phylum Proteobacteria
  - *Enterobacter, Escherichia, Klebsiella,* and *Shigella*
- Decreased relative abundance of genera containing beneficial bacteria
  - *Bifidobacterium, Butyrivibrio, Faecalibacterium, Lactobacillus,* and *Roseburia*
- Decreased microbial community richness (fewer unique organisms)
- Microbiome "immaturity," with delayed acquisition of age-specific microbes and microbial genes

Data from Velly H, Britton RA, Preidis GA. Mechanisms of cross-talk between the diet, the intestinal microbiome, and the undernourished host. Gut Microbes 2017;8(2):98–112.

---

subsets of commensal microbes may be eliminated by host-secreted antimicrobial peptides,[77] by disruption of the oxygen gradient at the mucosal surface[78–80] and by generation of reactive oxygen and nitrogen species.[81,82]

Recent preclinical studies demonstrate a causal link between the malnourished microbiome and growth impairment. Fecal microbes isolated from malnourished children can induce weight loss in gnotobiotic mice under specific conditions.[83–85] Similarly, mice iteratively challenged with a combination of nonpathogenic commensal microbes demonstrate impaired growth.[86] Intriguingly, the microbiota's effect on growth in each of these mouse models is dependent on administration of a low-protein, low-fat diet—if the animals consume standard chow, growth impairment is not observed. Furthermore, the presence of a malnourished microbiota can exacerbate weight loss due to pathogenic infection.[87] On the other hand, specific beneficial microbes have been positively linked to growth. For example, *Lactobacillus plantarum* increases IGF-1 expression and linear growth in a model of chronic malnutrition.[88]

Several large double-blind, randomized controlled trials have examined the role of microbiome-targeting therapies for SAM but have demonstrated conflicting results (**Table 1**).[89–94] Current WHO guidelines recommend treating all cases of complicated or uncomplicated SAM with broad-spectrum antibiotics because their use results in decreased mortality, and 1 study associated early-life antibiotic exposure with an increase in ponderal growth among children in low-income settings.[95] These guidelines are warranted, but vigilance must be kept for adverse events that may emerge as well.[96,97] Although trials of probiotics and prebiotics have not revealed growth benefits for malnourished children,[93,94] these microbiome-targeting therapies were not tailored to microbial species or functional deficiencies within the target populations; thus, the full potential of microbiome-targeting therapies for child malnutrition has not yet been realized.

PROSPECTUS

Although recovery rates in SAM treatment programs routinely exceed 85%, hundreds of thousands of children still die every year. The next generation of treatment modalities must reflect the growing knowledge of the pathogenesis of malnutrition and the comorbidities that affect multiple organ systems. There also exists, however, an enormous coverage gap, with less than 15%[98] of affected children globally, including less than 2% in East Asia and the Pacific,[99] having access to malnutrition treatment. Among the barriers to access are caretaker awareness of malnutrition and local

Table 1
Randomized, double-blind, placebo-controlled trials examining microbiome-targeting therapies in the treatment of malnourished children

Microbiome-Targeting Therapy	Study Population	Primary Outcome	Secondary Outcomes	Reference
(Super Synbiotics AB, Stockholm, Sweden)[a] in RUTF vs RUTF alone for treatment duration (mean 33 d)	N = 795, 5 mo–168 mo with WFH <70%, nutritional edema, or MUAC <11 cm, receiving inpatient treatment in Blantyre, Malawi	No effect on nutritional cure (WFH >80% on 2 consecutive outpatient visits): 53.9% treatment vs 51.3% placebo, $P = .40$	No effect on mortality, outpatient defaulting, treatment failures, hospital readmissions, loss to follow-up, rate of weight gain, or days to nutritional cure	Kerac et al,[93] 2009
Amoxicillin (80–90 mg/kg/d) vs cefdinir (14 mg/kg/d) vs placebo in 2 daily doses during the initial 7 d of RUTF	N = 2767, 6 mo–59 mo with nutritional edema or WHZ < -3 and able to consume RUTF as outpatient therapy at 18 feeding clinics in rural Malawi	Placebo increased risk of treatment failure vs amoxicillin (RR 1.32; 95% CI, 1.04–1.68) and vs cefdinir (RR 1.64; 95% CI, 1.27–2.11) and risk of death vs amoxicillin (RR 1.55; 95% CI, 1.07–2.24) and vs cefdinir (RR 1.80; 95% CI, 1.22–2.64)	Placebo decreased rate of weight gain vs cefdinir (3.1 ± 4.1 vs 3.9 ± 6.3 g/kg/d, $P = .002$); placebo decreased rate of MUAC gain (0.22±0.41 mm/d) vs amoxicillin (0.27 ± 0.42 mm/d, $P = .01$) and vs cefdinir (0.28 ± 0.42 mm/d, $P = .002$); no effect on time to recovery or rate of gain of length/height	Trehan et al,[89] 2013
Amoxicillin (80 mg/kg/d) vs placebo twice daily for 7 d	N = 2412, 6 mo–59 mo with WHZ < -3 or MUAC <115 mm (but no nutritional edema), in outpatient therapy at 4 health centers in rural Niger	No effect on nutritional recovery (WHZ ≥ -2 on 2 consecutive visits and MUAC ≥115 and no nutritional edema ≥7 d and all treatments completed) by 8 wk of follow-up, risk ratio for amoxicillin vs placebo 1.05; 95% CI, 0.99–1.12	Amoxicillin decreased risk of hospital admission by 14%; no effect on nonresponse rate at 8 wk, death from any cause, or default	Isanaka et al,[91] 2016

Intervention	Population	Outcome	Conclusion	Reference
Cotrimoxazole (120 mg/d for age <6 mo or 240 mg/d for age 6 mo to 5 y) vs placebo daily for 6 mo	N = 1778, 60 d–59 mo with MUAC <115 mm (≥6 mo) or <110 mm (2–5 mo) or nutritional edema, and HIV-antibody rapid test negative and completed initial stabilization phase of treatment at 2 rural and 2 urban hospitals in Kenya	No effect on mortality during the 365-d study period, hazard ratio for cotrimoxazole vs placebo 0.90; 95% CI, 0.71–1.16	Cotrimoxazole increased incidence of diarrhea and decreased incidence of confirmed malaria, skin or soft tissue infections, and positive urine culture; no effect on frequency of other nonfatal illness episodes, pathogens detected from blood culture, suspected toxic effects, or changes in anthropometric or hematological indices	Berkley et al,[92] 2016
Bifidobacterium animalis subsp *lactis* and *Lactobacillus rhamnosus* (10⁹ CFUs/d) vs placebo from admission to completion of outpatient treatment (range 8–12 wk)	N = 400, 6 mo–59 mo with MUAC <115 mm or WHZ/WLZ <−3 or nutritional edema, in inpatient therapy in Kampala, Uganda	No effect on mean duration of diarrhea, adjusted effect size for probiotics vs placebo during inpatient treatment +0.2; 95% CI, −0.8 d–1.2 d	Probiotics decreased duration of diarrhea vs placebo (−2.2 d; 95% CI −3.5–−0.3); no effect on incidence or severity of diarrhea, pneumonia incidence or duration or severity, nutritional recovery, weight gain, fever, vomiting, duration of hospitalization, or mortality	Grenov et al,[94] 2017

Abbreviations: CFUs, colony-forming units; RR, relative risk; WFH, weight-for-height as mean of National Center for Health Statistics data.

ᵃ Freeze-dried 10¹¹ CFUs *Pediococcus pentosaceus, Leuconostoc mesenteroides, Lactobacillus paracasei,* and *Lactobacillus plantarum;* 2.5 g each of oat bran, inulin, pectin, and resistant starch.

treatment programs, high opportunity costs of seeking treatment, and proximity.[98] Interventions that may reduce the coverage gap include educating and engaging mothers, integrating community-based management of SAM with existing health programs, and strengthening government involvement to increase coverage and data collection.[99] There is now a unique and extraordinary opportunity to work together—basic and clinical scientists, policymakers, and mothers of afflicted children—to ease the suffering from the most dire health problem plaguing children today.

REFERENCES

1. UNICEF/WHO/World Bank Group. Levels and Trends in Child Malnutrition: UNICEF/WHO/World Bank Group Joint Child Malnutrition Estimates: Key findings of the 2017 edition. Geneva (Switzerland): UNICEF/WHO/World Bank; 2017.
2. Black RE, Allen LH, Bhutta ZA, et al. Maternal and child undernutrition: global and regional exposures and health consequences. Lancet 2008;371(9608): 243–60.
3. Guerrant RL, DeBoer MD, Moore SR, et al. The impoverished gut–a triple burden of diarrhoea, stunting and chronic disease. Nat Rev Gastroenterol Hepatol 2013; 10(4):220–9.
4. World Health Organization. Guideline: updates on the management of severe acute malnutrition in infants and children. Geneva (Switzerland): World Health Organization; 2013.
5. Lenters LM, Wazny K, Webb P, et al. Treatment of severe and moderate acute malnutrition in low- and middle-income settings: a systematic review, meta-analysis and Delphi process. BMC Public Health 2013;13(Suppl 3):S23.
6. Schoonees A, Lombard M, Musekiwa A, et al. Ready-to-use therapeutic food for home-based treatment of severe acute malnutrition in children from six months to five years of age. Cochrane Database Syst Rev 2013;6:CD009000.
7. Katz J, Lee AC, Kozuki N, et al. Mortality risk in preterm and small-for-gestational-age infants in low-income and middle-income countries: a pooled country analysis. Lancet 2013;382(9890):417–25.
8. Christian P, Lee SE, Donahue Angel M, et al. Risk of childhood undernutrition related to small-for-gestational age and preterm birth in low- and middle-income countries. Int J Epidemiol 2013;42(5):1340–55.
9. Black RE, Victora CG, Walker SP, et al. Maternal and child undernutrition and overweight in low-income and middle-income countries. Lancet 2013; 382(9890):427–51.
10. Persson LA, Arifeen S, Ekstrom EC, et al. Effects of prenatal micronutrient and early food supplementation on maternal hemoglobin, birth weight, and infant mortality among children in Bangladesh: the MINIMat randomized trial. JAMA 2012; 307(19):2050–9.
11. Nguyen TP, Yong HE, Chollangi T, et al. Placental vitamin D receptor expression is decreased in human idiopathic fetal growth restriction. J Mol Med (Berl) 2015; 93(7):795–805.
12. Workalemahu T, Badon SE, Dishi-Galitzky M, et al. Placental genetic variations in vitamin D metabolism and birthweight. Placenta 2017;50:78–83.
13. Martin-Estal I, de la Garza RG, Castilla-Cortazar I. Intrauterine growth retardation (IUGR) as a novel condition of insulin-like growth factor-1 (IGF-1) deficiency. Rev Physiol Biochem Pharmacol 2016;170:1–35.
14. Tobi EW, Goeman JJ, Monajemi R, et al. DNA methylation signatures link prenatal famine exposure to growth and metabolism. Nat Commun 2014;5:5592.

15. Ding YX, Cui H. Integrated analysis of genome-wide DNA methylation and gene expression data provide a regulatory network in intrauterine growth restriction. Life Sci 2017;179:60–5.

16. Kyle UG, Pichard C. The Dutch Famine of 1944-1945: a pathophysiological model of long-term consequences of wasting disease. Curr Opin Clin Nutr Metab Care 2006;9(4):388–94.

17. Martorell R, Zongrone A. Intergenerational influences on child growth and undernutrition. Paediatr Perinat Epidemiol 2012;26(Suppl 1):302–14.

18. Gonzalez-Rodriguez P, Cantu J, O'Neil D, et al. Alterations in expression of imprinted genes from the H19/IGF2 loci in a multigenerational model of intrauterine growth restriction (IUGR). Am J Obstet Gynecol 2016;214(5):625.e1–11.

19. Dror DK. Vitamin D status during pregnancy: maternal, fetal, and postnatal outcomes. Curr Opin Obstet Gynecol 2011;23(6):422–6.

20. Charbonneau MR, O'Donnell D, Blanton LV, et al. Sialylated milk oligosaccharides promote microbiota-dependent growth in models of infant undernutrition. Cell 2016;164(5):859–71.

21. Vaitla B, Devereux S, Swan SH. Seasonal hunger: a neglected problem with proven solutions. PLoS Med 2009;6(6):e1000101.

22. Burza S, Mahajan R, Marino E, et al. Seasonal effect and long-term nutritional status following exit from a Community-Based Management of Severe Acute Malnutrition program in Bihar, India. Eur J Clin Nutr 2016;70(4):437–44.

23. Ghosh S. Protein quality in the first thousand days of life. Food Nutr Bull 2016; 37(Suppl 1):S14–21.

24. Mal-Ed Network Investigators. Childhood stunting in relation to the pre- and postnatal environment during the first 2 years of life: The MAL-ED longitudinal birth cohort study. PLoS Med 2017;14(10):e1002408.

25. Ghosh S. Assessment of protein adequacy in developing countries: quality matters. Food Nutr Bull 2013;34(2):244–6.

26. Semba RD, Shardell M, Sakr Ashour FA, et al. Child stunting is associated with low circulating essential amino acids. EBioMedicine 2016;6:246–52.

27. Laplante M, Sabatini DM. mTOR signaling in growth control and disease. Cell 2012;149(2):274–93.

28. Freemark M. Metabolomics in nutrition research: biomarkers predicting mortality in children with severe acute malnutrition. Food Nutr Bull 2015;36(1 Suppl): S88–92.

29. Wong SC, Dobie R, Altowati MA, et al. Growth and the growth hormone-insulin like growth factor 1 axis in children with chronic inflammation: current evidence, gaps in knowledge, and future directions. Endocr Rev 2016;37(1):62–110.

30. Bartz S, Mody A, Hornik C, et al. Severe acute malnutrition in childhood: hormonal and metabolic status at presentation, response to treatment, and predictors of mortality. J Clin Endocrinol Metab 2014;99(6):2128–37.

31. Semba RD, Trehan I, Li X, et al. Low serum omega-3 and omega-6 polyunsaturated fatty acids and other metabolites are associated with poor linear growth in young children from rural Malawi. Am J Clin Nutr 2017;106(6):1490–9.

32. DeBoer MD, Scharf RJ, Leite AM, et al. Systemic inflammation, growth factors, and linear growth in the setting of infection and malnutrition. Nutrition 2017;33: 248–53.

33. Doherty JF, Adam EJ, Griffin GE, et al. Ultrasonographic assessment of the extent of hepatic steatosis in severe malnutrition. Arch Dis Child 1992;67(11):1348–52.

34. van Zutphen T, Ciapaite J, Bloks VW, et al. Malnutrition-associated liver steatosis and ATP depletion is caused by peroxisomal and mitochondrial dysfunction. J Hepatol 2016;65(6):1198–208.

35. Preidis GA, Kim KH, Moore DD. Nutrient-sensing nuclear receptors PPARalpha and FXR control liver energy balance. J Clin Invest 2017;127(4):1193–201.

36. Ajouz H, Mukherji D, Shamseddine A. Secondary bile acids: an underrecognized cause of colon cancer. World J Surg Oncol 2014;12:164.

37. Preidis GA, Keaton MA, Campeau PM, et al. The undernourished neonatal mouse metabolome reveals evidence of liver and biliary dysfunction, inflammation, and oxidative stress. J Nutr 2014;144(3):273–81.

38. Stanfield JP, Hutt MS, Tunnicliffe R. Intestinal biopsy in kwashiorkor. Lancet 1965; 2(7411):519–23.

39. Welsh FK, Farmery SM, MacLennan K, et al. Gut barrier function in malnourished patients. Gut 1998;42(3):396–401.

40. Sampaio IC, Medeiros PH, Rodrigues FA, et al. Impact of acute undernutrition on growth, ileal morphology and nutrient transport in a murine model. Braz J Med Biol Res 2016;49(10):e5340.

41. Attia S, Feenstra M, Swain N, et al. Starved guts: morphologic and functional intestinal changes in malnutrition. J Pediatr Gastroenterol Nutr 2017;65(5):491–5.

42. Kvissberg MA, Dalvi PS, Kerac M, et al. Carbohydrate malabsorption in acutely malnourished children and infants: a systematic review. Nutr Rev 2016;74(1): 48–58.

43. Arsenault JE, Brown KH. Effects of protein or amino-acid supplementation on the physical growth of young children in low-income countries. Nutr Rev 2017;75(9): 699–717.

44. Manary M, Callaghan M, Singh L, et al. Protein quality and growth in malnourished children. Food Nutr Bull 2016;37(Suppl 1):S29–36.

45. Grenov B, Briend A, Sangild PT, et al. Undernourished children and milk lactose. Food Nutr Bull 2016;37(1):85–99.

46. Campbell DI, Elia M, Lunn PG. Growth faltering in rural Gambian infants is associated with impaired small intestinal barrier function, leading to endotoxemia and systemic inflammation. J Nutr 2003;133(5):1332–8.

47. Amadi B, Besa E, Zyambo K, et al. Impaired barrier function and autoantibody generation in malnutrition enteropathy in Zambia. EBioMedicine 2017;22:191–9.

48. Wada M, Tamura A, Takahashi N, et al. Loss of claudins 2 and 15 from mice causes defects in paracellular Na+ flow and nutrient transport in gut and leads to death from malnutrition. Gastroenterology 2013;144(2):369–80.

49. Denno DM, VanBuskirk K, Nelson ZC, et al. Use of the lactulose to mannitol ratio to evaluate childhood environmental enteric dysfunction: a systematic review. Clin Infect Dis 2014;59(Suppl 4):S213–9.

50. Harper KM, Mutasa M, Prendergast AJ, et al. Environmental enteric dysfunction pathways and child stunting: a systematic review. PLoS Negl Trop Dis 2018;12(1): e0006205.

51. Attia S, Versloot CJ, Voskuijl W, et al. Mortality in children with complicated severe acute malnutrition is related to intestinal and systemic inflammation: an observational cohort study. Am J Clin Nutr 2016;104(5):1441–9.

52. Rytter MJ, Kolte L, Briend A, et al. The immune system in children with malnutrition–a systematic review. PLoS One 2014;9(8):e105017.

53. Nakajima K, Crisma AR, Silva GB, et al. Malnutrition suppresses cell cycle progression of hematopoietic progenitor cells in mice via cyclin D1 down-regulation. Nutrition 2014;30(1):82–9.

54. Cunha MC, Lima Fda S, Vinolo MA, et al. Protein malnutrition induces bone marrow mesenchymal stem cells commitment to adipogenic differentiation leading to hematopoietic failure. PLoS One 2013;8(3):e58872.

55. Fock RA, Vinolo MA, Blatt SL, et al. Impairment of the hematological response and interleukin-1beta production in protein-energy malnourished mice after endotoxemia with lipopolysaccharide. Braz J Med Biol Res 2012;45(12):1163–71.

56. Ibrahim MK, Zambruni M, Melby CL, et al. Impact of Childhood Malnutrition on Host Defense and Infection. Clin Microbiol Rev 2017;30(4):919–71.

57. Bowman TA, Goonewardene IM, Pasatiempo AM, et al. Vitamin A deficiency decreases natural killer cell activity and interferon production in rats. J Nutr 1990; 120(10):1264–73.

58. Vissers MC, Wilkie RP. Ascorbate deficiency results in impaired neutrophil apoptosis and clearance and is associated with up-regulation of hypoxia-inducible factor 1alpha. J Leukoc Biol 2007;81(5):1236–44.

59. Hughes SM, Amadi B, Mwiya M, et al. Dendritic cell anergy results from endotoxemia in severe malnutrition. J Immunol 2009;183(4):2818–26.

60. Badr G, Sayed D, Alhazza IM, et al. T lymphocytes from malnourished infants are short-lived and dysfunctional cells. Immunobiology 2011;216(3):309–15.

61. Gonzalez-Torres C, Gonzalez-Martinez H, Miliar A, et al. Effect of malnutrition on the expression of cytokines involved in Th1 cell differentiation. Nutrients 2013; 5(2):579–93.

62. Williams L, Seki Y, Delahaye F, et al. DNA hypermethylation of CD3(+) T cells from cord blood of infants exposed to intrauterine growth restriction. Diabetologia 2016;59(8):1714–23.

63. Chatraw JH, Wherry EJ, Ahmed R, et al. Diminished primary CD8 T cell response to viral infection during protein energy malnutrition in mice is due to changes in microenvironment and low numbers of viral-specific CD8 T cell precursors. J Nutr 2008;138(4):806–12.

64. Saucillo DC, Gerriets VA, Sheng J, et al. Leptin metabolically licenses T cells for activation to link nutrition and immunity. J Immunol 2014;192(1):136–44.

65. Rodriguez L, Graniel J, Ortiz R. Effect of leptin on activation and cytokine synthesis in peripheral blood lymphocytes of malnourished infected children. Clin Exp Immunol 2007;148(3):478–85.

66. Bruno A, Conus S, Schmid I, et al. Apoptotic pathways are inhibited by leptin receptor activation in neutrophils. J Immunol 2005;174(12):8090–6.

67. Sefik E, Geva-Zatorsky N, Oh S, et al. MUCOSAL IMMUNOLOGY. Individual intestinal symbionts induce a distinct population of RORgamma(+) regulatory T cells. Science 2015;349(6251):993–7.

68. Czerkinsky C, Holmgren J. Vaccines against enteric infections for the developing world. Philos Trans R Soc Lond B Biol Sci 2015;370(1671).

69. Rho S, Kim H, Shim SH, et al. Protein energy malnutrition alters mucosal IgA responses and reduces mucosal vaccine efficacy in mice. Immunol Lett 2017;190: 247–56.

70. Guerrant RL, Oria RB, Moore SR, et al. Malnutrition as an enteric infectious disease with long-term effects on child development. Nutr Rev 2008;66(9):487–505.

71. Kotloff KL. The burden and etiology of diarrheal illness in developing countries. Pediatr Clin North Am 2017;64(4):799–814.

72. Platts-Mills JA, Taniuchi M, Uddin MJ, et al. Association between enteropathogens and malnutrition in children aged 6-23 mo in Bangladesh: a case-control study. Am J Clin Nutr 2017;105(5):1132–8.

73. Blanton LV, Barratt MJ, Charbonneau MR, et al. Childhood undernutrition, the gut microbiota, and microbiota-directed therapeutics. Science 2016;352(6293):1533.

74. Kane AV, Dinh DM, Ward HD. Childhood malnutrition and the intestinal microbiome. Pediatr Res 2015;77(1–2):256–62.

75. Velly H, Britton RA, Preidis GA. Mechanisms of cross-talk between the diet, the intestinal microbiome, and the undernourished host. Gut Microbes 2017;8(2):98–112.

76. De Filippo C, Cavalieri D, Di Paola M, et al. Impact of diet in shaping gut microbiota revealed by a comparative study in children from Europe and rural Africa. Proc Natl Acad Sci U S A 2010;107(33):14691–6.

77. Sanchez de Medina F, Romero-Calvo I, Mascaraque C, et al. Intestinal inflammation and mucosal barrier function. Inflamm Bowel Dis 2014;20(12):2394–404.

78. Marteyn B, West NP, Browning DF, et al. Modulation of Shigella virulence in response to available oxygen in vivo. Nature 2010;465(7296):355–8.

79. Albenberg L, Esipova TV, Judge CP, et al. Correlation between intraluminal oxygen gradient and radial partitioning of intestinal microbiota. Gastroenterology 2014;147(5):1055–63.e8.

80. Morris RL, Schmidt TM. Shallow breathing: bacterial life at low O(2). Nat Rev Microbiol 2013;11(3):205–12.

81. Winter SE, Thiennimitr P, Winter MG, et al. Gut inflammation provides a respiratory electron acceptor for Salmonella. Nature 2010;467(7314):426–9.

82. Winter SE, Winter MG, Xavier MN, et al. Host-derived nitrate boosts growth of E. coli in the inflamed gut. Science 2013;339(6120):708–11.

83. Smith MI, Yatsunenko T, Manary MJ, et al. Gut microbiomes of Malawian twin pairs discordant for kwashiorkor. Science 2013;339(6119):548–54.

84. Blanton LV, Charbonneau MR, Salih T, et al. Gut bacteria that prevent growth impairments transmitted by microbiota from malnourished children. Science 2016;351(6275):854–7.

85. Kau AL, Planer JD, Liu J, et al. Functional characterization of IgA-targeted bacterial taxa from undernourished Malawian children that produce diet-dependent enteropathy. Sci Transl Med 2015;7(276):276ra224.

86. Brown EM, Wlodarska M, Willing BP, et al. Diet and specific microbial exposure trigger features of environmental enteropathy in a novel murine model. Nat Commun 2015;6:7806.

87. Wagner VE, Dey N, Guruge J, et al. Effects of a gut pathobiont in a gnotobiotic mouse model of childhood undernutrition. Sci Transl Med 2016;8(366):366ra164.

88. Schwarzer M, Makki K, Storelli G, et al. Lactobacillus plantarum strain maintains growth of infant mice during chronic undernutrition. Science 2016;351(6275):854–7.

89. Trehan I, Goldbach HS, LaGrone LN, et al. Antibiotics as part of the management of severe acute malnutrition. N Engl J Med 2013;368(5):425–35.

90. Dubray C, Ibrahim SA, Abdelmutalib M, et al. Treatment of severe malnutrition with 2-day intramuscular ceftriaxone vs 5-day amoxicillin. Ann Trop Paediatr 2008;28(1):13–22.

91. Isanaka S, Langendorf C, Berthe F, et al. Routine amoxicillin for uncomplicated severe acute malnutrition in children. N Engl J Med 2016;374(5):444–53.

92. Berkley JA, Ngari M, Thitiri J, et al. Daily co-trimoxazole prophylaxis to prevent mortality in children with complicated severe acute malnutrition: a multicentre, double-blind, randomised placebo-controlled trial. Lancet Glob Health 2016;4(7):e464–73.

93. Kerac M, Bunn J, Seal A, et al. Probiotics and prebiotics for severe acute malnutrition (PRONUT study): a double-blind efficacy randomised controlled trial in Malawi. Lancet 2009;374(9684):136–44.
94. Grenov B, Namusoke H, Lanyero B, et al. Effect of probiotics on diarrhea in children with severe acute malnutrition: a randomized controlled study in uganda. J Pediatr Gastroenterol Nutr 2017;64(3):396–403.
95. Rogawski ET, Platts-Mills JA, Seidman JC, et al. Early antibiotic exposure in low-resource settings is associated with increased weight in the first two years of life. J Pediatr Gastroenterol Nutr 2017;65(3):350–6.
96. Cho I, Yamanishi S, Cox L, et al. Antibiotics in early life alter the murine colonic microbiome and adiposity. Nature 2012;488(7413):621–6.
97. Cox LM, Yamanishi S, Sohn J, et al. Altering the intestinal microbiota during a critical developmental window has lasting metabolic consequences. Cell 2014; 158(4):705–21.
98. UNICEF/Coverage Monitoring Network/ACF International. The State of Global SAM Management Coverage 2012. New York and London: (UNICE/CMN/ACF); 2012.
99. UNICEF. Annual Results Report 2016 Nutrition. New York: United Nations Children's Fund (UNICEF); 2017.

Infantile Colic
New Insights into an Old Problem

Tu Mai, MD, Nicole Y. Fatheree, BBA, Wallace Gleason, MD,
Yuying Liu, PhD, MEd, Jon Marc Rhoads, MD*

KEYWORDS

- Infant • Barr diary • Crying • Neutropenia • Microbiome

KEY POINTS

- Infant colic is a characteristic group of behaviors seen in young infants.
- The most prominent feature is prolonged crying.
- Additional characteristics, including clenching of the fists and flexion of the hips, have led to the suggestion that these behaviors are related to abdominal discomfort.
- Infant colic may represent gut inflammation and microbial dysbiosis that impacts brain function and even brain development.

So runs my dream, but what am I?
An infant crying in the night
An infant crying for the light
And with no language but a cry.

—Alfred, Lord Tennyson, 1849

DEFINITION AND BACKGROUND

Infant colic is a characteristic group of behaviors seen in young infants. The most prominent feature is prolonged crying. Additional characteristics, including clenching of the fists and flexion of the hips, have led to the suggestion that these behaviors are related to abdominal discomfort; thus the term "colic,"derived from *kolikos*, the Greek term for colon. A commonly used set of diagnostic criteria was proposed by Morris Wessel and colleagues,[1] based on observations of 98 infants in the newborn nursery at Yale, 25 of whom had inconsolable crying. These criteria are summarized by the frequently quoted "rule of 3s": crying by an otherwise healthy infant that lasts more than 3 hours per day on more than 3 days a week for more than 3 weeks.

Disclosure: Supported by the National Institutes of Health/National Center for Complementary and Integrative Health (R34 AT006727).
Department of Pediatrics, Division of Gastroenterology, Hepatology, and Nutrition, The University of Texas Health Science Center at Houston McGovern Medical School, 6431 Fannin Street, MSB 3.137, Houston, TX 77030, USA
* Corresponding author.
E-mail address: J.Marc.Rhoads@uth.tmc.edu

Gastroenterol Clin N Am 47 (2018) 829–844
https://doi.org/10.1016/j.gtc.2018.07.008
0889-8553/18/© 2018 Elsevier Inc. All rights reserved.

In a most informative article in the *New Yorker*, Groopman[2] quotes the British social anthropologist Sheila Kitzinger as stating the "sound of a crying baby...is just about the most disturbing, demanding, shattering noise we can hear." He goes on to point out that the US military has used the sound of wailing infants as an instrument of psychological stress, piping recordings of their cries into the cells of detainees at Guantanamo Bay.

Infant fussing and crying can be quantified by a "Barr diary" (**Fig. 1**),[3] which often shows increased crying after feedings. Crying occurs throughout the day but peaks in the hours between 6 AM to 12 PM and 6 PM to 12 AM (**Fig. 2**).[1] Colic may be a factor in child abuse and infanticide.[4,5] In one investigation of more than 100 cases of abusive head trauma to infants, forensic interrogation revealed that shaking was violent and repetitive in most cases. The parent, usually a father, reported that he shook the infant to stop the infant from crying in the most cases, without the intention of actually hurting the infant.[6] Recently, a systematic review by Wolke and colleagues[1] extracted Barr diary data from more than 8690 infants. They found that up to 25% of normal infants have colic at 6 weeks of age, compared to only 0.6% at 10–12 weeks of age.[7]

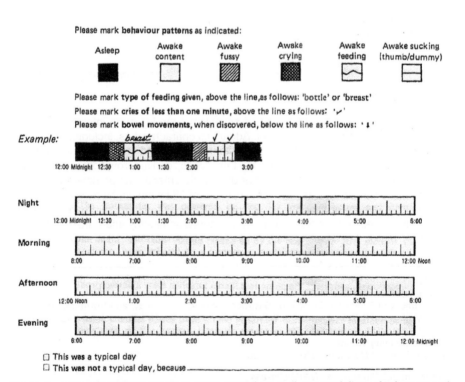

Fig. 1. Barr diary. (*From* Barr RG, Kramer MS, Boisjoly C, et al. Parental diary of infant cry and fuss behavior. Arch Dis Child 1988;63:384; with permission.)

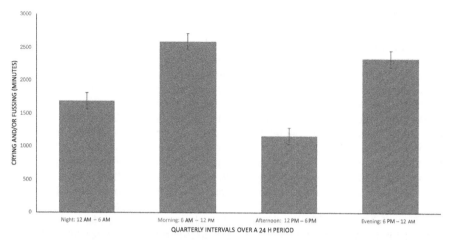

Fig. 2. Daily breakdown of crying time in infants with colic: crying and fussing in minutes (n = 27). Means +/− SEM. (*Adapted from* Rhoads JM, Collins J, Fatheree NY, et al. Infant colic represents gut inflammation and dysbiosis. J Pediatr, in press; with permission.)

ETIOLOGY

The etiology of infantile colic is unknown, but is likely to be multifactorial. Proposed etiologies include gastrointestinal, hormonal, neurodevelopmental, and psychosocial factors.

Gastrointestinal

Several gastrointestinal disorders have been suggested to cause colic, as the infants often lift their legs and pass gas during the crying episodes.[8] These factors, although controversial, include cow's milk protein allergy or allergy to other substances in the maternal diet, excessive gas production, lactose intolerance, poor feeding technique, and dysbiosis.[9]

Cow's milk protein allergy
The association between colic and cow's milk protein allergy is equivocal.[10] A previous study indicated that infantile colic is not associated with cow's milk protein intolerance, based on similar prevalence of colic in formula-fed versus breast-fed infants, as well as a lack of intestinal damage (as determined by fecal alpha-1-antitrypsin and fecal hemoglobin) in colicky infants.[11] In contrast, another study presented evidence of intestinal inflammation, with increased fecal calprotectin and less diverse fecal microflora in infants with colic; however, the difference could not be attributed to formula versus breast milk feeding.[12] Several systematic reviews of clinical trials or randomized controlled trials in infants with colic have shown that the use of protein hydrolysate formulas decrease crying time in these infants.[9,13,14] The limitations of most of these studies were an unclear method of randomization and/or inadequate blinding.[9]

Intolerance to other substances in the maternal diet
A maternal diet that consists of cruciferous vegetables (such as cauliflower, cabbage, garden cress, bok choy, broccoli, and brussels sprouts), cow's milk, onion, and chocolate have also been suggested as a cause for colic, in theory related to colonic gas

production.[15] Many pediatricians recommend that mothers reduce cruciferous vegetables in their diet, although there is little proof that this is beneficial.

Gas production

It has been suggested that colicky infants have more intestinal gas produced as a result of colonic bacterial fermentation. Thirty years ago, an Australian study by Moore and colleagues[16] suggested excessive H_2 gas production was a problem in many infants with colic, with an initially high level of breath hydrogen decreasing as the colic resolves. We, too, found that baseline breath H_2 was high in 25% to 50% of infants with colic,[12,17] supporting bacterial overgrowth or simply the inability to excrete colonic gas effectively at this age. Of note, breath H_2 level was also high in 25% of control infants without colic. Hyams and colleagues[18] showed that most infants with and without colic had a positive lactulose breath H_2 test, which is often used to diagnose bacterial overgrowth (defined by adult criteria of a rise of 10 parts per million after ingesting lactulose). They pointed out that many infants with massive rises in H_2 gas production following lactulose did not cry or show any signs of discomfort. Thus, the literature is not convincing that excessive gas causes colic, although it may be a contributing factor.[12,16,18–21]

Lactose intolerance

In the previously mentioned study by Moore and colleagues,[16] zero-time (baseline) breath H_2 values were significantly higher, by twofold to fourfold, in colicky compared with noncolicky infants at both 6 weeks and 3 months. After lactose-containing milk, there were significantly more positive breath H_2 tests (as defined by a breath hydrogen level that increased > 10 parts per million after milk ingestion) in colicky compared with noncolicky infants at 6 weeks (78% vs 36%) and 3 months (89% vs 45%).[15] The findings suggested that lactose malabsorption could be important in this condition. Our group, however, found no significant differences between the postprandial levels of breath hydrogen when we compared healthy and colicky infants using a similar protocol.[12] Randomized clinical trials of oral lactase administration to facilitate lactose hydrolysis have shown conflicting results in the treatment of infantile colic.[22,23] Hence, the association between lactose malabsorption and colic is unclear. Our interpretation is that there is a high level of colonic bacterial fermentation in most infants at this age, but lactose intolerance by itself is unlikely to cause colic.

Poor feeding technique

Improper feeding technique, such as underfeeding or overfeeding, or infrequent burping, has been suggested to be a cause for colic.[10] First-born infants have been reported to have an increased risk of colic in 2 studies.[24,25] However, in both these studies and in our experience, later birth-order infants are frequently seen with colic. Overreporting or hypervigilance by primiparous parents (rather than parental ineptitude) may be a factor.

Hormonal

A higher level of serotonin has also been suggested to be a cause of infantile colic. Serotonin made in the gut affects mood and social behavior.[26] According to one study, colicky infants had a higher level of random urinary 5-OH IAA, a metabolite of serotonin, as compared with the infants in the control group.[27]

Neurodevelopmental

Neurodevelopmental factors have also been proposed as one of the contributing etiologies.

Normal emotional development

Previous studies have shown that the crying pattern in colicky infants is similar to that of healthy infants (late afternoon and evening onset, peak crying at 2 months of age), although infants with colic have crying of longer duration and are harder to console. In one study, colic was described as a stage of normal emotional development, during which the infant has diminished capacity to regulate crying episodes.[28]

Migraine and colic

An association between maternal migraine and infantile colic has been shown in several case-control studies. It was shown that mothers with migraine were more than twice as likely to have infants with colic.[8]

"Missing fourth trimester" theory

According to this theory by Dr. Harvey Karp,[29] a developmental specialist, infants are born too "early" by approximately 3 months (or a trimester), which results in inconsolable episodes of crying. According to this theory, they miss out on pleasant womb sensations (which can be mimicked by keeping them warm and quiet, swaddling them tightly, carrying them prone, and shaking them with a jiggling motion). Newborns and horses are compared in this book, with the newborn human being helpless and unable to take care of himself or herself, whereas a newborn horse starts running the same day. The inconsolable crying episodes resolve in most infants at approximately 3 months of age, at which time the infants start to "wake up," accepting their environment, smiling, rolling over, and cooing.[30]

Psychosocial

Inadequate parent-infant interaction, parental anxiety, maternal smoking, and advanced maternal age have also been suggested as a potential contributors to or causes of colic.[9] Maternal depression and paternal depression have also been shown to be associated with colic.[31-33]

Inadequate parent-infant interaction

Father-infant and mother-infant interactions were less optimal in one colic group as compared with a control group. Also, there were more dysfunctional interactions between parents in the severe colic group.[34] These findings have not been noted in most other studies.

Parental anxiety

Infants born to mothers with high trait anxiety and mothers with a "spoil-fearing" attitude have higher risk of developing colic. In this study, trait anxiety was scored by the "trait" scale of the State-Trait Anxiety Inventory (STAI), and classified into the low, middle, and high score groups. "Spoil-fearing" participants answered "completely true" or "fairly true" to the statement, "If the infant is taken up into the arms (of the caregiver) too much, he/she can become spoiled or too dependent."[35]

Maternal smoking

Daily maternal smoking during pregnancy has been related to subsequent colic in infants, but the association with maternal smoking was reported when infants were approximately 5 weeks of age, ruling against infant dependency; and the association with colic did not reach statistical significance.[36]

Advanced maternal age

Advanced maternal age was shown to be the most important risk factor for infantile colic in one study, whereas another study did not confirm the association.[31,37]

Maternal and paternal depression

Maternal depression during early pregnancy has been clearly linked to subsequent infantile colic.[31,32] In one study, there was a threefold increased risk of infantile colic in mothers who reported distress during pregnancy.[32] Interestingly, after adjustment for maternal depressive symptoms, paternal depression has also been associated with colic, as suggested by a prospective population-based study in 4426 2-month-old infants by van den Berg.[33] This could be a direct association, or an indirect one through marital, familial, or economic distress.

Inflammation/Dysbiosis

Recently, we found that stools of infants with colic had increased fecal calprotectin, a marker for gut inflammation (**Fig. 3**A). Levels are known to be higher in breast-fed babies, but when breast-fed babies were separately analyzed from those on formula, fecal calprotectin was consistently higher in those with colic than in those without (**Fig. 3**B). We also found that the fecal microbial population was different in babies with colic, with fewer Actinobacteria (95% of which are Bifidobacteria) (**Fig. 3**C). Principal components analysis revealed that microbial ß-diversity differed significantly (**Fig. 3**D). This current hypothesis describing a relationship between the microbial composition of the colon, inflammation, and colic is described later in this article, in the section "Probiotic treatment."

Diagnosis

Most studies use the parental graphing on a Barr diary to quantify crying and fussing, but this is not convenient for most patients seen in the clinic. The diagnosis of colic is traditionally made on the basis of an infant 3 weeks to 3 months of age who has intermittent periods on most days of inconsolable crying and/or fussing. Most often, the periods of worst crying are in the evening and/or after feedings. Other entities to be considered in the differential diagnosis include cow milk protein allergy, urinary tract infection or nephrolithiasis, severe thrush, anal fissure, constipation, occult fracture, and neurologic problems (including seizure activity or maternal drug abuse).

TREATMENT

Conventional Approaches

Many therapies/techniques have arisen over the years, from acupuncture to changing feeding techniques (for example, nipple adjustment), swaddling while prone,[29] removing or giving environmental stimulation (white noise, soft sounds, and motion), switching formula, giving gripe water, and skin-to-skin bonding (closeness). These methods have not been scientifically studied, but are rational and anecdotally beneficial.

Acupuncture

Acupuncture is a method of systemic stimulation of neurotransmitters and hormones throughout the central nervous system.[38] It is has been shown that acupuncture in animals inhibits somatic and visceral pain and has an effect on the autonomous system.[39] Gastric motility and acid secretion can be affected by acupuncture[40]; jejunal motility can be stimulated[41]; and functional dyspepsia can be improved in adults.[42]

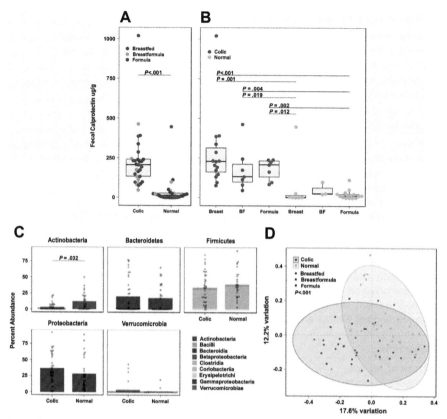

Fig. 3. (*A, B*): Relationship between fecal calprotectin, colic, and feeding modality in infants. (*C, D*): Fecal microbial community composition in infants with and without colic. (*A*) Infants with colic (n = 29) have significantly higher levels of fecal calprotectin than normal controls (n = 25) (P<.0001, Wilcoxon rank sum test). (*B*) Breastfed infants significantly higher levels of fecal calprotectin than Formula fed infants (P = .019, Kruskal-Wallis with post hoc Dunn's test and correction for multiple comparisons). (*C*) Phylum/Class level composition of colic (n = 37) vs control (n = 28) samples. Normal control samples have a significantly higher abundance of Actinobacteria, (P = .032, Wilcoxon rank sum tests with correction for multiple comparisons). (*D*) Microbial β-diversity composition of infants with and without colic is significantly different (P = .003, permutational multivariate analysis of variance). (*Adapted from* Rhoads JM, Collins J, Fatheree NY, et al. Infant colic represents gut inflammation and dysbiosis. J Pediatr, in press; with permission.)

Acupuncture features different points of optimal effect; in colic the most commonly used location would be LI4, which is associated with gastrointestinal symptoms.[43,44] A randomized controlled trial by Landgren and Hallstrom[45] in 80 infants showed a significant decrease of colicky symptoms (P = .03) in the acupuncture group versus controls. A larger multicenter British study showed reduction in crying duration and a shortening of the length of colic symptoms using 2 different types of acupuncture, compared with placebo treatment. Other studies have been completed showing benefit for light (systemic) or targeted (LI4) point stimulation,[46] with one study in disagreement these findings.[47] Additional randomized controlled trials should be undertaken.

Chiropractic

Chiropractic therapy focuses on the musculoskeletal system and nerves. This therapy makes adjustments to the alignment of the spine and connecting nerves, purportedly pressure areas causing pain. A Cochrane review by Dobson and colleagues[48] indicated that the trials have been generally "positive" but inconclusive, because of an inherent risk of performance bias because the assessors (parents) were not blind as to who had received chiropractic treatment. There is a need for further research with this technique.

Complementary Medicine

Alternative or complementary medical treatments are designed to treat the diseased body naturally. Common holistic approaches for colic are herbs, including fennel (*Foeniculum vulgare*), chamomile (*Matricaria recutita*), and lemon balm (*Melissa officinalis*); several of which have been effective in several randomized controlled trials for colic.[49] From 5 studies, 491 participants with colic were treated with herbal medicine; results were reviewed. Fennel extract, herbal tea, and fennel oil, as well as a herbal tea called ColiMil were shown to be better than placebo. Of the 5 studies, one reported nonsevere vomiting, sleepiness, and constipation; the other 4 did not report side effects. Multi-herbal treatments (such as Colic Calm) are available over-the-counter and currently not regulated. Fennel preparations were reviewed and found to have no severe adverse events.[50] In our opinion, herbal treatments are not recommended as first-line treatment, due to unproven safety and efficacy in infants, as well as unknown biological effects and dosing response.

Medications

Tincture of opium
The medical document *Papyrus Ebers* (ca. 1500 BCE) was purchased by Georg Ebers in 1873 and resides at the University of Leipzig. It cites a remedy for a colicky baby:

> *Pods of the poppy plant*
> *Fly dirt which is on the wall*
> *Make into one, strain, and take for four days*
> *It acts at once!*

The poppy seed would have provided opium for the cramps of colic, with fly dung added as a thickener. In the United States, paregoric was extensively used for many years for colic. Paregoric consists of 4% opium, benzoic acid, camphor, and anise oil. Before 1970, it was given over-the-counter, but it became a regulated (schedule III) drug thereafter, except as a component of Donnagel-PG (schedule V). Because of addictive properties, it was banned in 2011, only to be resumed in 2012, but is now only to be used for the purpose of weaning opiate-addicted newborns.[51]

Simethicone
Simethicone is an over-the-counter medication used to relieve gassiness, bloating, and discomfort in adults. Simethicone has been used widely, with outcomes no better than placebo.[52] We do not recommend simethicone for in the treatment of infant colic.[52]

Acid blockers
Most infants referred to subspecialists in pediatric gastroenterology have been treated with acid blockers, often at very high doses. There is evidence that neither omeprazole[53] nor lansoprazole[54] reduces infant irritability. Acid blocker treatment was successful in reducing acid exposure time but did not reduce crying,[53] suggesting that esophageal reflux is not relevant to infant colic. Concerns have been raised that these infants are overmedicated.[55]

Probiotic treatment

Dysbiosis describes a proven difference in microbial community composition when comparing a clinical group (eg, patients with irritable bowel syndrome[56] or inflammatory bowel disease[57]) with healthy controls. Dysbiosis is a term that is somewhat ambiguous, and it does not prove causality.[58] Microbial composition of the dysbiotic stool can be dominated by *pathobionts*, or commensal organisms that are known to have modestly proinflammatory characteristics. Fecal communities can be programmed by genetic defects, postnatal maturation, medications, dietary choices, antibiotics, life-style choices, and psychological stress.[59]

In the landmark article describing colic, Wessel and colleagues[1] suggested gastrointestinal distress, caused by "excessive proteoids like those of the bean which rapidly undergo gaseous decomposition… [which] causes violent peristalsis, " and/or "physiologic immaturity of the intestinal tract resulting in overdistension."They also pointed out that "enemas may decrease putrefactive fermentation" in this condition, thus implicating abnormal fecal composition in the seminal report.

Francesco Savino and his group[60,61] in Turin, Italy, were the first to investigate, using stool cultures and subsequently molecular techniques, whether colic is related to gut dysbiosis. His group found reduced lactobacilli and increased *Escherichia coli* using polymerase chain reaction to measure bacterial ribosomal DNA. Subsequently, our group's observations from infants in Houston, using denaturing gradient gel electrophoresis and sequencing, substantiated some of these findings, although we found an increase in a different member of genus Proteobacteria, *Klebsiella,* in half of 18 infants with colic.[12] We also suggested that there was reduced fecal microbial diversity, as well as gastrointestinal inflammation in these infants, as measured by an increase in fecal calprotectin, a cytoplasmic protein abundant in neutrophils.

The dysbiosis-inflammation theory proposes that aberrant colonization of the newborn creates a gut environment that affects brain function and the behavior of the infant. Colic represents an ideal model for understanding the effects of individual microbes and their associated microbial-brain interactions, inasmuch as these infants are colonized by only 1 to 3 dominant species, "dominant" referring to the 65% to 97% of the operational taxonomic units (OTUs, or species).[62] This limited diversity in infants (especially those with colic [see **Fig. 3**]) contrasts markedly with studies of the stools of adults, which have a much more balanced composition of approximately 400 OTUs, of which approximately 12% are stable components of a "temporal core."[63] Differential colonization of a relatively sterile gut with proinflammatory commensals, such as Gammaproteobacteria, also known as gram-negative rods, when not balanced by anti-inflammatory commensals (*Bifidobacterium, Lactobacillus, Bacteroides*) may underlie the gut inflammation that has been reported in our infants with colic.[60,64] **Fig. 3**C from our group shows that there was a significant decrease in the percentage composition of Actinobacteria (95% of which are Bifidobacteria) in infants with colic.

Reduced fecal bifidobacterial species in infants with colic compared with controls were reported by 2 groups,[64,65] although low levels were not confirmed by others.[66,67] Reduced lactobacilli were also found by Savino's group,[60] although recently a study by the same group using fluorescence in situ hybridization (FISH) techniques failed to find reduced lactobacilli.[66] We found that these 2 genera (*Lactobacillus* and *Bifidobacterium*) comprise a very small fraction of the gut microbiota in infants 3 weeks to 3 months old,[17,62] although bifidobacteria are known to bloom later during infancy. An imbalance between genera of Proteobacteria and Actinobacteria (mainly bifidobacilli) has been found in 2 prospective studies of necrotizing enterocolitis (NEC) in premature infants. Results indicated that those who developed NEC had fecal microbial populations that evolved to become different from those of infants who did not develop NEC.[68,69] In both studies, there was a progressive overgrowth of Proteobacteria in those who developed NEC compared with infants with stable gastrointestinal health. The recent study by Savino and colleagues[66] also showed an increase in Enterobacteriaceae, as assessed by FISH, in infants with colic compared with those without colic.

To probe gut inflammation in infants with colic, no studies have used colonoscopy to determine if there is a low-grade colitis. Olafsdottir and colleagues[70] reported no differences in fecal calprotectin when they compared healthy infants with those with colic. In fact, they noted very high levels of calprotectin in all infants this age. However, subsequently we and others have reported a much higher level of fecal calprotectin in infants with colic compared with age-matched controls.[12,67] Furthermore, in longitudinal studies, a dramatic decrease in calprotectin has been consistently seen, in parallel to the resolution of the colic[17,71,72] (see **Fig. 3**A). It should be noted, however, that there is currently no consensus as to whether gut inflammation causes colic.

Simultaneous with these case-control comparisons, Savino and colleagues[73] initially, and others subsequently, began to investigate the possibility that a normal fecal commensal, *Lactobacillus reuteri*, when given as probiotic drops, could modify the course of crying and irritability in these infants. LR ATCC 55730 and its offspring, strain DSM 17938 (the latter cured of an antibiotic-resistance plasmid), originally isolated from a Peruvian mother's breast milk, have been available commercially for >20 years as "colic drops" in sunflower oil. Each dose of 5 drops contains more than 20 million colony-forming units. To try to quantify outcome, many studies used the Barr diary created by Ronald Barr, a daily timeline that the parents can color in when the infants either cry or fuss (recorded as 5-minute intervals).[3,74] We and others have found the Barr diary to be an instrument that is user-friendly, quantitative, and often welcomed by the parents of infants with colic (see **Fig. 1**).

Subsequent studies of L reuteri DSM 17938 showed efficacy in studies conducted in Turin, Italy,[75] Warsaw, Poland,[76] Toronto, Canada,[77] and Hong Kong, China.[78] All (with one exception[78]) were investigator-masked and parent-masked, and all used Barr diaries. Meta-analyses concluded that a treatment effect was observed at 1, 2, and 3 weeks, with a weighted mean difference of crying + fussing time of 28 to 56 minutes daily, with the best effect at 2 and 3 weeks.[79–81] One meta-analysis compared LR 17938 with a variety of other treatments and concluded that only L reuteri DSM 17938 and fennel were effective.[79]

There were 2 studies that did not find a trend toward improvement in colicky infants treated with L reuteri, authored by Sung and colleagues[71] and Fatheree and colleagues.[62] The study by Sung and colleagues[71] was the largest trial, but it included children who were taking formula, as opposed to all other studies that included only breast-fed infants. There is evidence from rodent studies that stimulation by L reuteri of regulatory T cells is augmented by breast milk.[82] The latter trial of breast-fed infants was underpowered and demonstrated an unusually brisk cessation of fussing/crying in the placebo group. It is noted that this was 1 of only 2 trials that reimbursed the parents for multiple clinic visits, potentially augmenting the placebo response. Both of these (nonconfirmatory) trials also included children who were on acid blockers, which may have influenced an impact of the probiotic on crying time and the microbiota.

Nevertheless, the meta-analyses mentioned previously showed very promising results. It should be noted that in more than 350 infants studied in the various trials, no serious adverse events of probiotic, such as bacteremia, were reported. In fact, neutropenia (a condition associated with increased risk of infection) was noted in approximately 50% of children in a recent trial at enrollment, and it resolved in 70% of the infants after 2 months of treatment with the probiotic.[62]

Several studies investigated other probiotics for infants with colic. One showed that *Lactobacillus rhamnosus GG* reduced crying time,[83] whereas another smaller study (n = 20) looking at the effects of *L rhamnosus GG* in infants on a casein hydrolysate formula (compared with controls) did not show a difference.[17] In other small studies, a symbiotic formula with several species of *Lactobacillus* and *Bifidobacilluş* as well as *Streptococcus thermophilus* and fructooligosaccharides showed benefit,[84] as did a symbiotic with heat-killed *L reuteri, Brevibacillus brevis*, and xyloglucan.[85] Neither of these studies used the Barr diary.

One additional comment is that *L reuteri* DSM 17938 has also been shown to help to *prevent* the development of colic in 2 studies.[86,87]

PROGNOSIS

Generally, infants with colic are believed to have an excellent prognosis, as colic is often viewed as a temporary disorder, regardless of etiology. The vast majority of these infants stop crying by 4 to 5 months of age. However, there has always been a concern that "little belly achers" could grow up to become "big belly achers." A 10-year follow-up study by Savino and colleagues[88] recorded (by parental "anamnesis" [history]) gastrointestinal, allergic, and psychological symptoms in 52 children who were hospitalized for severe colic as infants. After age 10, they were compared with 51 who had been hospitalized during their infancy for other reasons. The survey showed that the children who had experienced colic were significantly more likely to develop recurrent abdominal pain, allergic disease (eczema, rhinitis, asthma, and food allergies), and sleeping disorders. Remarkably, 40% to 60% of the children with colic had also gone on to develop aggressiveness, fussiness, or feelings of supremacy, with a relative risk of each calculated to be 10-fold higher than controls.

A fascinating, seemingly outlandish theory in the emerging field of "psychobiotics" (coined by the group in Cork, Ireland) is that neonatal microbiota may regulate the development of the central nervous system.[89,90] This theory is mainly supported by observations in rodent models, but may have implications for the development in childhood of autism spectrum disorders and later in life, of schizophrenia. These neurologic disorders might be impacted by microbial manipulation. Examples include (1) development of stress behavior in the germ-free mouse is linked to an enlarged amygdala and hippocampus, rescued by *Bifidobacillus infantis* (reviewed in Vuong and colleagues[91]); (2) depression in humans has been linked to increased fecal Actinobacteria and *Bacteroides*, transmissible to the germ-free mouse[92]; and (3) functional bowel symptoms linked to high anxiety/depression scores improved symptomatically in response to a probiotic containing *Lactobacillus helveticus* and *Bifidobacterium longum*.[93]

SUMMARY

Parents caring for a miserable infant with colic may be reassured by the consistent finding that "time is on your side." These infants will recover over the next 2 to 3 months almost 100% of the time. Swaddling, white noise, gentle stimulation (jiggling), and *L reuteri* drops may be of benefit, in contrast to the traditional acid blockers, which have not been shown to affect infant fussiness and crying.[53]

In this article, we have shown emerging evidence to support the concept that infant colic could represent a dysbiosis that impacts brain function and even brain development. Recently, Partty and colleagues[94] performed a long-term follow-up study of infants treated with a probiotic. These infants (who did not have colic) were treated for the first 6 months of life with 10^{10} colony-forming units daily of *L rhamnosus GG*, alongside a control group of similarly normal infants who received a placebo (microcrystalline cellulose). Strikingly, 13 years later, 6 of 35 children who received placebo as infants had gone on to develop attention-deficit disorder or mild autism spectrum disorder (Asperger syndrome), whereas 0 of 40 children who had received the probiotic developed these disorders ($P<.01$). One might ponder the "unthinkable": that not only could the symptoms of colic respond favorably to probiotic treatment, but also (in severe cases) successful treatment of the dysbiosis might favorably impact future neurodevelopmental outcome.

REFERENCES

1. Wessel MA, Cobb JC, Jackson EB, et al. Paroxysmal fussing in infancy, sometimes called colic. Pediatrics 1954;14:421–35.
2. Groopman J. The colic conundrum: the crying that doctors can't stop. Ann Med. 2007. Available at: http://www.newyorker.com/magazine/2007-09/17/the-colic-conundrum. Accessed September 17, 2007.
3. Barr RG, Rotman A, Yaremko J, et al. The crying of infants with colic: a controlled empirical description. Pediatrics 1992;90:14–21.
4. Barr RG. Crying as a trigger for abusive head trauma: a key to prevention. Pediatr Radiol 2014;44(Suppl 4):S559–64.
5. Levitzky S, Cooper R. Infant colic syndrome—maternal fantasies of aggression and infanticide. Clin Pediatr (Phila) 2000;39:395–400.
6. Adamsbaum C, Grabar S, Mejean N, et al. Abusive head trauma: judicial admissions highlight violent and repetitive shaking. Pediatrics 2010;126:546–55.
7. Wolke D, Bilgin A, Samara M. Systematic review and meta-analysis: fussing and crying durations and prevalence of colic in infants. J Pediatr 2017;185:55–61.
8. Gelfand AA. Infant Colic. Semin Pediatr Neurol 2016;23:79–82.
9. Hall B, Chesters J, Robinson A. Infantile colic: a systematic review of medical and conventional therapies. J Paediatr Child Health 2012;48:128–37.
10. Parker S, Magee T, Colic. The Zuckerman Parker handbook of developmental and behavioral pediatrics for primary care. In: Augustyn M, Zucerkman B, Caronna EB, editors. 3rd edition. Philadelphia: Lippincott Williams & Wilkins; 2011. p. 182.
11. Thomas DW, McGilligan K, Eisenberg LD, et al. Infantile colic and type of milk feeding. Am J Dis Child 1987;141:451–3.
12. Rhoads JM, Fatheree NY, Norori J, et al. Altered fecal microflora and increased fecal calprotectin in infants with colic. J Pediatr 2009;155:823–8.
13. Garrison MM, Christakis DA. A systematic review of treatments for infant colic. Pediatrics 2000;106:184–90.
14. Lucassen PL, Assendelft WJ, Gubbels JW, et al. Effectiveness of treatments for infantile colic: systematic review. BMJ 1998;316:1563–9.
15. Lust KD, Brown JE, Thomas W. Maternal intake of cruciferous vegetables and other foods and colic symptoms in exclusively breast-fed infants. J Am Diet Assoc 1996;96:46–8.
16. Moore DJ, Robb TA, Davidson GP. Breath hydrogen response to milk containing lactose in colicky and noncolicky infants. J Pediatr 1988;113:979–84.
17. Fatheree NY, Liu Y, Ferris M, et al. Hypoallergenic formula with *Lactobacillus rhamnosus GG* for babies with colic: a pilot study of recruitment, retention, and fecal biomarkers. World J Gastrointest Pathophysiol 2016;7:160–70.
18. Hyams JS, Geertsma MA, Etienne NL, et al. Colonic hydrogen production in infants with colic. J Pediatr 1989;115:592–4.

19. Miller JJ, McVeagh P, Fleet GH, et al. Breath hydrogen excretion in infants with colic. Arch Dis Child 1989;64:725–9.
20. Treem WR. Infant colic. A pediatric gastroenterologist's perspective. Pediatr Clin North Am 1994;41:1121–38.
21. Barr RG, Wooldridge J, Hanley J. Effects of formula change on intestinal hydrogen production and crying and fussing behavior. J Dev Behav Pediatr 1991;12:248–53.
22. Kanabar D, Randhawa M, Clayton P. Improvement of symptoms in infant colic following reduction of lactose load with lactase. J Hum Nutr Diet 2001;14:359–63.
23. Liebman WM. Infantile colic. Association with lactose and milk intolerance. JAMA 1981;245:732–3.
24. Fazil M. Prevalence and risk factors for infantile colic in District Mansehra. J Ayub Med Coll Abbottabad 2011;23:115–7.
25. Talachian E, Bidari A, Rezaie MH. Incidence and risk factors for infantile colic in Iranian infants. World J Gastroenterol 2008;14:4662–6.
26. Young SN, Leyton M. The role of serotonin in human mood and social interaction. Insight from altered tryptophan levels. Pharmacol Biochem Behav 2002;71: 857–65.
27. Kurtoglu S, Uzum K, Hallac IK, et al. 5-Hydroxy-3-indole acetic acid levels in infantile colic: is serotoninergic tonus responsible for this problem? Acta Paediatr 1997;86:764–5.
28. Vartabedian B. Colic solved: the essential guide to infant reflux and the care of your crying, difficult-to-sooth baby. New York (NY): Ballantine Books; 2007. Version 3.1.
29. Karp HN. Safe swaddling and healthy hips: don't toss the baby out with the bathwater. Pediatrics 2008;121:1075–6.
30. Karp H. The happiest baby on the block: the new way to calm crying and help your newborn baby sleep longer. 2nd edition. New York (NY): Bantam Books; 2015.
31. Paradise JL. Maternal and other factors in the etiology of infantile colic. Report of a prospective study of 146 infants. JAMA 1966;197:191–9.
32. Sondergaard C, Olsen J, Friis-Hasche E, et al. Psychosocial distress during pregnancy and the risk of infantile colic: a follow-up study. Acta Paediatr 2003;92: 811–6.
33. van den Berg MP, van der Ende J, Crijnen AA, et al. Paternal depressive symptoms during pregnancy are related to excessive infant crying. Pediatrics 2009; 124:e96–103.
34. Raiha H, Lehtonen L, Huhtala V, et al. Excessively crying infant in the family: mother-infant, father-infant and mother-father interaction. Child Care Health Dev 2002;28:419–29.
35. Canivet CA, Ostergren PO, Rosen AS, et al. Infantile colic and the role of trait anxiety during pregnancy in relation to psychosocial and socioeconomic factors. Scand J Public Health 2005;33:26–34.
36. Canivet CA, Ostergren PO, Jakobsson IL, et al. Infantile colic, maternal smoking and infant feeding at 5 weeks of age. Scand J Public Health 2008;36:284–91.
37. Crowcroft NS, Strachan DP. The social origins of infantile colic: questionnaire study covering 76,747 infants. BMJ 1997;314:1325–8.
38. Carlsson C. Acupuncture mechanisms for clinically relevant long-term effects—reconsideration and a hypothesis. Acupunct Med 2002;20:82–99.
39. Madsen MV, Gotzsche PC, Hrobjartsson A. Acupuncture treatment for pain: systematic review of randomised clinical trials with acupuncture, placebo acupuncture, and no acupuncture groups. BMJ 2009;338:a3115.

40. Sato A, Sato Y, Suzuki A, et al. Neural mechanisms of the reflex inhibition and excitation of gastric motility elicited by acupuncture-like stimulation in anesthetized rats. Neurosci Res 1993;18:53–62.

41. Yuan M, Li Y, Wang Y, et al. Electroacupuncture at ST37 enhances jejunal motility via excitation of the parasympathetic system in rats and mice. Evid Based Complement Alternat Med 2016;2016:3840230.

42. Zeng F, Qin W, Ma T, et al. Influence of acupuncture treatment on cerebral activity in functional dyspepsia patients and its relationship with efficacy. Am J Gastroenterol 2012;107:1236–47.

43. Landgren K, Kvorning N, Hallstrom I. Acupuncture reduces crying in infants with infantile colic: a randomised, controlled, blind clinical study. Acupunct Med 2010; 28:174–9.

44. Reinthal M, Lund I, Ullman D, et al. Gastrointestinal symptoms of infantile colic and their change after light needling of acupuncture: a case series study of 913 infants. Chin Med 2011;6:28.

45. Landgren K, Hallstrom I. Effect of minimal acupuncture for infantile colic: a multicentre, three-armed, single-blind, randomised controlled trial (ACU-COL). Acupunct Med 2017;35:171–9.

46. Reinthal M, Andersson S, Gustafsson M, et al. Effects of minimal acupuncture in children with infantile colic—a prospective, quasi-randomised single blind controlled trial. Acupunct Med 2008;26:171–82.

47. Skjeie H, Skonnord T, Fetveit A, et al. Acupuncture for infantile colic: a blinding-validated, randomized controlled multicentre trial in general practice. Scand J Prim Health Care 2013;31:190–6.

48. Dobson D, Lucassen PL, Miller JJ, et al. Manipulative therapies for infantile colic. Cochrane Database Syst Rev 2012;12:CD004796.

49. Savino F, Ceratto S, De MA, et al. Looking for new treatments of infantile colic. Ital J Pediatr 2014;40:53.

50. Anheyer D, Frawley J, Koch AK, et al. Herbal medicines for gastrointestinal disorders in children and adolescents: a systematic review. Pediatrics 2017; 139 [pii:e20170062].

51. Paregoric. Available at: http://en.wikipedia.org/wiki/Paregoric. Accessed March 12, 2018.

52. Savino F, Tarasco V. New treatments for infant colic. Curr Opin Pediatr 2010;22: 791–7.

53. Moore DJ, Tao BS, Lines DR, et al. Double-blind placebo-controlled trial of omeprazole in irritable infants with gastroesophageal reflux. J Pediatr 2003;143: 219–23.

54. Orenstein SR, Hassall E, Furmaga-Jablonska W, et al. Multicenter, double-blind, randomized, placebo-controlled trial assessing the efficacy and safety of proton pump inhibitor lansoprazole in infants with symptoms of gastroesophageal reflux disease. J Pediatr 2009;154:514–20.

55. Hudson B, Alderton A, Doocey C, et al. Crying and spilling—time to stop the over-medicalisation of normal infant behaviour. N Z Med J 2012;125:119–26.

56. Ringel Y, Ringel-Kulka T. The intestinal microbiota and irritable bowel syndrome. J Clin Gastroenterol 2015;49(Suppl 1):S56–9.

57. Gevers D, Kugathasan S, Denson LA, et al. The treatment-naive microbiome in new-onset Crohn's disease. Cell Host Microbe 2014;15:382–92.

58. Olesen SW, Alm EJ. Dysbiosis is not an answer. Nat Microbiol 2016;1:16228.

59. Jandhyala SM, Talukdar R, Subramanyam C, et al. Role of the normal gut microbiota. World J Gastroenterol 2015;21:8787–803.

60. Savino F, Cresi F, Pautasso S, et al. Intestinal microflora in breastfed colicky and non-colicky infants. Acta Paediatr 2004;93:825–9.
61. Savino F, Cordisco L, Tarasco V, et al. Molecular identification of coliform bacteria from colicky breastfed infants. Acta Paediatr 2009;98:1582–8.
62. Fatheree NY, Liu Y, Taylor CM, et al. *Lactobacillus reuteri* for infants with colic: a double-blind, placebo-controlled, randomized clinical trial. J Pediatr 2017;191: 170–8.
63. Martinez I, Muller CE, Walter J. Long-term temporal analysis of the human fecal microbiota revealed a stable core of dominant bacterial species. PLoS One 2013;8:e69621.
64. de Weerth C, Fuentes S, Puylaert P, et al. Intestinal microbiota of infants with colic: development and specific signatures. Pediatrics 2013;131:e550–8.
65. Partty A, Kalliomaki M, Endo A, et al. Compositional development of *Bifidobacterium* and *Lactobacillus* microbiota is linked with crying and fussing in early infancy. PLoS One 2012;7:e32495.
66. Savino F, Quartieri A, De MA, et al. Comparison of formula-fed infants with and without colic revealed significant differences in total bacteria, Enterobacteriaceae and faecal ammonia. Acta Paediatr 2017;106:573–8.
67. Savino F, Garro M, Montanari P, et al. Crying time and RORgamma/FOXP3 expression in *Lactobacillus reuteri* DSM17938-treated infants with colic: a randomized trial. J Pediatr 2017;192:171–7.e1.
68. Mai V, Young CM, Ukhanova M, et al. Fecal microbiota in premature infants prior to necrotizing enterocolitis. PLoS One 2011;6:e20647.
69. Warner BB, Deych E, Zhou Y, et al. Gut bacteria dysbiosis and necrotising enterocolitis in very low birthweight infants: a prospective case-control study. Lancet 2016;387:1928–36.
70. Olafsdottir E, Aksnes L, Fluge G, et al. Faecal calprotectin levels in infants with infantile colic, healthy infants, children with inflammatory bowel disease, children with recurrent abdominal pain and healthy children. Acta Paediatr 2002;91: 45–50.
71. Sung V, Hiscock H, Tang ML, et al. Treating infant colic with the probiotic *Lactobacillus reuteri*: double blind, placebo controlled randomised trial. BMJ 2014; 348:g2107.
72. Savino F, De MA, Ceratto S, et al. Fecal calprotectin during treatment of severe infantile colic with *Lactobacillus reuteri* DSM 17938: a randomized, double-blind, placebo-controlled trial. Pediatrics 2015;135(Suppl 1):S5–6.
73. Savino F, Pelle E, Palumeri E, et al. *Lactobacillus reuteri* (American Type Culture Collection Strain 55730) versus simethicone in the treatment of infantile colic: a prospective randomized study. Pediatrics 2007;119:e124–30.
74. Barr RG, Kramer MS, Boisjoly C, et al. Parental diary of infant cry and fuss behaviour. Arch Dis Child 1988;63:380–7.
75. Savino F, Cordisco L, Tarasco V, et al. *Lactobacillus reuteri* DSM 17938 in infantile colic: a randomized, double-blind, placebo-controlled trial. Pediatrics 2010;126: e526–33.
76. Szajewska H, Gyrczuk E, Horvath A. *Lactobacillus reuteri* DSM 17938 for the management of infantile colic in breastfed infants: a randomized, double-blind, placebo-controlled trial. J Pediatr 2013;162:257–62.
77. Chau K, Lau E, Greenberg S, et al. Probiotics for infantile colic: a randomized, double-blind, placebo-controlled trial investigating *Lactobacillus reuteri* DSM 17938. J Pediatr 2015;166:74–8.

78. Mi GL, Zhao L, Qiao DD, et al. Effectiveness of *Lactobacillus reuteri* in infantile colic and colicky induced maternal depression: a prospective single blind randomized trial. Antonie Van Leeuwenhoek 2015;107:1547–53.
79. Harb T, Matsuyama M, David M, et al. Infant colic—what works: a systematic review of interventions for breast-fed infants. J Pediatr Gastroenterol Nutr 2016;62: 668–86.
80. Xu M, Wang J, Wang N, et al. The efficacy and safety of the probiotic bacterium *Lactobacillus reuteri* DSM 17938 for infantile colic: a meta-analysis of randomized controlled trials. PLoS One 2015;10:e0141445.
81. Sung V, Cabana MD, D'Amico F, et al. *Lactobacillus reuteri* DSM 17938 for managing infant colic: protocol for an individual participant data meta-analysis. BMJ Open 2014;4:e006475.
82. Liu Y, Fatheree NY, Dingle BM, et al. *Lactobacillus reuteri* DSM 17938 changes the frequency of Foxp3+ regulatory T cells in the intestine and mesenteric lymph node in experimental necrotizing enterocolitis. PLoS One 2013;8(2):e56547.
83. Partty A, Lehtonen L, Kalliomaki M, et al. Probiotic *Lactobacillus rhamnosus GG* therapy and microbiological programming in infantile colic: a randomized, controlled trial. Pediatr Res 2015;78:470–5.
84. Kianifar H, Ahanchian H, Grover Z, et al. Synbiotic in the management of infantile colic: a randomised controlled trial. J Paediatr Child Health 2014;50:801–5.
85. Vandenplas Y, Bacarea A, Marusteri M, et al. Efficacy and safety of APT198K for the treatment of infantile colic: a pilot study. J Comp Eff Res 2017;6:137–44.
86. Indrio F, Di MA, Riezzo G, et al. Prophylactic use of a probiotic in the prevention of colic, regurgitation, and functional constipation: a randomized clinical trial. JAMA Pediatr 2014;168:228–33.
87. Savino F, Ceratto S, Poggi E, et al. Preventive effects of oral probiotic on infantile colic: a prospective, randomised, blinded, controlled trial using *Lactobacillus reuteri* DSM 17938. Benef Microbes 2015;6:245–51.
88. Savino F, Castagno E, Bretto R, et al. A prospective 10-year study on children who had severe infantile colic. Acta Paediatr Suppl 2005;94:129–32.
89. Kelly JR, Minuto C, Cryan JF, et al. Cross talk: the microbiota and neurodevelopmental disorders. Front Neurosci 2017;11:490.
90. Rea K, Dinan TG, Cryan JF. The microbiome: a key regulator of stress and neuroinflammation. Neurobiol Stress 2016;4:23–33.
91. Vuong HE, Yano JM, Fung TC, et al. The microbiome and host behavior. Annu Rev Neurosci 2017;40:21–49.
92. Zheng P, Zeng B, Zhou C, et al. Gut microbiome remodeling induces depressive-like behaviors through a pathway mediated by the host's metabolism. Mol Psychiatry 2016;21:786–96.
93. Messaoudi M, Lalonde R, Violle N, et al. Assessment of psychotropic-like properties of a probiotic formulation (*Lactobacillus helveticus* R0052 and *Bifidobacterium longum* R0175) in rats and human subjects. Br J Nutr 2011;105:755–64.
94. Partty A, Kalliomaki M, Wacklin P, et al. A possible link between early probiotic intervention and the risk of neuropsychiatric disorders later in childhood: a randomized trial. Pediatr Res 2015;77:823–8.

Constipation
Beyond the Old Paradigms

Peter L. Lu, MD, MS[a],*, Hayat M. Mousa, MD[b]

KEYWORDS

- Pediatrics • Children • Fecal incontinence • Encopresis • Defecation disorder
- Antegrade continence enema • Sacral nerve stimulation • Sacral neuromodulation

KEY POINTS

- Although most children with constipation respond to conventional treatment, symptoms persist in a minority. Recent advancements offer promise in the management of these children.
- Identifying a rectal evacuation disorder or colonic motility disorder by performing anorectal and colonic manometry testing can guide subsequent management.
- Novel pharmacologic treatments used in adults with constipation are beginning to be used in children, with promising results.
- Biofeedback therapy and anal sphincter botulinum toxin injection can be considered for children with a rectal evacuation disorder.
- Surgical management of constipation includes the use of antegrade continence enemas, sacral nerve stimulation, colonic resection, and stoma creation.

INTRODUCTION

Constipation is commonly encountered in children and can result from several medical conditions, ranging from congenital abnormalities to metabolic disorders. However, most children with constipation do not have any underlying medical condition causing their constipation and therefore have functional constipation (FC).[1] The Rome criteria are the most widely used diagnostic criteria for FC, and the recently released Rome IV criteria define FC as experiencing 2 or more of the following at least once a week over the past month[2]:

1. Two or fewer bowel movements per week
2. At least 1 episode of fecal incontinence per week

Disclosures: The authors do not have any relevant disclosures.
[a] Division of Gastroenterology, Hepatology and Nutrition, Department of Pediatrics, Nationwide Children's Hospital, 700 Children's Drive, Columbus, OH 43205, USA; [b] Division of Gastroenterology, Hepatology and Nutrition, Department of Pediatrics, University of California, San Diego, Rady Children's Hospital, 3030 Children's Way, San Diego, CA 92123, USA
* Corresponding author.
E-mail address: peter.lu@nationwidechildrens.org

Gastroenterol Clin N Am 47 (2018) 845–862
https://doi.org/10.1016/j.gtc.2018.07.009
0889-8553/18/© 2018 Elsevier Inc. All rights reserved.

Abbreviations

ACE	Antegrade continence enema
FC	Functional constipation
SNS	Sacral nerve stimulation
TES	Transcutaneous electrical stimulation

3. History of retentive posturing or excessive volitional stool retention
4. History of hard or painful bowel movements
5. Presence of a large fecal mass in the rectum
6. History of large-diameter stools that can obstruct the toilet

Pediatric population-based studies on constipation from around the world describe a prevalence ranging from 0.7% to 29.6%, with a median of 12%.[3] The cost associated with the care of children with constipation is substantial. Using data from 2003 to 2004, it was estimated that medical care for children with constipation accounted for an additional $3.9 billion in medical costs per year in the United States.[4] This figure is likely now significantly higher, particularly because both the number of hospitalizations for children with constipation and the mean cost of each hospitalization in the United States have been steadily increasing.[5] However, despite how common constipation is in children, understanding of the prognosis of children with FC is limited. The studies available are few and heterogeneous, but one review found that, after 5 to 10 years of follow-up, only 56% of children had recovered and were no longer taking laxatives. Children who were treated by a specialist had a higher success rate, but more than a quarter continued to have symptoms requiring laxative treatment at follow-up.[6]

The North American and European societies of pediatric gastroenterology recently put forth evidence-based recommendations on the treatment of FC. Conventional treatment of FC includes education of the child and family, toilet training, and oral medications, including osmotic and stimulant laxatives. If the child's symptoms persist, assessment of treatment adherence and adjustment of laxative treatment may be needed.[1] However, a proportion of children have symptoms despite conventional treatment, and the management of this population can be challenging and varies widely among providers and institutions.[7]

For these children, the treatment paradigm is evolving. This article summarizes recent advancements in the evaluation and treatment of children with FC and discusses their clinical applications, particularly to children with continued symptoms despite conventional treatment. Identifying the mechanisms contributing to a child's presentation can allow more personalized and effective management.

EVALUATION

The diagnosis of FC is a clinical one made using the Rome criteria. However, further evaluation may still be needed after establishing the diagnosis of FC, particularly for children with refractory symptoms. The symptoms associated with FC can result from several underlying mechanisms. If a child's symptoms do not respond to conventional treatment, testing may be able to identify contributing factors for that individual patient, allowing a better understanding of the child's constipation and potentially guiding subsequent treatment.[1] This evaluation should begin by ensuring that a thorough history and physical examination have been completed.

Although this article discusses several diagnostic tests, it is important to remember that most children with FC do not need any of them. The primary role of a thorough history and physical examination is to exclude an underlying organic disorder, but the history may also guide the provider's management.[1] For example, a report of prolonged straining to pass soft stool could increase suspicion for pelvic floor dyssynergia. The history should also include an assessment of the impact of a child's symptoms on daily functioning and quality of life. For older children with daily retentive fecal incontinence who are wearing diapers and have withdrawn from school, the treatment plan would be more aggressive and include a plan to return to school.

For those who continue to have symptoms despite optimal conventional treatment, diagnostic testing may be able to identify a responsible mechanism that would guide subsequent treatment. In a broad sense, evaluation would aim to identify whether the child's constipation is secondary to a rectal evacuation disorder, a colonic motility disorder, or potentially both concurrently.

Evaluation for a Rectal Evacuation Disorder

Anorectal manometry

Anorectal manometry testing involves assessment of the neuromuscular function of the anus and rectum by using a manometric catheter placed through the anal canal and into the rectum. Anorectal manometry is the most commonly performed gastrointestinal motility test in children and has become more widely available over time. The North American societies for neurogastroenterology and motility and pediatric gastroenterology recently published a consensus document on anorectal and colonic manometry testing.[8]

The catheters used for anorectal manometry have evolved with time, from standard water-perfused catheters to solid-state high-resolution catheters to three-dimensional high-definition catheters that allow dynamic imaging of the anal canal (**Fig. 1**). Most of the experience with anorectal manometry testing in children thus far has been using water-perfused and solid-state catheters, and the utility of three-dimensional catheters in pediatrics, although promising, is still unclear.[9] For cooperative children, anorectal manometry testing involves measurement of resting anal pressure and the length of the anal canal, evaluation of squeeze and bear-down (or push) mechanisms, and evaluation of rectal sensation and for a rectoanal inhibitory reflex with progressive

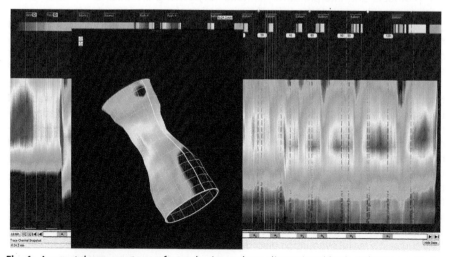

Fig. 1. Anorectal manometry performed using a three-dimensional high-definition catheter allows dynamic recreation of the anal canal.

rectal balloon inflation. Balloon expulsion testing can be informative as well.[8] A paradoxic increase in external anal sphincter pressure during the bear-down maneuver can be suggestive of an increase in anal pressure during attempts to defecate and pelvic floor dyssynergia.[10]

For younger or uncooperative children, anorectal manometry testing can be attempted under sedation. It is important to recognize that, even for older children, the test can be associated with significant anxiety in both the children and parents.[11] Sedation limits the test to assessment of resting anal pressure and evaluation for a rectoanal inhibitory reflex, and anesthetic agents such as propofol can decrease the ability to measure a useful resting anal pressure.[12] The primary utility in performing an anorectal manometry test under sedation is in evaluating for Hirschsprung disease or anal sphincter achalasia, which should be suspected if the rectoanal inhibitory reflux is absent.[8]

Defecography

Defecography is a radiologic test used to assess the pelvic floor during the act of defecation and can be useful in identifying pelvic floor dyssynergia and also structural abnormalities such as rectocele or rectal prolapse. Experience with defecography in children is limited, but the test is safe and generally well tolerated in children older than 4 to 5 years of age.[13,14] A small study of children with defecation disorders evaluated by fluoroscopic defecography reported that results directly influenced subsequent treatment in 67% of the cohort.[13] However, defecography involves radiation exposure and experience in adults has raised concerns regarding interobserver bias and variable methodology among centers.[15]

Evaluation for a Colonic Motility Disorder

Colonic transit testing

Measurement of colonic transit time can be helpful in the evaluation of children with refractory FC. The most commonly used method of colonic transit testing is by using radiopaque markers. After ingestion, the position of these markers in the colon is evaluated by abdominal radiographs (**Fig. 2**). Although inexpensive and simple to perform, test protocols and interpretative methods vary among institutions.[16,17] One of the more commonly used methods involves ingestion of a capsule containing a set number of markers on 3 consecutive days. This ingestion is followed by an abdominal radiograph on the fourth day and in some cases another radiograph on the seventh day. Using skeletal landmarks to divide the colon into segments, both segmental and total colonic transit time can be calculated and compared with normative data.[16]

Colonic scintigraphy involves measuring the transit of an ingested radioisotope through the colon. One study in children showed that colonic scintigraphy was well tolerated and showed fair agreement with colonic manometry in differentiating between normal transit, delay in the distal colon, and colonic inertia.[18] Wireless pH-motility capsule testing has been used to measure colonic transit time in adults, and measurements correlate well with results of radiopaque marker testing.[19] Wireless pH-motility capsule testing has been shown to be safe and well tolerated in children, but its use for measurement of colonic transit time in children remains untested.[20] Normal colonic transit and prompt evacuation of radiopaque markers or radioisotope in a child with frequent fecal incontinence should raise concern for nonretentive fecal incontinence.[1] Prompt transit to the rectum with retention of markers or radioisotope may suggest a rectal evacuation disorder. Slow colonic transit in a child with refractory FC benefits from assessment of segmental colonic function by colonic manometry evaluation when available.

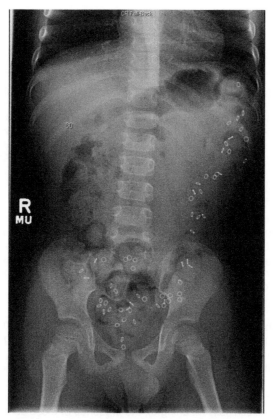

Fig. 2. An abdominal radiograph taken several days after ingestion of radiopaque markers shows retention of markers in the rectosigmoid and descending colon.

Colonic manometry

Colonic manometry testing involves assessment of colonic motor activity by using a manometry catheter placed in the lumen of the colon. Similar to the catheters used for anorectal manometry, the catheters used for colonic manometry have also evolved from primarily water-perfused catheters to solid-state high-resolution catheters.[21] Catheter placement is generally performed under general anesthesia during colonoscopy or with fluoroscopic guidance. Some centers use an endoscopic clip to attach the distal tip of the catheter to the colonic mucosa to reduce migration during the study (**Fig. 3**).[8] There is evidence that recent anesthesia can affect subsequent colonic manometry results, although the length of time needed for this effect to cease is unclear.[22,23]

Once the catheter is in place and time has been given for recovery after anesthesia, the colonic manometry test begins. Although testing protocols vary among providers and institutions, testing generally begins with assessment of colonic activity while fasting. This assessment is followed by a meal and assessment for a gastrocolic response, characterized by a physiologic increase in colonic contractions and tone after a meal. Series of high-amplitude propagating contractions can occur in all phases of the study but can be seen as part of the gastrocolic response. In some cases (ie, when high-amplitude propagating contractions are absent or limited after the meal),

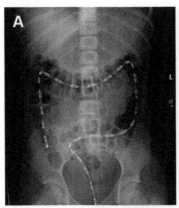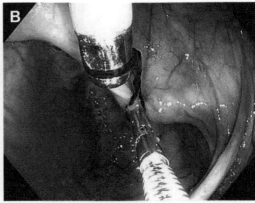

Fig. 3. (*A*) Abdominal radiograph taken after colonoscopy with colonic manometry catheter placement shows the catheter coursing through the colon. An endoscopic clip attached to the catheter is visible in the proximal colon. (*B*) The distal tip of the manometry catheter is visible extending down from the top of the image. A black suture has been tied to the tip of the catheter and an endoscopic clip is being placed to secure the catheter to the colonic mucosa. (*Courtesy of* Neetu Bali, MD, Columbus, OH.)

this is followed by provocative testing to assess the colonic response to drug challenge, most commonly by evaluating for high-amplitude propagating contractions after administration of bisacodyl (**Fig. 4**).[8]

For children with refractory FC, colonic manometry testing can identify a colonic motility disorder. Although there is growing evidence that colonic motor patterns observed during manometry testing other than high-amplitude propagating contractions are likely to be clinically meaningful, the presence of these contractions remains the most recognizable and clinically significant portion of the test.[24,25] Absence of high-amplitude propagating contractions throughout the colon suggests colonic inertia. Propagation that terminates prematurely (ie, before reaching the distal sigmoid colon) suggests segmental colonic dysmotility. By correlating manometry results with an abdominal radiograph taken after catheter placement, providers can estimate the length of dysmotile colon, which can be helpful if surgical resection is needed.[8,26] Normal colonic manometry is associated with an improved response to antegrade continence enema (ACE) treatment.[27–30]

However, the utility of colonic manometry is not limited to the measurement of colonic contractile activity alone. Clinical observation of the patient during the study can be revealing as well. Children with FC who deny the urge to defecate often show that they do sense high-amplitude propagating contractions through nonverbal communication such as grimacing or posturing. Children may also show evidence of volitional stool retention. For these children, it may be helpful for them to recognize that the sensation they felt at the time of propagating contractions should prompt them to have a bowel movement.[31]

TREATMENT

Treatment of children with FC begins with education of the child and family, toilet training, and oral medications, including traditional osmotic and stimulant laxatives. As discussed earlier, conventional treatment is sufficient for most children with FC.[1] Treatment options for children with symptoms refractory to optimal conventional

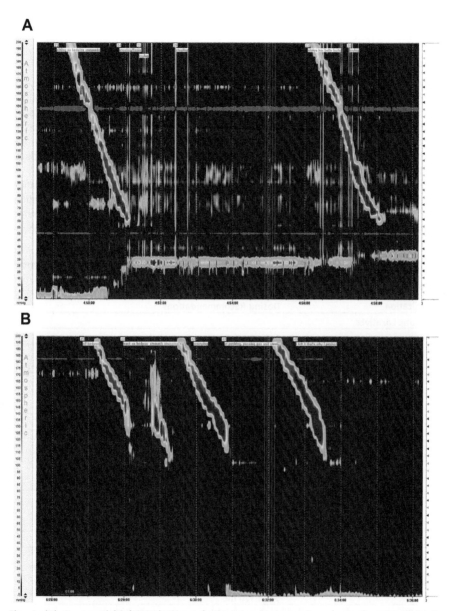

Fig. 4. (*A*) A normal high-resolution colonic manometry tracing shows 2 series of high-amplitude propagating contractions that terminate near the anal canal, presumably in the area of the rectum. (*B*) An abnormal colonic manometry tracing shows multiple series of high-amplitude propagating contractions that terminate prematurely, approximately halfway through the studied colon.

treatment have traditionally been limited, but recent advancements offer promise. Several novel pharmacologic treatments have emerged for adults with constipation and constipation-predominant irritable bowel syndrome that are beginning to be used in the pediatric population. For children with FC and an identified rectal evacuation disorder and/or colonic motility disorder, nonpharmacologic treatment options beyond conventional treatment can be chosen based on the mechanisms contributing to the child's presentation.

Novel Pharmacologic Treatments

Traditional pharmacologic treatment of children with FC generally begins with use of osmotic laxatives such as polyethylene glycol, followed by use of stimulant laxatives or lubricants if symptoms persist.[17] Evidence-based recommendations on laxative treatment of children with FC have been published (**Table 1**).[1] However, newer pharmacologic treatments have been used successfully in adults with constipation and constipation-predominant irritable bowel syndrome. Experience with these medications remains limited in children with FC but is growing with time.

Lubiprostone is a prostaglandin E1 derivative that promotes intestinal fluid secretion by acting on the type 2 chloride channel, softening stool and promoting intestinal motility in response to luminal distention.[17] Lubiprostone is approved in the United States for treatment of chronic idiopathic constipation in adults and irritable bowel

---

Table 1
Dosing recommendations for commonly used oral and rectal laxatives

Medication	Dosing Recommendations
Osmotic Laxatives	
Lactulose	1–2 g/kg, once or twice per day
PEG 3350	Maintenance: 0.2–0.8 g/kg/d Fecal disimpaction: 1–1.5 g/kg/d (up to 6 consecutive days)
Milk of magnesia	2–5 y: 0.4–1.2 g/d, once or divided 6–11 y: 1.2–2.4 g/d, once or divided 12–18 y: 2.4–4.8 g/d, once or divided
Stool Softeners	
Mineral oil	1–18 y: 1–3 mL/kg/d, once or divided, maximum 90 mL/d
Stimulant Laxatives	
Bisacodyl	3–10 y: 5 mg/d >10 y: 5–10 mg/d
Senna	2–6 y: 2.5–5 mg once or twice per day 6–12 y: 7.5–10 mg/d >12 y: 15–20 mg/d
Rectal Laxatives/Enemas	
Bisacodyl	2–10 y: 5 mg once per day >10 y: 5–10 mg once per day
Sodium docusate	<6 y: 60 mL >6 y: 120 mL
Sodium phosphate	1–18 y: 2.5 mL/kg, maximum 133 mL/dose
Sodium chloride	Neonate <1 kg: 5 mL Neonate >1 kg: 10 mL >1 y: 6 mL/kg once or twice per day 2–11 y: 30–60 mL once per day >11 y: 60–150 mL once per day
Mineral oil	2–11 y: 30–60 mL once per day >11 y: 60–150 mL once per day

Adapted from Tabbers MM, DiLorenzo C, Berger MY, et al. Evaluation and treatment of functional constipation in infants and children: evidence-based recommendations from ESPGHAN and NASPGHAN. J Ped Gastro Nutr 2014;58(2):269; with permission.

syndrome with constipation in adult women.[32] Several randomized controlled studies have shown the efficacy and safety of lubiprostone in adults with constipation.[33–35] In a multicenter, open-label study of children with FC, lubiprostone led to a significant increase in bowel movement frequency and was generally well tolerated, with nausea, vomiting, and diarrhea as the most common adverse events.[32] A randomized controlled trial in children is underway.[17]

Linaclotide is a peptide agonist of the intestinal guanylate cyclase-C receptor, promoting intestinal fluid secretion. Linaclotide not only softens stool and promotes intestinal motility but also reduces visceral sensitivity in animal models. Linaclotide is approved in the United States for treatment of chronic intestinal constipation and irritable bowel syndrome with constipation in adults.[36] Randomized controlled studies in adults have shown significant improvement in bowel movement frequency and abdominal pain. Treatment was generally well tolerated, with diarrhea as the most common adverse event.[36–38] No studies have yet been completed in children.

Prucalopride is a highly selective 5-hydroxytryptamine receptor 4 serotonergic agent that increases acetylcholine release and subsequently increases intestinal motility, particularly in the lower gastrointestinal tract.[39] Multiple randomized controlled studies in adults with chronic idiopathic constipation have shown significant improvement in bowel movement frequency.[40–42] In an initial open-label study of children with FC, prucalopride led to improvements in bowel movement frequency, fecal incontinence, and stool consistency. Prucalopride was generally well tolerated in children.[43] However, a multicenter, randomized controlled study did not find any difference in clinical response or perceived benefit compared with placebo.[44]

Treatment of a Rectal Evacuation Disorder

Biofeedback therapy

The purpose of biofeedback therapy is to restore a normal pattern of defecation using visual and verbal feedback techniques. For children with pelvic floor dyssynergia, this involves training children to relax the external anal sphincter while increasing abdominal pressure during attempts to defecate. Visual feedback is provided either by placing an anorectal manometry catheter to show abdominal and anal pressures or by applying surface electromyography leads externally. The duration of biofeedback therapy (ie, number of training sessions required) varies depending on the child's response. Although the North American and European societies for neurogastroenterology and motility recommend biofeedback therapy for adults with pelvic floor dyssynergia based on high-quality evidence, the efficacy of biofeedback therapy in children for the same indication is less clear and routine treatment with biofeedback therapy was not recommended.[45]

Studies of children with FC treated with biofeedback therapy have shown variable results. Although some studies have found clinical improvement in as many as 90% of children with FC treated with biofeedback therapy, several controlled studies have not found any significant long-term improvement compared with conventional treatment.[1,45–47] Two large randomized controlled studies did not find biofeedback therapy to be helpful compared with conventional treatment (education, toilet training, and laxatives) or in addition to conventional treatment.[48,49] However, a recent randomized controlled study evaluating the addition of biofeedback therapy to conventional treatment did show a significant advantage in symptomatic improvement and ability to discontinue laxative treatment.[46] Studies have not shown an association between improvement and normalization of defecation dynamics based on anorectal manometry.[47,49]

The role that biofeedback therapy plays in the management of children with FC therefore remains unclear. For children with a rectal evacuation disorder and persistent symptoms despite optimal conventional treatment, biofeedback therapy is an option that can be considered, particularly given its lack of adverse effects. However, biofeedback therapy is only feasible in older, cooperative children, and the training is labor intensive and requires practitioners with specialized training.[45]

Anal sphincter botulinum toxin injection

Injection of botulinum toxin into the anal sphincter has been used for children with impaired rectal evacuation secondary to Hirschsprung disease, anal sphincter achalasia, or anal fissure, generally with good response.[50–55] Injection is performed under sedation, often by dividing the administered toxin into the 4 quadrants of the internal anal sphincter. Injection is typically well tolerated, with transient fecal incontinence, rectal pain, and pelvic muscle paresis as potential side effects.[52,54]

Evidence of the efficacy of anal sphincter botulinum toxin injection for children with FC and a normal rectoanal inhibitory reflex remains limited. A randomized study of children with refractory FC found that improvement after anal sphincter botulinum toxin was comparable with internal anal sphincter myectomy. Children who had low anal resting pressures were excluded, but the cohort included children with normal and increased resting pressures.[56] In a cohort study that included children who had a high-threshold rectoanal inhibitory reflex, investigators reported symptomatic improvement after injection.[57] In a recent survey of pediatric gastroenterologists and surgeons, more than half of respondents reported that they would use anal sphincter botulinum toxin injection to treat a child with refractory FC who had an intact rectoanal inhibitory reflex and an increased resting anal pressure, suggesting that the use of botulinum toxin injection for treatment of FC may be more common than the literature suggests.[7] Further studies are needed to clarify the role of anal sphincter botulinum toxin injection in the treatment of children with FC and a rectal evacuation disorder.

Surgical Treatment of Functional Constipation

Antegrade continence enemas

ACE treatment involves the administration of an enema into the proximal colon through surgical creation of an appendicostomy or cecostomy. The choice of procedure is based in part on patient and surgeon preference. Although appendicostomy creation offers some cosmetic advantage with the ability to hide the site at the umbilicus (with access obtained by cannulation), a minority of children experience stricture formation. Cecostomy creation requires placement of a tube used for access.[26] Complications of appendicostomy and cecostomy are common, particularly minor complications such as pain with catheterization, skin irritation or granulomata, stomal leakage, and stomal stenosis.[58]

Although several case series describing outcomes of ACE treatment have been published over the past 2 decades, few have been prospective.[58] Studies have also been variable in both the definition of successful treatment and rate of success.[59] A review of the existing literature found that positive outcomes were reported in 82% of children treated with ACE, but resolution of symptoms allowing appendicostomy or cecostomy closure was reported only in 9.5%.[58] A larger, prospective cohort study that included children with both functional and organic causes of constipation reported that 93% of children had a positive response, and that approximately a quarter of children were no longer using ACE after a mean follow-up duration of 5.5 years. Children with FC were more likely to no longer require ACE treatment.[60] A recent retrospective review supports the finding that children with FC may be more likely to discontinue ACE treatment, estimating that, after 5 years of ACE treatment, approximately a third of children have their ostomy closed.[61]

Colonic manometry may play a role in predicting children's responses to ACE treatment. Several studies have found that normal colonic manometry before ACE treatment is associated with a better response to ACE treatment.[27,28] In children with colonic dysmotility before ACE treatment, repeat colonic manometry after ACE treatment often shows improvement in colonic motility.[62] A more recent retrospective review of children with FC who completed colonic manometry testing before and after ACE treatment initiation reported that the baseline manometry was not predictive of outcome, but high-amplitude propagating contractions on repeat manometry after ACE treatment were associated with a decreased need for ACE treatment.[29]

Neurostimulation
Over the last 2 decades, there has been increasing interest in the use of neurostimulation for treatment of children with refractory FC as an alternative to more invasive surgical procedures. Although pediatric experience with neurostimulation for gastrointestinal disorders remains limited, several modalities have shown promise and warrant further investigation.

Sacral nerve stimulation (SNS) is perhaps the most established form of neurostimulation used in children with defecation disorders. SNS involves the delivery of low-amplitude electrical stimulation to the sacral nerve root via an electrode placed in the sacral foramen (**Fig. 5**). This electrode is connected to a pulse generator and battery that may remain external to the child during an initial temporary stimulation trial before permanent implantation into a subcutaneous pocket in the buttock.[63] The initial reports of SNS for treatment of children with bladder dysfunction described

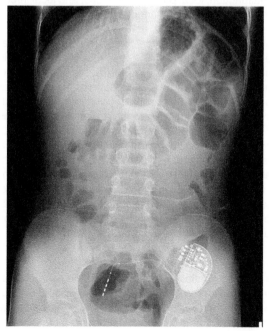

Fig. 5. An abdominal radiograph shows a sacral nerve stimulator lead and implanted pulse generator and battery.

improvement in not only urinary symptoms but in constipation and fecal incontinence as well.[64–66] Two institutions have recently published long-term outcomes of SNS treatment of children with severe constipation. In one study of girls with FC, significant improvement in constipation continued after a median follow-up of 22 months. However, 56% were considered not to have had a successful response to SNS based on bowel movement frequency.[67] The authors recently described the 2-year outcomes of a group of children treated with SNS for constipation, of which most had refractory FC. Although bowel movement frequency did not change significantly, durable improvement was seen in fecal incontinence and associated quality of life. Nearly all families surveyed reported health-related benefit.[68]

The role of SNS in relation to other surgical treatment options for FC (eg, ACE or colonic resection) remains unclear. In a study of children with continued constipation despite ACE treatment, SNS allowed a steady decrease in ACE usage. At a median of 18 months of follow-up, 45% had not only discontinued ACE usage but had undergone appendicostomy or cecostomy closure. SNS can be considered for children with FC who have persistent symptoms despite ACE treatment.[69] A recent study comparing children with FC treated with ACE or SNS showed that ACE leads to greater improvement in bowel movement frequency and abdominal pain but SNS may lead to greater improvement in fecal incontinence.[70] This finding is consistent with the adult experience with SNS, in which randomized controlled studies have shown significant improvement in adults with fecal incontinence but not FC.[71,72]

When considering SNS treatment, it is important to recognize the likelihood of complications requiring further surgery. In the largest cohort of children treated with SNS, 49% of children experienced complications requiring further surgery.[73] In addition to the 2 procedures required for SNS initiation, a proportion of children require lead revision, device removal, or device replacement, most often performed because of lead displacement or malfunction, local pain or numbness, and local infection.[67,68] However, attempts to identify factors predictive of complications after SNS have not been successful.[74]

Noninvasive forms of neurostimulation for FC are therefore needed. Abdominal transcutaneous electrical stimulation (TES) is the best-studied noninvasive modality and involves placement of 2 surface electrodes on the anterior abdomen at the level of the umbilicus and 2 on the lower back at the level of the upper lumbar spine. These electrodes are used to generate 2 sinusoidal currents that cross within the abdomen and apply interferential electrical current to the abdomen at an intensity less than the motor threshold.[75,76] Preliminary studies showed improvement in constipation, but a recent review reported that results of a randomized controlled study did not show significant differences in clinical response between abdominal TES and sham stimulation.[77] Nonetheless, given the advantages conferred by the noninvasive nature of abdominal TES, which are particularly relevant to the pediatric population, further investigation is needed. A recent cohort study showed that home-based abdominal TES was feasible for children with FC and led to significant improvement in bowel movement frequency, fecal incontinence, and abdominal pain.[78]

Colonic resection

For children with FC and continued severe, debilitating symptoms despite optimal medical management, colonic resection may be beneficial. Careful evaluation and consideration are needed before surgery, particularly because the available literature in children remains limited and specific indications for surgery unclear. A variety of procedures have been described, with the general aim of removing dilated, dysmotile colon thought to be responsible for the child's persistent symptoms.[26,58] Colonic manometry, particularly in cases in which manometry shows segmental dysmotility, may be useful to guide surgical decision making.[7,26] Colonic resection can be combined with creation of an appendicostomy to allow for administration of ACE postoperatively, which can decrease the need for oral laxatives and limit postoperative fecal incontinence.[79]

Stoma formation and bowel diversion

Temporary or permanent stoma formation and bowel diversion may be needed in certain situations. The literature on this topic is sparse and of limited quality. Based on small case series, almost half of children treated with stoma formation are able to undergo delayed restoration of intestinal continuity with good outcomes.[26,58] Stoma formation, specifically by creation of an ileostomy, may be beneficial for young children (<3 years of age) with colonic manometry testing showing diffuse colonic dysmotility, particularly in those with resulting failure to thrive. In these children, evaluation for chronic intestinal pseudo-obstruction, which almost invariably involves the small bowel as well, is critical because a positive diagnosis has therapeutic and prognostic implications.[26]

SUMMARY

Most children with constipation respond to education, toilet training, and laxatives and do not require any testing aside from a thoughtful history and physical examination. However, for the minority of children who continue to have symptoms despite conventional treatment, advancements over the past decade promise to improve their management beyond the old paradigms. Constipation is the end result of several potential contributing mechanisms, and diagnostic testing to identify the mechanism relevant to the individual child can guide subsequent treatment. Manometry testing is becoming more precise and results more meaningful. New medications will undoubtedly soon be available for children with refractory constipation. Measurement of anorectal function and colonic motility can inform the use of an array of nonpharmacologic treatment options, including biofeedback therapy, anal sphincter botulinum toxin injection, ACE treatment, neurostimulation, and colonic resection.

REFERENCES

1. Tabbers MM, DiLorenzo C, Berger MY, et al. Evaluation and treatment of functional constipation in infants and children: evidence-based recommendations from ESPGHAN and NASPGHAN. J Pediatr Gastroenterol Nutr 2014;58(2): 258–74.
2. Hyams JS, Di Lorenzo C, Saps M, et al. Functional disorders: children and adolescents. Gastroenterology 2016;150(6):1456–68.
3. Mugie SM, Benninga MA, Di Lorenzo C. Epidemiology of constipation in children and adults: a systematic review. Best Pract Res Clin Gastroenterol 2011;25(1): 3–18.
4. Liem O, Harman J, Benninga M, et al. Health utilization and cost impact of childhood constipation in the United States. J Pediatr 2009;154(2):258–62.
5. Park R, Mikami S, LeClair J, et al. Inpatient burden of childhood functional GI disorders in the USA: an analysis of national trends in the USA from 1997 to 2009. Neurogastroenterol Motil 2015;27(5):684–92.
6. Pijpers MA, Bongers ME, Benninga MA, et al. Functional constipation in children: a systematic review on prognosis and predictive factors. J Pediatr Gastroenterol Nutr 2010;50(3):256–68.

7. Koppen IJ, Kuizenga-Wessel S, Lu PL, et al. Surgical decision-making in the management of children with intractable functional constipation: What are we doing and are we doing it right? J Pediatr Surg 2016;51(10):1607–12.

8. Rodriguez L, Sood M, Di Lorenzo C, et al. An ANMS-NASPGHAN consensus document on anorectal and colonic manometry in children. Neurogastroenterol Motil 2017;29(1):1–8.

9. Ambartsumyan L, Rodriguez L, Morera C, et al. Longitudinal and radial characteristics of intra-anal pressures in children using 3D high-definition anorectal manometry: new observations. Am J Gastroenterol 2013;108(12):1918–28.

10. Belkind-Gerson J, Surjanhata B, Kuo B, et al. Bear-down maneuver is a useful adjunct in the evaluation of children with chronic constipation. J Pediatr Gastroenterol Nutr 2013;57(6):775–9.

11. Lamparyk K, Mahajan L, Debeljak A, et al. Anxiety associated with high-resolution anorectal manometry in pediatric patients and parents. J Pediatr Gastroenterol Nutr 2017;65(5):e98–100.

12. Tran K, Kuo B, Zibaitis A, et al. Effect of propofol on anal sphincter pressure during anorectal manometry. J Pediatr Gastroenterol Nutr 2014;58(4):495–7.

13. Mugie SM, Bates DG, Punati JB, et al. The value of fluoroscopic defecography in the diagnostic and therapeutic management of defecation disorders in children. Pediatr Radiol 2015;45(2):173–80.

14. Zhang SC, Wang WL, Liu X. Defecography used as a screening entry for identifying evacuatory pelvic floor disorders in childhood constipation. Clin Imaging 2014;38(2):115–21.

15. Rao SS, Ozturk R, Laine L. Clinical utility of diagnostic tests for constipation in adults: a systematic review. Am J Gastroenterol 2005;100(7):1605–15.

16. Southwell BR, Clarke MC, Sutcliffe J, et al. Colonic transit studies: normal values for adults and children with comparison of radiological and scintigraphic methods. Pediatr Surg Int 2009;25(7):559–72.

17. Koppen IJ, Di Lorenzo C, Saps M, et al. Childhood constipation: finally something is moving! Expert Rev Gastroenterol Hepatol 2016;10(1):141–55.

18. Mugie SM, Perez ME, Burgers R, et al. Colonic manometry and colonic scintigraphy as a diagnostic tool for children with severe constipation. J Pediatr Gastroenterol Nutr 2013;57(5):598–602.

19. Camilleri M, Thorne NK, Ringel Y, et al. Wireless pH-motility capsule for colonic transit: prospective comparison with radiopaque markers in chronic constipation. Neurogastroenterol Motil 2010;22(8):874–82, e233.

20. Green AD, Belkind-Gerson J, Surjanhata BC, et al. Wireless motility capsule test in children with upper gastrointestinal symptoms. J Pediatr 2013;162(6):1181–7.

21. Liem O, Burgers RE, Connor FL, et al. Solid-state vs water-perfused catheters to measure colonic high-amplitude propagating contractions. Neurogastroenterol Motil 2012;24(4):345–e167.

22. Ammoury RF, Emhardt JD, Aitchison WB, et al. Can colonic manometry studies be done on the day of colonic motility catheter placement? J Pediatr Gastroenterol Nutr 2012;55(3):278–82.

23. Arbizu RA, Nurko S, Heinz N, et al. Prospective evaluation of same day versus next day colon manometry results in children with medical refractory constipation. Neurogastroenterol Motil 2017;29(7):1–6.

24. Sood MR, Mousa H, Tipnis N, et al. Interobserver variability in the interpretation of colon manometry studies in children. J Pediatr Gastroenterol Nutr 2012;55(5):548–51.

25. Wessel S, Koppen IJ, Wiklendt L, et al. Characterizing colonic motility in children with chronic intractable constipation: a look beyond high-amplitude propagating sequences. Neurogastroenterol Motil 2016;28(5):743–57.

26. Wood RJ, Yacob D, Levitt MA. Surgical options for the management of severe functional constipation in children. Curr Opin Pediatr 2016;28(3):370–9.

27. van den Berg MM, Hogan M, Caniano DA, et al. Colonic manometry as predictor of cecostomy success in children with defecation disorders. J Pediatr Surg 2006; 41(4):730–6 [discussion: 730–6].

28. Mugie SM, Machado RS, Mousa HM, et al. Ten-year experience using antegrade enemas in children. J Pediatr 2012;161(4):700–4.

29. Rodriguez L, Nurko S, Flores A. Factors associated with successful decrease and discontinuation of antegrade continence enemas (ACE) in children with defecation disorders: a study evaluating the effect of ACE on colon motility. Neurogastroenterol Motil 2013;25(2):140-e81.

30. Gomez-Suarez RA, Gomez-Mendez M, Petty JK, et al. Associated factors for antegrade continence enemas for refractory constipation and fecal incontinence. J Pediatr Gastroenterol Nutr 2016;63(4):e63–8.

31. Firestone Baum C, John A, Srinivasan K, et al. Colon manometry proves that perception of the urge to defecate is present in children with functional constipation who deny sensation. J Pediatr Gastroenterol Nutr 2013;56(1):19–22.

32. Hyman PE, Di Lorenzo C, Prestridge LL, et al. Lubiprostone for the treatment of functional constipation in children. J Pediatr Gastroenterol Nutr 2014;58(3): 283–91.

33. Johanson JF, Morton D, Geenen J, et al. Multicenter, 4-week, double-blind, randomized, placebo-controlled trial of lubiprostone, a locally-acting type-2 chloride channel activator, in patients with chronic constipation. Am J Gastroenterol 2008; 103(1):170–7.

34. Johanson JF, Ueno R. Lubiprostone, a locally acting chloride channel activator, in adult patients with chronic constipation: a double-blind, placebo-controlled, dose-ranging study to evaluate efficacy and safety. Aliment Pharmacol Ther 2007;25(11):1351–61.

35. Barish CF, Drossman D, Johanson JF, et al. Efficacy and safety of lubiprostone in patients with chronic constipation. Dig Dis Sci 2010;55(4):1090–7.

36. Schoenfeld P, Lacy BE, Chey WD, et al. Low-dose linaclotide (72 μg) for chronic idiopathic constipation: A 12-week, randomized, double-blind, placebo-controlled trial. Am J Gastroenterol 2018;113(1):105–14.

37. Lembo AJ, Kurtz CB, Macdougall JE, et al. Efficacy of linaclotide for patients with chronic constipation. Gastroenterology 2010;138(3):886–95.e1.

38. Lembo AJ, Schneier HA, Shiff SJ, et al. Two randomized trials of linaclotide for chronic constipation. N Engl J Med 2011;365(6):527–36.

39. Diederen K, Mugie SM, Benninga MA. Efficacy and safety of prucalopride in adults and children with chronic constipation. Expert Opin Pharmacother 2015; 16(3):407–16.

40. Camilleri M, Kerstens R, Rykx A, et al. A placebo-controlled trial of prucalopride for severe chronic constipation. N Engl J Med 2008;358(22):2344–54.

41. Quigley EM, Vandeplassche L, Kerstens R, et al. Clinical trial: the efficacy, impact on quality of life, and safety and tolerability of prucalopride in severe chronic constipation–a 12-week, randomized, double-blind, placebo-controlled study. Aliment Pharmacol Ther 2009;29(3):315–28.

42. Tack J, van Outryve M, Beyens G, et al. Prucalopride (Resolor) in the treatment of severe chronic constipation in patients dissatisfied with laxatives. Gut 2009;58(3): 357–65.
43. Winter HS, Di Lorenzo C, Benninga MA, et al. Oral prucalopride in children with functional constipation. J Pediatr Gastroenterol Nutr 2013;57(2):197–203.
44. Mugie SM, Korczowski B, Bodi P, et al. Prucalopride is no more effective than placebo for children with functional constipation. Gastroenterology 2014;147(6): 1285–95.e1.
45. Rao SS, Benninga MA, Bharucha AE, et al. ANMS-ESNM position paper and consensus guidelines on biofeedback therapy for anorectal disorders. Neurogastroenterol Motil 2015;27(5):594–609.
46. van Engelenburg-van Lonkhuyzen ML, Bols EM, Benninga MA, et al. Effectiveness of pelvic physiotherapy in children with functional constipation compared with standard medical care. Gastroenterology 2017;152(1):82–91.
47. Jarzebicka D, Sieczkowska J, Dadalski M, et al. Evaluation of the effectiveness of biofeedback therapy for functional constipation in children. Turk J Gastroenterol 2016;27(5):433–8.
48. Loening-Baucke V. Biofeedback treatment for chronic constipation and encopresis in childhood: long-term outcome. Pediatrics 1995;96(1 Pt 1):105–10.
49. van der Plas RN, Benninga MA, Buller HA, et al. Biofeedback training in treatment of childhood constipation: a randomised controlled study. Lancet 1996; 348(9030):776–80.
50. Church JT, Gadepalli SK, Talishinsky T, et al. Ultrasound-guided intrasphincteric botulinum toxin injection relieves obstructive defecation due to Hirschsprung's disease and internal anal sphincter achalasia. J Pediatr Surg 2017;52(1):74–8.
51. Wester T, Granstrom AL. Botulinum toxin is efficient to treat obstructive symptoms in children with Hirschsprung disease. Pediatr Surg Int 2015;31(3):255–9.
52. Han-Geurts IJ, Hendrix VC, de Blaauw I, et al. Outcome after anal intrasphincteric Botox injection in children with surgically treated Hirschsprung disease. J Pediatr Gastroenterol Nutr 2014;59(5):604–7.
53. Husberg B, Malmborg P, Strigard K. Treatment with botulinum toxin in children with chronic anal fissure. Eur J Pediatr Surg 2009;19(5):290–2.
54. Chumpitazi BP, Fishman SJ, Nurko S. Long-term clinical outcome after botulinum toxin injection in children with nonrelaxing internal anal sphincter. Am J Gastroenterol 2009;104(4):976–83.
55. Irani K, Rodriguez L, Doody DP, et al. Botulinum toxin for the treatment of chronic constipation in children with internal anal sphincter dysfunction. Pediatr Surg Int 2008;24(7):779–83.
56. Keshtgar AS, Ward HC, Sanei A, et al. Botulinum toxin, a new treatment modality for chronic idiopathic constipation in children: long-term follow-up of a double-blind randomized trial. J Pediatr Surg 2007;42(4):672–80.
57. Ahmadi J, Azary S, Ashjaei B, et al. Intrasphincteric botulinum toxin injection in treatment of chronic idiopathic constipation in children. Iran J Pediatr 2013; 23(5):574–8.
58. Siminas S, Losty PD. Current surgical management of pediatric idiopathic constipation: a systematic review of published studies. Ann Surg 2015;262(6):925–33.
59. Kuizenga-Wessel S, Mousa HM, Benninga MA, et al. Lack of agreement on how to use antegrade enemas in children. J Pediatr Gastroenterol Nutr 2016;62(1): 71–9.

60. Randall J, Coyne P, Jaffray B. Follow up of children undergoing antegrade continent enema: experience of over two hundred cases. J Pediatr Surg 2014;49(9): 1405–8.
61. Khoo AK, Askouni E, Basson S, et al. How long will I have my ACE? The natural history of the antegrade continence enema stoma in idiopathic constipation. Pediatr Surg Int 2017;33(11):1159–66.
62. Aspirot A, Fernandez S, Di Lorenzo C, et al. Antegrade enemas for defecation disorders: do they improve the colonic motility? J Pediatr Surg 2009;44(8): 1575–80.
63. Thaha MA, Abukar AA, Thin NN, et al. Sacral nerve stimulation for faecal incontinence and constipation in adults. Cochrane Database Syst Rev 2015;8: CD004464.
64. Humphreys MR, Vandersteen DR, Slezak JM, et al. Preliminary results of sacral neuromodulation in 23 children. J Urol 2006;176(5):2227–31.
65. Roth TJ, Vandersteen DR, Hollatz P, et al. Sacral neuromodulation for the dysfunctional elimination syndrome: a single center experience with 20 children. J Urol 2008;180(1):306–11 [discussion: 311].
66. Haddad M, Besson R, Aubert D, et al. Sacral neuromodulation in children with urinary and fecal incontinence: a multicenter, open label, randomized, crossover study. J Urol 2010;184(2):696–701.
67. van der Wilt AA, van Wunnik BP, Sturkenboom R, et al. Sacral neuromodulation in children and adolescents with chronic constipation refractory to conservative treatment. Int J Colorectal Dis 2016;31(8):1459–66.
68. Lu PL, Koppen IJN, Orsagh-Yentis DK, et al. Sacral nerve stimulation for constipation and fecal incontinence in children: long-term outcomes, patient benefit, and parent satisfaction. Neurogastroenterol Motil 2018;30(2):1–7.
69. Lu PL, Asti L, Lodwick DL, et al. Sacral nerve stimulation allows for decreased antegrade continence enema use in children with severe constipation. J Pediatr Surg 2017;52(4):558–62.
70. Vriesman MH, Lu PL, Diefenbach KA, et al. Sacral nerve stimulation or antegrade continence enema treatment for children with intractable constipation and fecal incontinence. J Pediatr Gastroenterol Nutr 2017;65(Supplement 2):S30–1.
71. Dinning PG, Hunt L, Patton V, et al. Treatment efficacy of sacral nerve stimulation in slow transit constipation: a two-phase, double-blind randomized controlled crossover study. Am J Gastroenterol 2015;110(5):733–40.
72. Zerbib F, Siproudhis L, Lehur PA, et al. Randomized clinical trial of sacral nerve stimulation for refractory constipation. Br J Surg 2017;104(3):205–13.
73. Dwyer ME, Vandersteen DR, Hollatz P, et al. Sacral neuromodulation for the dysfunctional elimination syndrome: a 10-year single-center experience with 105 consecutive children. Urology 2014;84(4):911–7.
74. Fuchs ME, Lu PL, Vyrostek SJ, et al. Factors predicting complications after sacral neuromodulation in children. Urology 2017;107:214–7.
75. Chase J, Robertson VJ, Southwell B, et al. Pilot study using transcutaneous electrical stimulation (interferential current) to treat chronic treatment-resistant constipation and soiling in children. J Gastroenterol Hepatol 2005;20(7):1054–61.
76. Clarke MC, Catto-Smith AG, King SK, et al. Transabdominal electrical stimulation increases colonic propagating pressure waves in paediatric slow transit constipation. J Pediatr Surg 2012;47(12):2279–84.
77. Ng RT, Lee WS, Ang HL, et al. Transcutaneous electrical stimulation (TES) for treatment of constipation in children. Cochrane Database Syst Rev 2016;(7):CD010873.

78. Yik YI, Stathopoulos L, Hutson JM, et al. Home transcutaneous electrical stimulation therapy to treat children with anorectal retention: a pilot study. Neuromodulation 2016;19(5):515–21.

79. Gasior A, Brisighelli G, Diefenbach K, et al. Surgical management of functional constipation: preliminary report of a new approach using a laparoscopic sigmoid resection combined with a Malone appendicostomy. Eur J Pediatr Surg 2017; 27(4):336–40.

Integration of Biomedical and Psychosocial Treatments in Pediatrics Functional Gastrointestinal Disorders

Miranda A.L. van Tilburg, PhD[a,b,c,*],
Charles A. Carter, BS, PharmD, MBA[a]

KEYWORDS

- Functional gastrointestinal disorders • Pediatrics • Irritable bowel syndrome
- Functional abdominal pain • Functional constipation • Biopsychosocial model
- Psychological treatments • Cognitive behavioral treatment

KEY POINTS

- Pediatric functional gastrointestinal disorders (FGIDs) are common childhood disorders.
- Treatment goals are centered around reduction of symptoms and disability, rather than finding a cure.
- Some evidence is available for the efficacy of various biomedical, nutritional and psychological approaches.
- Given the biopsychosocial nature of FGIDs integrative treatments are likely beneficial to a large number of patients.
- Integrative treatment approaches require collaboration of clinicians across disciplines and organizations, and tips are discussed on their implementation.

INTRODUCTION

Functional gastrointestinal disorders (FGIDs) are common childhood disorders affecting approximately 1 in 4 children.[1–3] They are associated with increased disability, such as school absences, decreased quality of life, and increased health care utilization.[1,3,4] The most common and most studied FGIDs are functional

Disclosure Statement: Authors have nothing to disclose.
[a] Department of Clinical Research, College of Pharmacy & Health Sciences, Campbell University, PO Box 1090, 180 Main Street, Buies Creek, NC 27506, USA; [b] Department of Medicine, Division of Gastroenterology and Hepatology, University of North Carolina, 130 Mason Farm road, Chapel Hill, NC 27599, USA; [c] Behavioral Medicine Research Group, School of Social Work, University of Washington, 4101 15th Avenue NE, Seattle, WA 98105, USA
* Corresponding author. Campbell University, PO Box 1090, 180 Main Street, Buies Creek, NC 27506.
E-mail address: vantilburg@campbell.edu

Gastroenterol Clin N Am 47 (2018) 863–875
https://doi.org/10.1016/j.gtc.2018.07.010
0889-8553/18/© 2018 Elsevier Inc. All rights reserved.

Abbreviations	
CBT	Cognitive behavioral therapy
FAPD	Functional abdominal pain disorders
FC	Functional constipation
FGID	Functional gastrointestinal disorders
FODMAP	Fermentable oligosaccharides, disaccharides, monosaccharides and polyols
IBS	Irritable bowel syndrome
PEG	Polyethylene glycol

constipation and functional abdominal pain disorders (FAPDs), such as irritable bowel syndrome (IBS).[1,3,4] As little is known about less common disorders, most of the information presented in this article comes from studies on functional constipation (FC) and FAPD.

FGIDs are disorders of the brain-gut axis. Complex pathophysiology is involved, including alterations in gut motility, microbiota, immune system, and central nervous system involvement.[5,6] Besides these biomedical aspects, psychosocial factors have long been recognized as important in the etiology, maintenance, and disability of FGIDs.[7] The brain-gut axis is explained in more detail in the article by Julie Khlevner and colleagues, "Brain-gut Axis—Clinical Implications," elsewhere in this issue. The exact pathophysiological factors involved in FGIDs vary by disorder but also by patient. Many patients are in need of integrative treatment approaches that may include a combination of biomedical, nutritional, and psychological approaches. In this article, we examine goals of treatment, give a brief overview of biomedical, nutritional, and psychological approaches, and finally discuss the integrative management of pediatric FGIDs.

GOALS OF TREATMENT/MANAGEMENT

Before deciding on a treatment plan, goals of treatment have to be clear for the physician, the patient, and the patient's family. For some diseases, the primary goal of treatment may be clear, such as reducing blood sugar in diabetic patients; however, this is not the case for FGIDs, given that these are complex disorders with varying symptom presentation and pathophysiology. Furthermore, these are usually chronic disorders and a complete remission of symptoms may not always be achievable.

Although our understanding of the pathophysiology of FGIDs has been growing, we are still lacking treatments to address many of these factors. For example, approximately two-thirds of patients with FAPD have visceral hypersensitivity,[8] and this has consistently been found to be associated with pain.[9] Numerous studies have shown that visceral hypersensitivity is mainly driven by central nervous system processes (the brain) rather than peripheral nerve dysregulation (the gut). Despite being one of the most common pathophysiological factors of FAPDs, there are currently no validated tests or efficacious treatments to reduce visceral hypersensitivity. Hence, not only are we limited in finding the correct pathophysiological factor to address, we have no access to treatments for these underlying pathophysiological factors.

Furthermore, many different FGIDs may have overlapping symptoms. For example, FC and IBS may both be characterized by pain and infrequent bowel movements. Despite similar symptoms, pathophysiology and, hence, treatments vary. FC, for example, is often caused by stool retention out of fear of painful or stressful bowel movements. Hence, stool softening reduces pain with defecation and subsequent stool retention. For IBS, pain may be the hallmark of the symptoms, but giving laxatives to soften stool, by definition, will not alleviate all pain. The picture becomes more complex when trying to address overlapping symptoms of FGIDs for which information from rigorous studies are largely lacking. One such symptom is nausea, which can afflict patients with multiple FGIDs, such as IBS, functional nausea, and FC. In this situation, it is not clear if nausea is caused by a similar mechanism for each FGID or what would be an effective course of treatment. Even if a pathophysiological factor can be directly treated, FGIDs are multifactorial disorders, and reducing one factor often does not result in significant symptomatic changes. Treatment should therefore always address multiple pathophysiological factors.

To complicate setting treatment goals, FGIDs are bothersome but not associated with increased morbidity or mortality. Many patients are able to fold the symptoms into their lives and not in need of physician guidance or treatment. Hence, affecting the pathophysiological underpinnings of symptoms is not needed as long as the patient leads a happy and full life with minor disruptions. However, FGIDs are known to cause extensive disability and reductions in quality of life for many patients. The latter may become the most hampering and "damaging" part of living with an FGID. Hence, treatment goals should not only be focused on symptom reduction but also on reducing the impact of the symptoms on a child's life and the child's family's life.

Patients and physicians also do not always agree on what the treatment goals should be. Many patients and their families are focused on finding a cause and cure for the child's symptoms and will reject the diagnosis of an FGID. These families often get second, third, or fourth medical opinions and the children are subjected to multiple medical tests. The value of medical testing in FGIDs is limited[10] and seldom yields results that will change the diagnosis. Furthermore, negative testing does not reassure the family. Rather it communicates that the real cause is elusive and more testing is needed.[11] Physicians therefore need to educate and reassure families before a discussion of appropriate treatment goals can begin. It is important to realize that many patients and their families have been frustrated with previous physicians who suggested the child's symptoms are all "in his/her head" and may not easily trust the physician.

Thus, treatment goals of FGIDs should focus on symptom reduction as well as reducing the impact of the symptoms on a child's life. What works for an individual patient may not be clear at the start of treatment and is often determined by trial and error. Families need to feel supported by the physician during this time. To regain trust and establish an effective doctor-patient relationship, a physician should remain available and involved during treatment, even when the patient is referred to an outside clinician, such as a psychologist. For this to work, families need to "buy in" to the treatment goals and plans. If this important work is not done, both physicians and families can become frustrated. Families will continue to request frequently for help and more testing, as they continue to focus on finding a cure rather than reducing the impact of the symptoms. It is important to reassure and educate families that an FGID diagnosis is a positive diagnosis (not one based on exclusion), has a known pathophysiological origin (brain-gut axis), and that many treatments exist that can help to reduce the (impact) of symptoms. It may also reassure families that many patients improve with time, and as many as 60% to 70% of patients may be without FGID within a year, although relapse is common.[12,13] Given that recovery is possible, a focus on supporting the child while the child is symptomatic, rather than finding a cure, may be more acceptable to parents.

BIOMEDICAL AND NUTRITIONAL THERAPY FOR FUNCTIONAL GASTROINTESTINAL DISORDERS

Hampered by lack of good clinical trials, there is no evidence to suggest dietary or pharmacologic treatments are efficacious for FAPD. However, this is mostly due to a lack of randomized controlled trials. For example, the FODMAP diet (discussed later in this article) has been found to be efficacious in adults with IBS but there is only one small trial in children.[14] At the same time, when appropriately used, most possess a low risk to produce harm to the child and use on a short-term basis is reasonable. Under this pretense, biomedical and nutritional treatments in children for FAPDs may be considered as adjunctive therapies to be combined with psychosocial strategies.

Probiotics

Although it is unclear how probiotics provide a beneficial effect in the management of abdominal pain, it is theorized they may restore the microbial balance in the gut through metabolic competition with pathogens, by augmenting the intestinal mucosal barrier, or by altering the intestinal inflammatory response.[15] Probiotics can be helpful in the management of abdominal pain in children regardless of the underlying mechanism of action and even with limited clinical evidence of substantial beneficial effect.

A recent Cochrane Systematic Review[16] on dietary interventions for FGIDs evaluated the evidence for efficacy of several probiotics, including *Lactobacillus rhamnosus GG*, *Lactobacillus reuteri*, *Bacillus coagulans*, *Lactobacillus plantarum* (LP299V), VSL#3 (combination probiotic), and *Bifidobacterium* species. The analyses produced a low to moderate quality level of evidence that probiotics are efficacious in reducing pain in children with FAPD. Nevertheless, probiotics generally do not produce significant adverse events. Considering the broad variety of probiotics available today, the selection of probiotic should be based on weighing potential benefits with costs and child preferences. A meta-analysis of 6 studies found evidence that *Lactobacillus rhamnosus GG* is efficacious for reducing abdominal pain in children with FAPD[17] and hence may be a good strain to consider.

Soluble Fiber Products

Soluble fiber products are typically derived from psyllium seed husk, also known as psyllium hydrophilic mucilloid, psyllium hydrocolloid, and psyllium seed gum. Soluble fiber-based products are not digested by the body and are useful as laxatives for the management of constipation in both children and adults. They absorb liquids from the intestines and swell to form a soft, bulky stool that stimulates the bowel, leading to defecation. For children with FAPDs, the use of soluble fiber may be useful when used with general management strategies. The exact mechanism by which fiber mitigates abdominal pain is not well understood, but may include modification of intestinal microbiota, altered composition of stool and gas, and/or accelerated gastrointestinal transit.[18,19] Benefits of soluble fiber supplementation should be weighed against the potential risk of increased bloating and pain that develops in some children. The ability of the child to swallow adequately should be a consideration when using powder forms of soluble fiber products because they swell and may cause choking. Taste, flavor, and sugar content of the various available products also should be considered. For children 6 to 12 years of age, soluble fiber products can be used 1 to 3 times a day for constipation, but the optimal dose and treatment duration for abdominal pain is unknown.

Peppermint Oil

Peppermint oil capsules are readily available without a prescription. Peppermint oil is thought to decrease smooth muscle spasms in the gastrointestinal tract,[20] and although the evidence is limited, has received some support as being helpful in the management of abdominal pain in children with FAPD.[21,22] Side effects are generally not reported.[23] It should be pointed out, that although generally well tolerated, peppermint oil may cause an exacerbation of gastroesophageal reflux, but despite early animal studies, there is no evidence it is related to renal damage or liver failure in humans.[24,25]

Other Antispasmodics

Antispasmodics are a broad class of medications that act on the neurotransmitter acetylcholine. Examples of antispasmodics include hyoscyamine and dicyclomine. They are clinically used for a variety of gastrointestinal conditions including IBS in adults. In childhood FAPD, there have been only a few studies reported and they generally demonstrated suboptimal results.[20] In addition, the use of antispasmodics in children poses the risk of anticholinergic adverse events, including dry mouth, blurred vision, decreased sweating, headache, dizziness, weakness, sleep problems, nausea, vomiting, constipation, and bloating. Before recommending the use of antispasmodics in children for FAPD, additional studies of safety and efficacy are necessary.

Cyproheptadine

Cyproheptadine is an interesting medication with both antihistaminic and antiserotonergic properties. Approved for use in a variety of allergic conditions, it has been studied in a variety of other conditions, including appetite stimulation, cyclic vomiting syndrome, dyspeptic syndrome, and migraine prophylaxis. Two studies performed retrospectively examined cyproheptadine for either pediatric FAPD or management of refractory upper gastrointestinal symptoms and found cyproheptadine promising.[26,27] Nevertheless, these results should be confirmed with well-designed prospective trials before recommending cyproheptadine for managing pediatric FAPD.

Other Dietary Approaches

Perceived food intolerances are frequent in patients with FAPDs with common culprits being lactose and gluten. There is no evidence that dietary intolerances such as lactose intolerance and gluten sensitivities are increased in these children or that exclusion diets are helpful, although the data are limited.[16,28]

In adults with IBS, there is convincing evidence of the role of fermentable carbohydrate intolerances.[16] FODMAPs (short for fermentable oligosaccharides, disaccharides, monosaccharides, and polyols) are poorly absorbed in the small intestine and produce gas that may cause symptoms of bloating, which is one of the hallmark symptoms of IBS. A low-FODMAP diet has been found helpful in adults with IBS but limited evidence is available in children and adolescents.[16] In a double-blind crossover trial, children reported fewer symptoms during 48 hours on a low-FODMAP diet compared with 48 hours on a typical American diet.[14] Some evidence exists for 2 of the FODMAPs: fructose and fructans. Increased fructose malabsorption has been described in children with FAPDs, but under double-blind challenges, symptoms often cannot be replicated.[28] In 2 randomized trials, fructose/fructan restriction was helpful for children with FAPDs independent of fructose malabsorption or gas production.[29,30] This may suggest that children with FAPDs may not malabsorb fructose, but are more likely to perceive gas production caused by fructose as painful (ie, visceral hypersensitivity). A recent double-blind crossover trial suggested that fructans also are capable of exacerbating abdominal pain in some children with IBS.[30] At this moment, there is insufficient evidence to suggest a low-FODMAP or fructose/fructan restricted diet in children with FAPD. These diets exclude many child favorite and healthy food choices, such as fruits and vegetables, which may affect a growing child. They should be only initiated under strict dietitian guidance to monitor for dietary insufficiencies and child rejection of the diet.

BIOMEDICAL AND NUTRITIONAL APPROACHES FOR FUNCTIONAL CONSTIPATION

Typically, treatment of FC requires the limited use of biomedical products in conjunction with behavior changes and dietary modifications. The approach to management should consider the child's clinical presentation, severity of constipation, age, and developmental stage. Deliberately engaging the parents and child in educational activities pertaining to FC is important to support successful outcomes. The goals of intervention include the ability of the child to begin to pass soft stools on a regular frequency. In addition, careful attention to preventing, or treating, fecal impaction is important. It is worthwhile to note that guidelines for management of FC in children are available from the North American Society for Pediatric Gastroenterology, Hepatology, and Nutrition, and the European Society for Pediatric Gastroenterology, Hepatology and Nutrition.[31] Clinicians should consult with these guidelines, and any potential updates. See the article by Peter L. Lu and Hayat M. Mousa, "Constipation: Beyond the Old Paradigms,"elsewhere in this issue, for further information.

Laxatives

The use of laxatives has been a traditional approach to treat FC for several decades. There are varieties of laxatives available that can be used in children by either oral or rectal administration. Oral medications are preferred in the United States because they are noninvasive and less emotionally compromising to the child, but rectal laxatives may be acceptable to children and parents in other cultures. In a child with severe impactions, the use of rectally administered laxatives is a real consideration based on their more rapid effect. Typical enemas for children contain sodium phosphate, mineral oil, or saline. After achieving disimpaction, a maintenance regimen combining oral laxatives, behavior changes, and dietary modification should be implemented to avoid another episode of impaction.

From the osmotic laxatives, polyethylene glycol or PEG is best supported by clinical experience and controlled trials.[31,32] Products containing PEG with or without electrolytes (eg, Miralax and GoLYTELY) have been shown efficacious in clinical studies of children.[33] These products are preferred and generally well tolerated when dosed properly. The advantage of PEG for use in children is its complete lack of taste and ability to be dissolved in a favorite drink.

Mineral oil has also been used in children. However, there is a higher risk of gastroesophageal reflux that can lead to dangerous pneumonitis because of it being an oil-based product. Other oral laxatives, such as magnesium citrate, sorbitol, senna, and bisacodyl, are also effective, but lack the evidence from controlled trials in children seen with the PEG products.

Fiber

Fiber supplements have been used in children with constipation in the presence of weak and conflicting data to support it.[31,34] In children particularly, fiber can have both a beneficial and an adverse impact. Although fiber is intended to add bulk and water content to the stool and make defecation easier, the bulkier stool may cause greater distension of the rectum and colon and fecal retention. This can potentially interfere with the child's ability to sense the need to defecate. In addition, maintaining adequate fluid intake to avoid the future impactions can be challenging in a child. One should seriously consider obviating the need for fiber supplements by dietary modifications. A balanced diet containing whole grains, fruits, and vegetables should be ample to provide adequate fiber and a necessary aspect of the treatment plan of FC in children.

Probiotics

Probiotic use for the treatment of constipation is based on data demonstrating differences in the intestinal microbiota between healthy individuals and patients with chronic constipation.[35] However, there are few well-controlled clinical studies with conflicting results. Nevertheless, there is a tremendous amount of research ongoing to understand the microbiota and the potential therapeutic use of probiotics. However, at the current time, systematic reviews and established guidelines conclude the evidence is insufficient to support the use of probiotics for FC in children.

PSYCHOSOCIAL APPROACHES

Given that FGIDs are brain-gut axis disorders, the value of psychological treatments for these disorders has long been recognized. Most of the evidence for psychological treatment comes from studies in FAPDs and FC and each is discussed in the following sections. Other therapies, such as yoga, deep breathing, and expressive writing, have been tested in small studies, but little evidence is available for their effectiveness and hence these are not discussed here.

Psychosocial Approaches for Functional Constipation

Most children develop FC because of stool withholding due to fear of having a painful or stressful bowel movement.[5] Hence, FC is primarily a behavioral disorder. It is common medical practice to prescribe laxatives in combination with behavioral techniques, such as toilet sitting after meals, to encourage defecation. In addition, parents often have misconceptions about the causes of their child's constipation (eg, child is being recalcitrant), and addressing these helps in improving the parents' appropriate management of their child's symptoms.[36] These techniques can be applied in the office by the treating physician and do not require a referral for psychological treatment. In fact, there is no evidence to suggest that additional treatment is beneficial, although Enhanced Toilet Training may benefit children with fecal incontinence.[37] Enhanced Toilet Training focuses on educating parents and children, increasing parent-child collaboration around symptoms, reducing fear of bowel movements, and teaching defecation skills.

A subgroup of children with FC may have difficulty passing stool because they suffer from dyssynergia.[38] Children with dyssynergic defecation have problems with coordinating their abdominal and pelvic floor muscles to evacuate stools. Defecation requires a coordinated contraction and relaxation of pelvic, rectal, anal, and abdominal muscles. In dyssynergic defecation, children may fail to notice the urge to defecate due to a hyposensitive rectum and/or the anal muscles may paradoxically contract, or fail to relax, which prevents evacuation. The appropriate coordination of the muscles can be taught through biofeedback. In anorectal biofeedback, intra-anal sensors are placed to measure sphincter pressures and muscular activity. Visual or auditory feedback is provided to the patient, who is then asked to change his or her muscle activity. The focus is on strengthening muscles as well as learning appropriate muscle coordination. Although biofeedback improves defecation dynamics, there is little evidence of long-term effects in children with constipation.[38] Therefore, it is currently not recommended for routine treatment but may be helpful for some children with chronic refractory symptoms.

Psychosocial Approaches for Functional Abdominal Pain Disorders

Psychological therapies for FAPDs can be focused on reducing pain itself or on reducing disability associated with pain. Several trials have suggested the benefits of psychological treatments, including cognitive behavioral therapy (CBT) and hypnosis,[39] for both outcomes. Many physicians suggest the use of psychological therapy as a way to reduce anxiety or stress in children with FAPDs. However, there is little evidence that the effects of psychological therapies work through the reduction of anxiety or stress.[37] Rather, most therapy focuses on improving maladaptive thoughts and coping with symptoms in order to reduce symptoms and impact of FAPDs.

Cognitive behavioral therapy for functional abdominal pain disorders

CBT combines cognitive (how do you think about your pain) and behavioral (how do you cope with your pain) techniques to improve the child's experience of and functioning while in pain. For example, many patients with pain confuse hurt with harm and patients are taught how to recognize and replace these maladaptive cognitions with more helpful ones. Behavioral techniques may include new ways to act when in pain (eg, going to school in a school avoidant child) and often include relaxation techniques, such as deep breathing, to cope with the discomfort these new ways of thinking and behaving may bring. In children, it is best practice to include both the parent and child in therapy. Parents are taught how their own thinking, emotions, and behaviors influence their child and are taught appropriate responses to their child's pain. There is good evidence that CBT is efficacious in reducing both pain and disability in FAPD.[37] In one study, the effect of CBT on gastrointestinal symptoms was explained by reductions in child pain catastrophizing (expecting the worst and feeling unable to do anything about it) and reductions in parent assessment of pain threat.[40]

A new type of CBT is exposure therapy. Children with FAPDs often fear gastrointestinal symptoms and avoid situations in which they may occur. In exposure therapy, children are guided in cognitive restructuring and relaxation to be able to tolerate gut sensations in a stepwise provocation of symptoms (eg, by eating symptom-inducing foods). There is evidence from one study that compared it with wait-list control that this type of therapy reduces gastrointestinal symptoms and increases quality of life in teens with FAPD.[41] Further studies are needed, but the initial results look promising.

Hypnosis and functional abdominal pain disorders

Hypnosis, also called guided imagery in some studies, has been used for controlling pain for hundreds of years. Only a few studies have tested the efficacy of hypnosis in treating FAPD, but the results in general show larger effect sizes than for CBT.[42] Hypnosis in particular has good evidence it can reduce pain intensity and frequency.[39] One study has shown long-term effects of hypnosis: after 5 years, 68% of children were in remission versus only 20% in the control group.[43] The mechanism by which hypnosis reduces pain is unclear. One study did not find hypnosis affected rectal visceral hypersensitivity in children with FAPD.[44] The effect may be through brain activation alteration from hypnosis. Studies have shown that modulation of pain during hypnosis is associated with activation of the left frontal, right cingulate, and right insular cortices, which are part of the brain "pain matrix," as well as deactivations in the thalamus, which could indicate a top-down inhibition of pain signals in the brain.[45] This suggests hypnosis may directly affect brain dysregulation in FAPD.

INTEGRATION OF BIOMEDICAL AND PSYCHOSOCIAL APPROACHES

Given the biopsychosocial nature of FGIDs, a treatment approach in which psychological, dietary, and medical approaches are integrated is often recommended.[5,46]

Although data in FGIDs are largely lacking, integrated treatment in general has been associated with improved outcomes, such as better access to treatments, increased patient satisfaction with treatment, and reduced health care costs.[46] In integrated care, psychologists, dietitians, medical doctors, and other clinicians as applicable, should ideally treat the patient holistically. All clinicians will work together on a comprehensive treatment plan and the patient will see each provider in a joint consultation to emphasize the unity of the approach. In the patient's eye, there is no distinction between the individual providers; they act as a team to address his or her biopsychosocial needs.

Although it is recognized that team approaches to care are ideal, often site-specific limitations reduce the feasibility of on-site integrated treatment teams. Medical facilities may not have access to an on-site psychologist or dietitian, or cannot coordinate visits between these providers. In addition, patients may lack insurance coverage for these services or live too far away from the medical center to make the regular visits that these treatments require. In most of these situations, integrated care can still be established, even if not all clinicians can be physically present at the same time and place. This will make it more challenging for the patient to participate in treatment, but in essence, the most important part of integrative care is the team-based approach and treatment plan.

It is important to realize that integrated treatment starts in the physician office. For most patients with FGIDs, the physician can provide education, reassurance, and easily implementable dietary or psychosocial approaches. The Rome IV committee developed a detailed psychosocial assessment plan that can be used to determine what kind of psychological care to offer to patients with FGIDs.[47] The physician should assess the role of psychosocial factors such as stress and psychiatric comorbidity and the impact of symptoms on a child's life to determine which level of care is needed. Level 1 care can be delivered in the physician office and consists of reassurance, education, and providing simple lifestyle or dietary changes. If level 1 does not provide relief, prescribing low doses of centrally acting drugs, such as antidepressants, should be considered (level 2) before a referral to a psychologist is made (level 3). Integrated treatment approaches are recommended by the Rome IV committee only for the most psychosocially affected patients. Although these guidelines were developed with both adults and children in mind, they are mostly geared toward the adult care model in which care is generally more separated by disciplines and integrative care is usually found only in specialized pain centers. In contrast, team-based approaches are common in pediatrics for various chronic diseases. Therefore, we would argue that integrated care could be offered earlier to children and teens (level 2). Even at lower levels of psychosocial distress and impact, children and their families can benefit from integrated care approaches. In addition, the prescription of centrally acting agents probably should be preserved for treatment-resistant pediatric patients, especially given black-box warnings for antidepressants in teens. A similar tiered model could be envisioned for nutritional care.

If involvement of providers with different expertise is desired, the optimal approach would be to integrate psychologists and dietitians in medical practices and schedule joint visits. If this is impractical or impossible, independent visits can be scheduled with joint planning of treatment goals and plans. Ideally, psychologists and dietitians should be in the same medical practice as the physicians, as this reduces stigma and barriers to access, and communicates the team approach. If this is impossible, physicians can work with community providers. In that case, it is important to set up times to communicate often with each provider to make sure treatment goals align and the provider understands FGIDs. Most dietitians and psychologists are not trained to treat this patient population. A simple referral may result in treatment for general problems (eg, anxiety or increase of vegetable and fruit intake), which generally are not efficacious for FGIDs. Furthermore, the provider needs to know when to refer back to the physician, such as when red flag symptoms are presented during therapy. In addition, referral to a psychologist or dietitian without follow-up and continued availability of the physician may communicate to patients that the physician does not believe their symptoms and is trying to get rid of them. For this reason, many patients will not follow-up on the referral. Therefore, the physician should always remain available and part of the treatment team.

Whether psychologists or dietitians are part of the medical team or work in private practice outside of the medical center where the physicians resides, working out some practical challenges will increase the likelihood for the integrative care model to be successful. First, a shared understanding of FGIDs and their assessment and treatment needs to be developed. For this to work, each clinician should be open to learn from each other and perhaps aid teaching as well as participating in professional workshops to learn about specific treatments, such as the FODMAP diet or hypnosis. Second, physicians should partner with dietitians and psychologists to develop a workable practice model that includes communications between each other, communications with the patient and the patient's family, as well as addressing potential billing challenges.

No matter the lofty goals, many well-intended attempts at integrative care stand in the unavailability of well-trained providers who can either be hired or who are willing to collaborate. In many communities, there is no access to psychologists or dietitians, and this complicates a biopsychosocial approach to treatment. E-treatments are being developed and tested, such as Internet-delivered CBT, Web-based FODMAP diet, as well as audio-recorded hypnosis.[41,48,49] Unfortunately, these are not currently available outside of research studies, but it is the hope they will become available in the near future. Of note, these e-treatments are likely somewhat less effective than in-person treatments, but they may increase access to these treatments to many more patients and create more availability of psychologists and dietitians who can focus on more complicated cases in need of individualized treatment.

In summary, the nature of FGIDs requires a focus on integrative care. Often this care can be provided by the physician through education, reassurance, and providing simple tools. However, the need of many patients requires that psychological and dietary therapies are integrated into traditionally medically oriented care and this is challenging. However, increasingly centers are making it work and find that a coordinated approach improves outcomes and saves costs.

REFERENCES

1. Lewis ML, Palsson OS, Whitehead WE, et al. Prevalence of functional gastrointestinal disorders in children and adolescents. J Pediatr 2016;177:39–43.e3.
2. van Tilburg MA, Levy RL, Walker LS, et al. Psychosocial mechanisms for the transmission of somatic symptoms from parents to children. World J Gastroenterol 2015;21:5532–41.
3. Robin SG, Keller C, Zwiener R, et al. Prevalence of pediatric functional gastrointestinal disorders according to the Rome IV criteria. J Pediatr 2018;195:134–9.
4. van Tilburg MA, Hyman PE, Walker L, et al. Prevalence of functional gastrointestinal disorders in infants and toddlers. J Pediatr 2015;166:684–9.
5. Hyams JS, Di Lorenzo C, Saps M, et al. Childhood Functional Gastrointestinal Disorders: Child/Adolescent. Gastroenterology 2016;150(6):1456–68.

6. Benninga MA, Faure C, Hyman PE, et al. Childhood functional gastrointestinal disorders: neonate/toddler. Gastroenterology 2016. [Epub ahead of print].
7. Van Oudenhove L, Crowell MD, Drossman DA, et al. Biopsychosocial aspects of functional gastrointestinal disorders. Gastroenterology 2016. [Epub ahead of print].
8. van Tilburg MAL. Integration of biomedical and psychosocial issues in pediatric functional gastrointestinal and motility disorders. In: Faure C, Thapar N, DiLorenzo C, editors. Neurogastroenterology: gastrointestinal motility and functional disorders in children. New York: Springer; 2017. p. 71–80.
9. Simren M, Tornblom H, Palsson OS, et al. Visceral hypersensitivity is associated with GI symptom severity in functional GI disorders: consistent findings from five different patient cohorts. Gut 2018;67(2):255–62.
10. Dhroove G, Chogle A, Saps M. A million-dollar work-up for abdominal pain: is it worth it? J Pediatr Gastroenterol Nutr 2010;51:579–83.
11. van Tilburg MAL, Venepalli NK, Freeman KL, et al. Parents' fears and worries about RAP. Gastroenterology 2003;124:A–528.
12. Walker LS, gler-Crish CM, Rippel S, et al. Functional abdominal pain in childhood and adolescence increases risk for chronic pain in adulthood. Pain 2010;150: 568–72.
13. de Lorijn F, van Wijk MP, Reitsma JB, et al. Prognosis of constipation: clinical factors and colonic transit time. Arch Dis Child 2004;89:723–7.
14. Chumpitazi BP, Cope JL, Hollister EB, et al. Randomised clinical trial: gut microbiome biomarkers are associated with clinical response to a low FODMAP diet in children with the irritable bowel syndrome. Aliment Pharmacol Ther 2015;42: 418–27.
15. Quigley EM. Probiotics in functional gastrointestinal disorders: what are the facts? Curr Opin Pharmacol 2008;8:704–8.
16. Newlove-Delgado TV, Martin AE, Abbott RA, et al. Dietary interventions for recurrent abdominal pain in childhood. Cochrane Database Syst Rev 2017;(3):CD010972.
17. Horvath A, Dziechciarz P, Szajewska H. Meta-analysis: *Lactobacillus rhamnosus GG* for abdominal pain–related functional gastrointestinal disorders in childhood. Aliment Pharmacol Ther 2011;33(12):1302–10.
18. Horvath A, Dziechciarz P, Szajewska H. Systematic review of randomized controlled trials: fiber supplements for abdominal pain-related functional gastrointestinal disorders in childhood. Ann Nutr Metab 2012;61:95–101.
19. Shulman RJ, Hollister EB, Cain K, et al. Psyllium fiber reduces abdominal pain in children with irritable bowel syndrome in a randomized, double-blind trial. Clin Gastroenterol Hepatol 2017;15(5):712–9.
20. Chiou E, Nurko S. Functional abdominal pain and irritable bowel syndrome in children and adolescents. Therapy 2011;8:315–31.
21. Ruepert L, Quartero AO, de Wit NJ, et al. Bulking agents, antispasmodics and antidepressants for the treatment of irritable bowel syndrome. Cochrane Database Syst Rev 2011;(8):CD003460.
22. Anheyer D, Frawley J, Koch AK, et al. Herbal medicines for gastrointestinal disorders in children and adolescents: a systematic review. Pediatrics 2017;139 [pii: e20170062].
23. Asgarshirazi M, Shariat M, Dalili H. Comparison of the effects of pH-dependent peppermint oil and synbiotic lactol (*Bacillus coagulans* + Fructooligosaccharides) on childhood functional abdominal pain: a randomized placebo-controlled study. Iran Red Crescent Med J 2015;17:e23844.

24. Charrois TL, Hrudey J, Gardiner P, et al. Peppermint oil. Pediatr Rev 2006;27: e49–51.
25. Chumpitazi BP, Kearns GL, Shulman RJ. Review article: the physiological effects and safety of peppermint oil and its efficacy in irritable bowel syndrome and other functional disorders. Aliment Pharmacol Ther 2018;47(6):738–52.
26. Madani S, Cortes O, Thomas R. Cyproheptadine use in children with functional gastrointestinal disorders. J Pediatr Gastroenterol Nutr 2016;62:409–13.
27. Rodriguez L, Diaz J, Nurko S. Safety and efficacy of cyproheptadine for treating dyspeptic symptoms in children. J Pediatr 2013;163:261–7.
28. van Tilburg MA, Felix CT. Diet and functional abdominal pain in children and adolescents. J Pediatr Gastroenterol Nutr 2013;57:141–8.
29. Wirth S, Klodt C, Wintermeyer P, et al. Positive or negative fructose breath test results do not predict response to fructose restricted diet in children with recurrent abdominal pain: results from a prospective randomized trial. Klin Padiatr 2014; 226:268–73.
30. Chumpitazi BP, McMeans AR, Vaughan A, et al. Fructans exacerbate symptoms in a subset of children with irritable bowel syndrome. Clin Gastroenterol Hepatol 2018;16(2):219–25.e1.
31. Tabbers MM, DiLorenzo C, Berger MY, et al. Evaluation and treatment of functional constipation in infants and children: evidence-based recommendations from ESPGHAN and NASPGHAN. J Pediatr Gastroenterol Nutr 2014;58:258–74.
32. Gordon M, MacDonald JK, Parker CE, et al. Osmotic and stimulant laxatives for the management of childhood constipation. Cochrane Database Syst Rev 2016;(8):CD009118.
33. Youssef NN, Peters JM, Henderson W, et al. Dose response of PEG 3350 for the treatment of childhood fecal impaction. J Pediatr 2002;141:410–4.
34. Tabbers MM, Boluyt N, Berger MY, et al. Nonpharmacologic treatments for childhood constipation: systematic review. Pediatrics 2011;128:753–61.
35. Zoppi G, Cinquetti M, Luciano A, et al. The intestinal ecosystem in chronic functional constipation. Acta Paediatr 1998;87:836–41.
36. van Tilburg MA, Squires M, Blois-Martin N, et al. Parental knowledge of fecal incontinence in children. J Pediatr Gastroenterol Nutr 2012;55:283–7.
37. van Tilburg MAL. Cognitive behavioral therapy for functional gastrointestinal disorders. In: Faure C, Thapar N, DiLorenzo C, editors. Neurogastroenterology: gastrointestinal motility and functional disorders in children. New York: Springer; 2017. p. 507–13.
38. Rao SS, Benninga MA, Bharucha AE, et al. ANMS-ESNM position paper and consensus guidelines on biofeedback therapy for anorectal disorders. Neurogastroenterol Motil 2015;27:594–609.
39. Abbott RA, Martin AE, Newlove-Delgado TV, et al. Psychosocial interventions for recurrent abdominal pain in childhood. Cochrane Database Syst Rev 2017;(1):CD010971.
40. Levy RL, Langer SL, Romano JM, et al. Cognitive mediators of treatment outcomes in pediatric functional abdominal pain. Clin J Pain 2014;30:1033–43.
41. Bonnert M, Olen O, Lalouni M, et al. Internet-delivered cognitive behavior therapy for adolescents with irritable bowel syndrome: a randomized controlled trial. Am J Gastroenterol 2017;112:152–62.
42. Rutten JM, Korterink JJ, Venmans LM, et al. Nonpharmacologic treatment of functional abdominal pain disorders: a systematic review. Pediatrics 2015;135: 522–35.

43. Vlieger AM, Rutten JM, Govers AM, et al. Long-term follow-up of gut-directed hypnotherapy vs. standard care in children with functional abdominal pain or irritable bowel syndrome. Am J Gastroenterol 2012;107:627–31.

44. Vlieger AM, van den Berg MM, Menko-Frankenhuis C, et al. No change in rectal sensitivity after gut-directed hypnotherapy in children with functional abdominal pain or irritable bowel syndrome. Am.J Gastroenterol 2010;105:213–8.

45. Del Casale A, Ferracuti S, Rapinesi C, et al. Hypnosis and pain perception: An Activation Likelihood Estimation (ALE) meta-analysis of functional neuroimaging studies. J Physiol Paris 2015;109:165–72.

46. Reed-Knight B, Claar RL, Schurman JV, et al. Implementing psychological therapies for functional GI disorders in children and adults. Expert Rev Gastroenterol Hepatol 2016;10:981–4.

47. Levy RL, Crowell MD, Drossman DA. Biopsychosocial aspects of functional gastrointestinal disorders. In: Drossman DA, editor. Rome IV: functional gastrointestinal disorders: disorders of gut-brain interaction, Vol. I. Raleigh (NC): The Rome Foundation; 2016. p. 443–548.

48. Ankersen DV, Carlsen K, Marker D, et al. Using eHealth strategies in delivering dietary and other therapies in patients with irritable bowel syndrome and inflammatory bowel disease. J Gastroenterol Hepatol 2017;32(Suppl 1):27–31.

49. van Tilburg MA, Chitkara DK, Palsson OS, et al. Audio-recorded guided imagery treatment reduces functional abdominal pain in children: a pilot study. Pediatrics 2009;124:e890–7.

Gastrointestinal Neuropathies

New Insights and Emerging Therapies

Marcella Pesce, MD[a,b], Osvaldo Borrelli, MD, PhD[a],
Efstratios Saliakellis, MD, PhD[a],
Nikhil Thapar, BM, MRCP(UK), FRCPCH, PhD[a,c],*

KEYWORDS

- Enteric nervous system • Enteric neuropathies • Gut motility disorders • Stem cell
- Transplantation

KEY POINTS

- Enteric neuropathies represent a heterogeneous and challenging group of gastrointestinal disorders with high long-term morbidity and mortality rates.
- They arise from congenital defects that primarily disrupt enteric nervous system development or acquired disorders that alter its structure/function, although the precise etiopathophysiologic basis remains elusive.
- Currently available therapy is largely limited to palliation of symptoms and/or to provide nutrition for growth and development, with intestinal transplantation remaining the only definitive treatment for the most severe conditions.
- New emerging therapies include newly developed drugs, electrical pacing, manipulation of intestinal microbiota, and gene and neural stem cell therapy.
- These have the potential for ameliorating outcomes or indeed providing cure, but are largely experimental and need to be informed by improved understanding of the target diseases themselves.

Disclosure Statement: N. Thapar has participated as clinical investigator, and/or advisory board member, and/or consultant, and/or speaker for Danone, Nutricia ELN, and Mead Johnson Nutritionals. All other authors have no conflict of interests to declare.
[a] Neurogastroenterology and Motility Unit, Department of Pediatric Gastroenterology, Great Ormond Street Hospital, London WC1N 3JH, UK; [b] Department of Clinical Medicine and Surgery, 'Federico II' University of Naples, Via Pansini 5, Naples 80131, Italy; [c] Stem Cells and Regenerative Medicine, UCL Institute of Child Health, 30 Guilford Street, London WC1N 1EH, UK
* Corresponding author. Stem Cells and Regenerative Medicine, UCL Great Ormond Street Institute of Child Health, 30 Guilford Street, London WC1N 1EH, UK.
E-mail address: n.thapar@ucl.ac.uk

INTRODUCTION: THE ENTERIC NERVOUS SYSTEM AND GASTROINTESTINAL NEUROPATHIES

The critical functions of the gastrointestinal (GI) tract and in turn, the well-being of the individual, are underpinned by the appropriate sensing and propagation of luminal contents along of the length of the GI tract.[1] This intestinal motility function depends on components of the enteric neuromusculature, namely, the effectors of intestinal motility (smooth muscle cells), the regulators of neuronal firing or pacemaker cells (interstitial cells of Cajal [ICCs]) and the neurons of the GI tract's intrinsic nervous system (enteric nervous system [ENS]), which is designed to control intestinal motor function and integrate it with central inputs.[2]

In this intricate scenario, the ENS has been coined the second brain, a term that reflects its ability to function as a largely independent neuronal network with a complexity comparable with that of the central nervous system.[3] Nonetheless, this complexity presents as much of a blessing as a curse, given that it also accounts for the intrinsic vulnerability of the ENS to develop a wide array of motor and sensory disorders, collectively labeled enteric neuropathies.[4] These conditions may arise from congenital defects that primarily disrupt ENS development or, alternatively, by acquired disorders that distort its normal functioning. The resultant conditions, which include esophageal achalasia, gastroparesis, chronic intestinal pseudoobstruction (CIPO), Hirschsprung disease (HSCR), and slow transit constipation (STC), represent an extremely challenging and heterogeneous group of GI disorders. Curative and pathophysiology-oriented therapies are still lacking and available therapeutic options for most of these conditions are indeed limited to palliation of symptoms or to provide nutrition, thus relieving their burden in terms of morbidity and mortality.

For the sake of brevity, we provide a general overview of the contemporary understanding of key intestinal neuropathies and current failings in management before focusing on emerging and novel therapeutic strategies. An extensive review of the pathophysiology and clinical management of intestinal neuropathies is beyond the scope of this article and reference is, therefore, made to more extensive and high-quality reviews on this topic.[5,6] **Table 1** provides an overview of enteric neuropathies and their main proposed pathophysiologic mechanisms.

ENTERIC NEUROPATHIES: A BRIEF OVERVIEW
Esophagus: Esophageal Achalasia

The esophagus can be affected in the context of a number of primary or secondary neuropathies, namely esophageal atresia/trachea–esophageal fistula, Chagas diseases, and esophageal achalasia. Esophageal achalasia is a classic example of an enteric neuropathy and is one of the most common primary motility disorders of the GI tract, characterized by partial/absent relaxation of the lower esophageal sphincter

Table 1
Enteric neuropathies and their main proposed pathophysiologic mechanisms, histopathologic features and current failings in the management

Enteric Neuropathy	Proposed Pathophysiologic Mechanism	Histopathologic Features	Comments	Reference
Esophageal achalasia	Autoimmune-driven inflammation of the myenteric plexus Circulating autoantibodies against myenteric neurons owing to molecular mimicry driven by viral infections	Myenteric ganglionitis with $CD3^+$ and $CD8^+$ T cells infiltrating the myenteric plexus in early stages Depletion of nitrergic neurons with fibrosis of myenteric plexus in end-stage achalasia	Common postoperative GERD-related symptoms and residual dysphagia owing to uncoordinated or absent peristalsis.	7–13
Gastroparesis	Idiopathic (70% of pediatric cases) Secondary (diabetic, postviral, postoperative, mitochondrial disease, drug-related)	Decreased number and/or structural abnormalities in ICCs network Hypoganglionosis and features of neuronal dysplasia	Sudden cardiac arrest and extrapyramidal side effects after therapy with prokinetics	14–18
Chronic (pediatric) intestinal pseudoobstruction	Primary (congenital, familial and sporadic) owing to abnormalities in genes involved in structure and/or function of the neuromusculature. Secondary (metabolic, muscular, neurologic and infectious diseases)	Absent/aberrant protein expression owing to identified genetic mutations (FLNA, ACTG2, TYMP/POLG1) Autoimmune-driven neuropathy with $CD3^+$ T lymphocytes in myenteric and submucosal plexuses Neurotropic virus infections (herpesviruses or polyomaviruses)	Long-term side effects related to parenteral nutrition (line sepsis, end stage liver disease, malnourishment). Palliative measures that do not act on the underlying pathophysiologic mechanisms	19–22

(continued on next page)

Table 1
(continued)

Enteric Neuropathy	Proposed Pathophysiologic Mechanism	Histopathologic Features	Comments	Reference
HSCR	Disruption of rostrocaudal colonization by the ENS precursors during the embryonic development of the GI tract	Defective formation of the ENS with absence of enteric ganglion cells in a variable region of the hindgut	Long-term morbidity with frequent need of reintervention in early childhood and adolescence	23–32
	RET gene (10q11.2) involved in HSCR in ≤50% of familial cases and up to 35% of sporadic ones	Narrowing of the aganglionic segment and distension of the proximal bowel		
Slow transit constipation	Depletion of enteric ganglion cells and ICCs	Abnormal enteric innervation with reduction of enteric ganglion cells and ICCs	Frequently reported tachyphylaxis with stimulant laxatives with loss of efficacy. Significant postoperative complications (dehiscence, infections, failure owing to relapse of constipation).	33–37
	Subtle changes in enteric neurotransmitters or neuropeptides (excessive production of nitric oxide)	Enteric neuronal loss partially attributable to apoptosis		

Abbreviations: ACTG2, actin G2; ENS, enteric nervous system; FLNA, filamin A; GERD, gastroesophageal reflux disease; GI, gastrointestinal; HSCR, Hirschsprung disease; ICCs, interstitial cells of Cajal; POLG1, polymerase gamma; TYMP, thymidine phosphorylase.

upon swallowing and defective esophageal peristalsis. This translates clinically into symptoms of dysphagia and regurgitation of undigested food that limits oral feeding. From a pathophysiologic standpoint, the disorder is characterized by defective inhibitory innervation with a consequent imbalance in the number of excitatory (cholinergic and tachinergic neurons) and inhibitory (nitrergic) neurons of the lower esophageal sphincter and lower esophageal body.[7] The loss of nitrergic neurons seems to be related to the activation of the immune system with the presence of an inflammatory infiltrate into the myenteric plexus and circulating autoantibodies in at least a proportion of patients.[7] Histopathologic examination from early stage achalasia esophageal specimens revealed features of myenteric ganglionitis with CD3[+] and CD8[+] T cells infiltrating the myenteric plexuses. This, in turn, results in the progressive depletion of nitrergic neurons and progressive fibrosis, as observed in patients with end-stage achalasia.[8] It is proposed that the interaction between autoimmune and inflammatory responses that seems to underlie achalasia is possibly triggered by viral infections occurring in genetically susceptible individuals.[9] A number of virus candidates have been proposed (eg, herpes simplex, varicella zoster, measles, human papilloma, and JC virus), with evidence of viral infections preceding the development of achalasia in a significant number of patients.[10] In only a minority of patients with achalasia is a defined genetic mutation implicated (eg, *ALADIN* 12q13 gene in Triple-A syndrome), with more recent studies focusing on a predisposition to autoimmunity and suggesting that variants within the HLA class II loci may play a role, although the association of these with achalasia is not absolute.[10,11] The current therapeutic management of this disorder includes either surgical or endoscopic interventions (botulinum toxin injection, pneumatic dilatation, per-oral endoscopic myotomy, laparoscopic Heller's myotomy) aiming at reducing LES resting pressure. Although some data suggest an improvement in esophageal motor activity after these interventions,[12] the therapeutic aim of these procedures is to primarily improve LES relaxation and thus postoperative dysphagia owing to residual uncoordinated esophageal peristalsis is a common finding in treated children.[13]

Stomach: Gastroparesis

Gastroparesis is the final endpoint of a series of conditions affecting the integrity of the neuromusculature of the stomach, which ultimately results in a significant delay in gastric emptying rates for both liquids and solids.[14] In adults, it is mainly an acquired condition secondary to diabetic neuropathy, whereas in children almost 70% of cases are idiopathic.[15] Although its underlying pathophysiology remains unclear, recent histopathologic data have demonstrated a decreased number and/or structural abnormalities in ICC networks in nearly 40% of patients with idiopathic gastroparesis.[16] Histopathologic examination of patients undergoing total gastrectomy for gastroparesis revealed, however, a more generalized process comprising hypoganglionosis and features of neuronal dysplasia, alongside with ICC abnormalities. Samples from adult patients with gastroparesis (idiopathic and diabetic) have shown significant disruption in nNOS[+] innervation alongside a reduction in the number ICCs.[17] Furthermore, in at least a subset of patients, neurodegenerative changes were associated with florid lymphocytic infiltrates, suggesting a causative role for myenteric ganglionitis in determining these alterations in ICC and neuronal networks.[18]

Available therapeutic strategies involve dietary and nutritional interventions alongside with prokinetic agents, whereas surgical interventions (ie, pyloroplasty or jejunostomy) are reserved for patients who are refractory to medical treatment. However, the most commonly used prokinetic agents must be carefully used in children because of the nonnegligible risk of sudden cardiac arrest and of extrapyramidal side effects.[14]

Small Bowel: Chronic Intestinal Pseudoobstruction

CIPO is a potentially life-threatening disorder clinically characterized by impaired GI motility, escalating to episodes of overt obstruction in the absence of any mechanical lesion accounting for these symptoms.[19] It often presents a challenging condition to diagnose with an erratic clinical presentation, ranging from subtle and nonspecific symptoms to severe and disabling intestinal failure. As a result, in a nonspecialist setting, there is often a delay of several years before a definitive diagnosis is made.[20] Although rare, CIPO represents one of the main causes of chronic intestinal failure, accounting for almost 15% of all pediatric cases.[19]

Rather than being a single clinical entity, the term CIPO embodies a spectrum of conditions, which may variably affect the structure and/or function of the neuromusculature of the GI tract. In childhood, it is more likely to be primary, congenital (>80% of cases presenting at <1 year of age) and sporadic, although familial cases have been described. In a small proportion of children, the disease is secondary to other systemic conditions (including metabolic, muscular, neurologic, and infectious diseases) or alternatively seems to be related to immune-mediated disruption of the ENS[21] or neurotrophic viruses.[22] Given the different pathogenetic background in adult and pediatric settings, a recent position and expert consensus paper from the European Society for Pediatric Gastroenterology, Hepatology, and Nutrition proposes to introduce the term pediatric intestinal pseudoobstructive (PIPO) disorders to emphasize the differences from adult-onset CIPO.[20] The as yet poorly characterized pathophysiology of PIPO no doubt accounts for the lack of targeted or curative treatments for the disorder and, in turn, the significant levels of both morbidity and mortality. Indeed, most of the available treatments are aimed at supporting nutrition (through parenteral and, when suitable, enteral nutrition) and at palliating symptoms (prokinetics, antibiotics for bacterial overgrowth, and nonopioid analgesics) with a substantially poor long-term outcome for the disease.[20]

Large Bowel: Hirschsprung Disease and Slow Transit Constipation

Hirschsprung disease

HSCR is the ultimate paradigmatic model of an enteric neuropathy, being one of the most frequently and effectively diagnosed, as well as best-characterized congenital neuropathies predominantly affecting the large bowel. HSCR derives from a defective formation of the ENS resulting in the absence of enteric ganglion cells in a variable region of the hindgut.[23] This in turn reflects the disruption in the rostrocaudal colonization by the ENS precursors during the embryogenic development of the GI tract. The lack of ganglionic cells ultimately results in unopposed tonic muscular contraction and thus narrowing of the aganglionic segment, causing symptoms of large bowel obstruction (ie, delayed passage of meconium and constipation) and consequent distension of the proximal ganglionic bowel. The RET gene (10q11.2) has been identified as the key gene to be involved in the pathogenesis of HSCR and mutations account for up to 50% of familial cases and up to 35% of sporadic ones.[5,24] Although RET mutations are the major identified risk factor for HSCR, evidence suggests that in the vast majority of patients the disease is likely to be multigenic, affecting both RET gene and genetic abnormalities in other loci, including EDNRB signaling and SOX10.[24–26] Recent initiatives have suggested a potential role for somatic mutations in RET[27] and for epigenetics[28] as well as novel approaches to identify genes implicated in HSCR.[29]

Although the disease is limited to the rectosigmoid region (short segment HSCR) in nearly 80% of cases, the disorder may also involve proximal segments of the large bowel (long segment HSCR) or even the entire gut in a small proportion of patients. Current therapeutic management is the surgical resection of the aganglionic region as assessed intraoperatively by histopathologic examination. However, surgical interventions have significant long-term morbidity, with nearly 20% of patients reporting soiling and 35% of patients suffering from postoperative constipation with the need of reintervention (eg, redo pull through, ostomies) in early childhood and adolescence.[30,31] A number of authors have reported persisting dysmotility of the retained ganglionic segment or indeed loss of a distal rectal brake[32,33] with the reported incidence of fecal incontinence in adolescence and adulthood ranging from 8% to 71%.[34] HSCR provides a key disease in which an improved understanding of basic science has the real prospect of being translated into clinical practice[35]

Slow transit constipation
Constipation is a common functional GI disorder, occurring in nearly 30% of children and is characterized clinically by infrequent bowel motions (<3 per week) and/or by symptoms of incomplete defecation.[36]

Based on the main underlying pathophysiologic mechanism, constipated patients can be subcategorized as having STC or outlet obstruction depending on evidence of prolonged colonic transit time or abnormal expulsion of luminal contents from the distal bowel, respectively.[37] Most of the data in the literature reporting abnormal enteric innervation in constipated patients derive from patients with severe STC (colonic inertia). In particular, a recent study on a cohort of severely constipated children has shown several histopathologic abnormalities involving enteric neurons, smooth muscle cells, and ICCs.[38] More interestingly, these abnormalities seemed to significantly correlate with the abnormal motor patterns identified by colonic manometry and with the lack of quiescence between the high-amplitude propagating contractions induced by bisacodyl.[38] Findings of discrete defects in neuronal subtypes and neurotransmitters in patients with STC are contradictory and better designed and more robust studies are needed.[5]

Current therapeutic management involves both oral and rectal treatment with laxatives (fiber supplementation, stool softeners, hyperosmotic agents, and stimulants). More recently, the use of transanal irrigation has been validated in pediatric cohorts with promising results.[39] However, a nonnegligible group of patients may experience symptoms despite the current state-of-the-art approach and surgery may, as well, be considered in a very selected subset of these patients. In children, many surgical interventions have been proposed, including appendicostomy for antegrade continence enemas, subtotal or even total colectomy with ileorectal anastomosis. However, these therapies carry a significant risk in terms of intraoperative (anesthesia) and postoperative complications (dehiscence, infections, failure owing to relapse of constipation).[40] See Drs Peter L. Lu and Hayat M. Mousa's article, "Constipation: Beyond the Old Paradigms," in this issue, for further details.

EMERGING THERAPEUTIC STRATEGIES
Pharmacotherapy

The role of pharmacotherapy in enteric neuropathies is strongly limited by their intrinsic heterogeneity and is largely oriented at controlling their symptoms by either stimulating GI motility or counteracting complications that may further compromise it (eg, bacterial overgrowth).[41] Aside from traditionally used medications comprising antiemetics, prokinetics, laxatives, and antibiotics, several new agents have been proposed for the treatment of enteric neuropathies in children. However, most of the data on the efficacy of newly developed drugs arises from adult studies with evidence of very limited quality from pediatric populations, often in the form of anecdotal case reports or studies in samples too small to draw clear conclusions.

Prucalopride is a selective 5HT4-agonist that has been previously shown to improve symptoms and is licensed for use in adult patients with chronic constipation. Its limited efficacy in the pediatric age group, albeit evidenced only in the context of functional constipation, has prevented the drug from being licensed for use in chronic constipation in children.[42] The success of the drug in adults has suggested its potential in STC and other neuropathies. Emmanuel and colleagues[43] showed that prucalopride accelerated colonic transit time and improved symptoms in a cohort of adults with chronic constipation. In a small-sized randomized controlled trial in patients with CIPO, prucalopride significantly ameliorated several symptoms, especially nausea and pain, without showing any significant laxative effects, thus implying a positive effect on upper GI transit. The putative beneficial effects of prucalopride in STC or PIPO have not been investigated so far.[44]

Octreotide, a somatostatin analogue, has been shown to modulate GI motility by inducing phase III-like activity in the small bowel and decreasing antral contractility in the fasting period. In a study by Di Lorenzo and colleagues,[45] 23 children with abnormal GI motility (8 with PIPO, 6 patients with dyspepsia, 6 with gastroesophageal reflux disease, and 3 with chronic refractory constipation) underwent antroduodenal manometry during the subcutaneous administration of 0.5 or 1.0 μg/kg of octreotide. Although only 13 of the 23 patients presented a phase III activity of the motor migrating complex at baseline recordings, octreotide administration was able to induce phase III activity in 21 children ($P<.02$). Furthermore, a more recent study on 16 PIPO patients reported an overall improvement in enteral feeding tolerance in nearly 70% of studied patients following octreotide administration.[46]

Lubiprostone is a selective activator of type 2 chloride channel, that has shown prokinetic effects, accelerating GI motility and enhancing the strength of GI contractions in response to the meal in preclinical studies.[47] Lubiprostone has been tested in an open-label study in children with refractory constipation with promising results[48]; however, at the present time, the results of a current large multicenter trial in children with functional constipation are awaited and the role of the drug in other conditions, for example, needs to be elucidated.

Finally, newly developed prokinetic agents (ghrelin agonist [relamorelin], motilin agonist [camicinal], 5-HT4 receptor agonist [velusetrag], and neurokinin-1 receptor antagonists [aprepitant]) have all shown promising results in severe upper GI dysmotility, and warrant further investigations in pediatric clinical trials.[49]

Electrical Pacing

Techniques that have shown more recent potential for the treatment of GI neuropathies involve the surgical implantation of devices able to deliver electrical inputs to override abnormal motor patterns and stimulate normal GI contractility (electrical pacing). Small intestinal and colonic pacing are recently born methods that deserve further study to draw conclusions about their safety, efficacy, and clinical applicability in pediatrics. In contrast, gastric pacing represents a suitable therapeutic option in severe gastroparesis that is refractory to medical treatment.[50] The rationale for using gastric pacing in gastroparesis lies on the evidence that most patients with idiopathic gastroparesis have a decreased number of ICCs (gastric pacemaker cells) rather than appreciable defects in gastric innervation.[16] Accumulating evidence shows a beneficial effect of this technique in children with an acceptable safety and tolerability profile. In the largest series to date of the systematic application of gastric electrical stimulation in children, it was found to be a safe and effective therapy for selected children with intractable gastroparesis with continued symptomatic improvement at 1 year and beyond.[51] However, it has to be noted that the symptomatic improvement of patients is not strictly related to the improvement of gastric emptying rates and might be greater than the real effect on gastric motility, similar to what has been observed with several prokinetic agents. Other studies are needed to confirm its long-term efficacy and safety in pediatric populations.[52]

Increasing attention has recently been drawn to the use of electrical stimulation in segments of the intestine beyond the stomach. The relative mobility of the small intestine has limited any such interventions, with studies focused on the effect of large bowel abdominal transcutaneous electrical stimulation as a noninvasive pain-free form of electrical stimulation that is believed to neuromodulate the GI motor activity by using interferential electrical current delivered by skin electrodes attached to the abdominal wall. Studies from 1 center have shown that transcutaneous electrical stimulation improved the quality of life, increased the frequency of bowel movement, and decreased the frequency of fecal incontinence, which parallels an increase in colonic propagating contractions and improvement of colonic transit. However, despite this promising evidence randomized placebo-controlled studies are warranted to confirm the effectiveness of transcutaneous electrical stimulation in children with chronic constipation and fecal incontinence.[53–58] Sacral nerve stimulation is a relatively new invasive neuromodulation method used in the treatment of children with constipation and fecal incontinence involving low-voltage stimulation of the sacral nerve roots by positioning an electrode via a sacral foramen. Studies in children have shown that sacral nerve stimulation decreases fecal incontinence, decreases the need for concurrent oral laxative or antegrade cecostomy enema use, and improves quality of life at 2 years after treatment initiation, suggesting its efficacy as a long-term therapeutic option in children with medically unresponsive refractory constipation. Current limiting factors include a high rate of postoperative complications, with up to one-quarter of patients requiring additional surgery, necessitating the need for randomized trials.[59–61]

Surgery and Intestinal Transplantation

With the notable exception of HSCR, in theory, surgical interventions in enteric neuropathies should be reserved for selected patients who are refractory to medical treatment. In practice, the relatively paucity of effective medical therapies has often meant the application of surgical treatments as first line across a range of enteric neuropathies (eg, PIPO). Classical surgical interventions for these patients focus on ensuring an alternative route to deliver enteral nutrition, via ostomies (ie, gastrostomies, jejunostomies) and to allow GI decompression (ileostomies, colostomies).[62] All these measures are not curative and should only be performed where unavoidable, because they carry an unquestionable risk of adhesions that could, in turn, worsen GI motility and consequently the overall clinical picture.

Undoubtedly, the role of intestinal transplantation (either isolated small bowel or multivisceral) in children with severe GI dysmotility deserves a separate article. To date, intestinal transplantation remains the only curative technique for children with severe motility disorders, that, as a group, represent the second most common indication for intestinal transplant, accounting for almost 18% of all cases.[63,64]

Four different types of surgical techniques have been developed so far: isolated intestinal transplant, combined liver and bowel transplantation, modified multivisceral transplantation (ie, inclusion of stomach, duodenum and pancreas along with the small intestine), and multivisceral transplantation (ie, inclusion of stomach, duodenum, pancreas and liver along with the small intestine with or without the large intestine).

The decision as to which surgical technique to apply is determined by a multidisciplinary discussion, involving different professionals (pediatric gastroenterologist and/or hepatologist, pediatric surgeon, dietitian, urologist, psychologist, social worker, etc) and is based on the presence or absence of end-stage liver disease associated with intestinal failure and the extent of the dysmotile GI tract. For these reasons, an extensive preoperative workup aimed at assessing the motor function of the foregut and hindgut is essential in evaluating which type of transplant should be performed (ie, inclusion of the stomach with or without the large intestine along with the small intestine).[65]

Overall, this multidisciplinary approach in highly specialized services and the recent advances in immunosuppressive treatments have contributed to sensibly improve the outcomes and survival rates after intestinal transplantation from an initially reported graft survival of 10 days to 49 months to the 60% survival rate at 5 years during the last decade.[66] Notwithstanding this progress, pediatric transplant programs remain strongly limited by the paucity of organs and high mortality rates. Therefore, intestinal transplantation should be reserved only for patients with severe dysmotility suffering from parenteral nutrition-associated complications (end-stage liver disease, recurrent episodes of central line sepsis, central venous catheter-related thrombosis) and/or a poor quality of life with a high risk of morbidity and mortality.[63–67]

Neural Stem Cell and Gene Therapies

The term stem cells is often used loosely to represent heterogenous populations of progenitors, encountered throughout the body, capable of unlimited self-renewal and of generating highly specialized functional progeny. The recent progress made in stem cell biology has allowed the introduction in clinical practice of several techniques, namely autologous and/or heterologous transplantation of stem cells, aimed at replenishing absent or defective specialized cells with their undifferentiated counterparts. In neurogastroenterology, however, these techniques are still in their infancy, given that a clear recognition of the type of resident enteric stem cells dates back only to the last decade, building on the progress made in better elucidating ENS development.

In fact, the mature ENS is mainly derived from a unique population of neural crest-derived cells able to migrate in a rostrocaudal fashion[68] and to fully colonize the gut at approximately 7 weeks, during embryogenesis.[69] The demonstration that multipotent cells, retaining the ability to form mature neural and glial cells,[70] are present during human development and even in postnatal life, has paved the way to consider transplantation of enteric neural stem cells (ENSC) as a viable alternative therapy to treat enteric neuropathies. More intriguingly from a translational standpoint to therapy is the evidence that ENSC could be potentially collected from mucosal biopsies during routine endoscopy, allowing in vivo autologous transplantation of either embryonic or even postnatal ENSC.[71–74] However, it has to be noted that, even though both types of ENSC have been shown to successfully engraft and colonize in vivo the colon,[75] embryonic ENSC were found to occupy a greater area as compared with postnatal ENSC after transplantation, thus, likely reflecting an inverse correlation between increasing developmental age and decreasing ENSC proliferative activity (**Fig. 1**).

Early studies from groups including those of the authors have provided proof of principle for the existence of adult ENSC, the ability to harvest them and propagate them in vitro within spherical cell aggregates (termed neurospheres or neurosphere-like bodies) and ultimately to transplant them into recipient intestine where they successfully engraft and colonize the gut, giving rise to mature enteric and glial cells at appropriate sites.[70] These preliminary observations in animal models has led to subsequent

DAPI GFP TuJ1

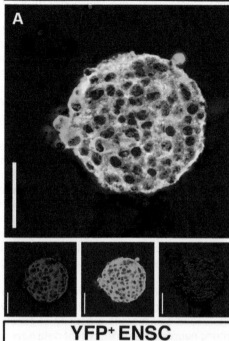

YFP⁺ENSC Transplanted Colon

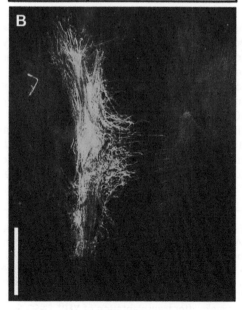

experiments in humans. In particular, more recently, neurosphere-like bodies were generated from ex vivo cultures obtained from full-thickness samples of nonneuropathic and patients with HSCR or from mucosal biopsy samples obtained during endoscopies.[73] Once again, when neurosphere-like bodies were transplanted into either embryonic or aganglionic gut explants from patients with HSCR, they have shown the ability to colonize the gut and differentiate into the appropriate enteric neuronal phenotypes.[73] More interestingly, ENSC transplantation into the distal bowel of nNOS[−/−] mice resulted in the restoration of nitrergic neuron function, leading to the in vivo rescue of impaired colonic motility.[75] This study was a landmark because it provided, for the first time, proof that neural stem cell transplantation was capable of rescuing whole organ function in a model of an enteric neuropathy. Altogether, there is increasing support for the use of gut-derived stem cells and the practicability of autologous transplantation.

Ideally, a number of conditions should be satisfied for successful stem cell therapy[76]; however, it is important to emphasize that the putative target disease needs to be well-characterized to understand what structural and/or functional deficits have occurred and consequently what type of replacement cells and strategies are required. Furthermore, stem cells isolated from patients with genetically driven enteric neuropathies might be defective as well, sharing the same genotype of their specialized counterpart. Given the complex underlying genetic abnormalities of these disorders, combining gene therapy and stem cell transplantation will probably be extremely challenging, particularly in disorders with a poorly characterized genetic background, like PIPO.

Indeed, there are a number of limitations preventing the use of gene therapy in enteric neuropathies. These conditions are indeed extremely heterogeneous in terms of genotypic alterations and there is a paucity of genetic data available for the vast majority of enteric neuropathies. Yet, recent data have shown that the combination of gene therapy and neuronal stem cell transplantation might be feasible as a novel therapeutic approach in HSCR. As reported elsewhere in this article, stem cell transplantation in genetically driven enteric neuropathies is not recommended because the autologous stem cells display the same genotype and hence might be defective too. However, Sun and colleagues[77] have recently constructed a recombinant adenovirus carrying the *GDNF* and *EDNRB* genes and have shown the coexpression of these genes in neural stem cells. *GDNF* and *EDNRB* genes are both recognized to participate in ganglion cells growth and, therefore, their transfection into neural stem cells might represent a feasible novel approach for combining gene therapy in HSCR.

Finally, motility disorders in which an immune-mediated pathophysiology has been hypothesized (esophageal achalasia and secondary PIPO) might not be suitably treated with stem cell therapy, given that inflammatory changes might negatively impact on the viability and survival of transplanted cells. Improving

◀─────────────────────────────────────

Fig. 1. Integration of enteric neural stem cell (ENSC)-derived cells after transplantation of YFP[+] neurospheres. (A) *Wnt1[cre/+];R26R[YFP/YFP]* derived neurospheres contain enteric neurons. Representative confocal images of a *Wnt1[cre/+];R26R[YFP/YFP]* derived neurosphere. YFP[+] (*green*) neurospheres colabel with the neuronal marker TuJ1 (*red*). DAPI was used to label nuclei. Scale bars in A represent 50 μm. (B) Transplanted ENSC extensively colonize and integrate within the nNOS[−/−] mouse colon. Representative stereoscopic montage image of nNOS[−/−] distal colon 4 weeks after transplantation of YFP[+] ENSC. Scale bar in B represents 1 mm. (*Courtesy of* Conor McCann, PhD, London, United Kingdom.)

our understanding of the pathophysiologic mechanisms and elucidating the structural/functional ENS deficits of these disorders is, therefore, pivotal to evaluate the long-term feasibility and efficacy of neural stem cell therapies in GI motility disorders.

Microbiome Manipulation and Fecal Transplantation

Enteric neuropathies are characterized by impaired GI transit and by subsequent qualitative and quantitative alterations in intestinal microbiota composition, leading to small intestinal bacterial overgrowth.[78] Small intestinal bacterial overgrowth may interfere with the absorption of nutrients and in turn worsen malnutrition.[79]

Interestingly, intestinal microbiota were shown to contribute in the regulation of intestinal motility.[80,81] Furthermore, clinical data have demonstrated the efficacy of nonabsorbable (eg, rifaximin) and systemically absorbed antibiotics (macrolides, metronidazole, etc) in improving GI symptoms reported by patients with gut dysmotility.[78] Altogether, these results have pointed toward the plausible involvement of intestinal microbiota in enteric neuropathies' pathophysiology and its potential role as a novel therapeutic tool in GI motility disorders.

In particular, fecal microbiota transplantation (FMT) is a recently developed technique involving the transplantation of intestinal microbiota from healthy donors to patients with intestinal dysbiosis to restore the phylogenetic diversity of intestinal microbiota.[82] The vast majority of clinical data available on the putative effects of FMT arises from patients with pseudomembranous colitis, inflammatory bowel disorders, and irritable bowel syndrome.[82,83] Although the precise mechanism underlying the efficacy of FMT remains controversial, it seems to be related to the relative changes in the composition of bacterial community.[84]

Consistent data about the efficacy of FMT in gut motor disorder are still lacking at present. A recent pilot study on 9 PIPO patients has demonstrated that FMT may relieve symptoms of abdominal pain and bloating and, more important, may improve tolerance to enteral feeding. The administration of serial FMT on consecutive days via nasojejunal tube was indeed able to increase enteral feeding tolerance in 6 patients and 4 of 9 subjects were established on a liquid oral diet, thus suggesting that serial FMT may be a candidate treatment for PIPO.[85]

Moreover, the efficacy of FMT has been recently tested against conventional treatment (behavioral strategies and oral laxatives) in a randomized clinical trial in 60 adult patients with chronic constipation.[86] The authors found that constipation subsided in almost 40% of patients in the FMT arm as compared with 13% of the control group. Among the remaining patients of the FMT group, nearly one-half (53%) reported an average increase of 1 or more bowel movements per week and this finding seemed to be significantly correlated with a faster transit, as shown by the colonic transit time assessment. Nonetheless, patients in the conventional treatment arm had fewer adverse events, compared with the FMT group. Indeed, 22 of 30 FMT patients had respiratory difficulties and discomfort when the nasointestinal tube was inserted and reported more commonly mild to moderate adverse events (fever, flatulence, and need to vent/decompress the bowel via the nasointestinal tube).[86] Despite the advances in this therapeutic modality, there are areas that warrant further investigation, such as the design of a standardized protocol when preparing the fecal suspension for FMT, the delivery methods of the treatment (nasojejunal vs endoscopic route of delivery), and, last, the long-term impact on the intestinal microbiota composition. Therefore, at present, evidence on the efficacy and safety of FMT in enteric neuropathies is limited and FMT cannot be recommended as a therapeutic approach in nonspecialized settings.

SUMMARY

The past decades have seen significant efforts in understanding enteric neuropathies as well as developing new techniques for their treatment. Several strategies have shown promising results in highly specialized clinical settings. In particular, intestinal transplantation, electrical stimulation/pacing, and microbiota manipulation have all been tested as potential treatments for these challenging disorders, with variable experience and success. Stem cell and gene therapies are arguably at the cusp of the first human trials; however, much more information is needed with regard to the genetics and precise pathology of target enteric neuropathies as well as experimental data on their practicability and safety before these novel methods can be applied to patients. Despite these limitations, the evidence produced so far attests to real progress in neurogastroenterology and the possibility of moving these treatments from purely experimental settings into real clinical practice is at hand.

ACKNOWLEDGMENTS

The authors thank Dr Conor McCann for his help with figures and legends.

REFERENCES

1. Furness JB. The enteric nervous system and neurogastroenterology. Nat Rev Gastroenterol Hepatol 2012;9:286–94.
2. Knowles CH, De Giorgio R, Kapur RP, et al. The London Classification of gastrointestinal neuromuscular pathology: report on behalf of the Gastro 2009 International Working Group. Gut 2010;59:882–7.
3. Gershon MD. The enteric nervous system: a second brain. Hosp Pract 1999;34: 31–42.
4. Knowles CH, De Giorgio R, Kapur RP, et al. Gastrointestinal neuromuscular pathology: guidelines for histological techniques and reporting on behalf of the Gastro 2009 International Working Group. Acta Neuropathol 2009;118:271–301.
5. Goldstein AM, Thapar N, Karunaratne TB, et al. Clinical aspects of neuro intestinal disease: pathophysiology, diagnosis, and treatment. Dev Biol 2016;417: 217–28.
6. Furness JB. The enteric nervous system: normal functions and enteric neuropathies. Neurogastroenterol Motil 2008;20:32–8.
7. Walzer N, Hirano I. Achalasia. Gastroenterol Clin North Am 2008;37:807–25.
8. Goldblum JR, Rice TW, Richter JE. Histopathologic features in esophagotomy specimens from patients with achalasia. Gastroenterology 1996;111:648–54.
9. Furuzawa-Carballeda J, Torres-Landa S, Valdovinos MA, et al. New insights into the pathophysiology of achalasia and implications for future treatment. World J Gastroenterol 2016;22(35):7892–907.
10. Becker J, Niebisch S, Ricchiuto A, et al. Comprehensive epidemiological and genotype-phenotype analyses in a large European sample with idiopathic achalasia. Eur J Gastroenterol Hepatol 2016;28:689–95.
11. Gockel I, Becker J, Wouters MM, et al. Common variants in the HLA-DQ region confer susceptibility to idiopathic achalasia. Nat Genet 2014;46:901–4.
12. Bielefeldt K, Enck P, Erckenbrecht JF. Motility changes in primary achalasia following pneumatic dilatation. Dysphagia 1990;5:152–8.
13. Boeckxstaens GE, Annese V, desVarannes SB, et al. European Achalasia Trial Investigators. Pneumatic dilation versus laparoscopic Heller's myotomy for idiopathic achalasia. N Engl J Med 2011;364:1807–16.

14. Patrick A, Epstein O. Review article: gastroparesis. Aliment Pharmacol Ther 2008; 27:724–40.
15. Waseem S, Islam S, Kahn G, et al. Spectrum of gastroparesis in children. J Pediatr Gastroenterol Nutr 2012;55:166–72.
16. Grover M, Bernard CE, Pasricha PJ, et al, NIDDK Gastroparesis Clinical Research Consortium (GpCRC). Clinical-histological associations in gastroparesis: results from the Gastroparesis Clinical Research Consortium. Neurogastroenterol Motil 2012;24:531–9.
17. Faussone-Pellegrini MS, Grover M, Pasricha PJ, et al. Ultrastructural differences between diabetic and idiopathic gastroparesis. J Cell Mol Med 2012;16(7): 1573–81.
18. De Giorgio R, Barbara G, Stanghellini V, et al. Idiopathic myenteric ganglionitis underlying intractable vomiting in a young adult. Eur J Gastroenterol Hepatol 2000;12:613–6.
19. De Giorgio R, Cogliandro RF, Barbara G, et al. Chronic intestinal pseudo-obstruction: clinical features, diagnosis, and therapy. Gastroenterol Clin North Am 2011;40:787–807.
20. Thapar N, Saliakellis E, Benninga MA, et al. Paediatric intestinal pseudo-obstruction: evidence and consensus-based recommendations from an ESPGHAN-led expert group. J Pediatr Gastroenterol Nutr 2018;66(6):991–1019.
21. Knowles CH, Lindberg G, Panza E, et al. New perspectives in the diagnosis and management of enteric neuropathies. Nat Rev Gastroenterol Hepatol 2013;10: 206–18.
22. De Giorgio R, Ricciardiello L, Naponelli V, et al. Chronic intestinal pseudo-obstruction related to viral infections. Transplant Proc 2010;42:9–14.
23. Heanue TA, Pachnis V. Enteric nervous system development and Hirschsprung's disease: advances in genetic and stem cell studies. Nat Rev Neurosci 2007;8: 466–79.
24. Brosens E, Burns AJ, Brooks AS, et al. Genetics of enteric neuropathies. Dev Biol 2016;417(2):198–208.
25. Carrasquillo MM, McCallion AS, Puffenberger EG, et al. Genome-wide association study and mouse model identify interaction between RET and EDNRB pathways in Hirschsprung disease. Nat Genet 2002;32:237–44.
26. Cantrell VA, Owens SE, Chandler RL, et al. Interactions between Sox10 and EdnrB modulate penetrance and severity of aganglionosis in the Sox10 Dom mouse model of Hirschsprung disease. Hum Mol Genet 2004;13:2289–301.
27. Brosens E, MacKenzie KC, Alves MM, et al. Do RET somatic mutations play a role in Hirschsprung disease? Genet Med 2018. https://doi.org/10.1038/gim.2018.6.
28. Torroglosa A, Alves MM, Fernández RM, et al. Epigenetics in ENS development and Hirschsprung disease. Dev Biol 2016;417(2):209–16.
29. Gui H, Schriemer D, Cheng WW, et al. Whole exome sequencing coupled with unbiased functional analysis reveals new Hirschsprung disease genes. Genome Biol 2017;18(1):48.
30. Catto -Smith AG, Trajanovska M, Taylor RG. Long-term continence after surgery for Hirschsprung's disease. J Gastroenterol Hepatol 2007;22:2273–82.
31. Pini Prato A, Gentilino V, Giunta C, et al. Hirschsprung disease: do risk factors of poor surgical outcome exist? J Pediatr Surg 2008;43:612–9.
32. Kaul A, Garza JM, Connor FL, et al. Colonic hyperactivity results in frequent fecal soiling in a subset of children after surgery for Hirschsprung disease. J Pediatr Gastroenterol Nutr 2011;52(4):433–6.

33. Di Lorenzo C, Solzi GF, Flores AF, et al. Colonic motility after surgery for Hirschsprung's disease. Am J Gastroenterol 2000;95(7):1759–64.
34. Wester T, Granström AL. Hirschsprung disease—Bowel function beyond childhood. Semin Pediatr Surg 2017;26:322–7.
35. Heuckeroth RO. Hirschsprung disease - integrating basic science and clinical medicine to improve outcomes. Nat Rev Gastroenterol Hepatol 2018;15(3): 152–67.
36. Tabbers MM, Di Lorenzo C, Berger MY, et al. European Society for Pediatric Gastroenterology, Hepatology, and Nutrition. North American Society for Pediatric Gastroenterology Evaluation and treatment of functional constipation in infants and children: evidence-based recommendations from ESPGHAN and NASPGHAN. J Pediatr Gastroenterol Nutr 2014;58(2):258–74.
37. Wald A. Constipation: pathophysiology and management. Curr Opin Gastroenterol 2015;31:45–9.
38. Giorgio V, Borrelli O, Smith VV, et al. High-resolution colonic manometry accurately predicts colonic neuromuscular pathological phenotype in pediatric slow transit constipation. Neurogastroenterol Motil 2013;25:70–7.
39. Koppen IJ, Kuizenga-Wessel S, Voogt HW, et al. Transanal irrigation in the treatment of children with intractable functional constipation. J Pediatr Gastroenterol Nutr 2017;64(2):225–9.
40. Cheng LS, Goldstein AM. Surgical Management of Idiopathic Constipation in Pediatric Patients. Clin Colon Rectal Surg 2018;31(2):89–98.
41. Di Lorenzo C, Youssef NN. Diagnosis and management of intestinal motility disorders. Semin Pediatr Surg 2010;19:50–8.
42. Mugie SM, Korczowski B, Bodi P, et al. Prucalopride is no more effective than placebo for children with functional constipation. Gastroenterology 2014;147: 1285–95.
43. Emmanuel AV, Cools M, Vandeplassche L, et al. Prucalopride improves bowel function and colonic transit time in patients with chronic constipation: an integrated analysis. Am J Gastroenterol 2014;109(6):887–94.
44. Emmanuel AV, Kamm MA, Roy AJ, et al. Randomised clinical trial: the efficacy of prucalopride in patients with chronic intestinal pseudo-obstruction–a double-blind, placebo-controlled, cross-over, multiple n = 1 study. Aliment Pharmacol Ther 2012;35:48–55.
45. Di Lorenzo C, Lucanto C, Flores AF, et al. Effect of octreotide on gastrointestinal motility in children with functional gastrointestinal symptoms. J Pediatr Gastroenterol Nutr 1998;27:508–12.
46. Ambartsumyan L, Flores A, Nurko S, et al. Utility of octreotide in advancing enteral feeds in children with chronic intestinal pseudo-obstruction. Paediatr Drugs 2016;18:387–92.
47. Song J, Yin J, Xu X, et al. Prokinetic effects of large-dose lubiprostone on gastrointestinal transit in dogs and its mechanisms. AM J Transl Res 2015;7:513–21.
48. Hyman PE, Di Lorenzo C, Prestridge LL, et al. Lubiprostone for the treatment of functional constipation in children. J Pediatr Gastroenterol Nutr 2014;58:283–91.
49. Stein B, Everhart KK, Lacy BE. Gastroparesis: a review of current diagnosis and treatment options. J Clin Gastroenterol 2015;49:550–8.
50. Islam S, Vicka LR, Runnels MJ, et al. Gastric electrical stimulation for children with intractable nausea and gastroparesis. J Pediatr Surg 2008;43(3):437–42.
51. Islam S, McLaughlin J, Pierson J, et al. Long-term outcomes of gastric electrical stimulation in children with gastroparesis. J Pediatr Surg 2016;51(1):67–71.

52. Teich S, Mousa HM, Punati J, et al. Efficacy of permanent gastric electrical stimulation for the treatment of gastroparesis and functional dyspepsia in children and adolescents. J Pediatr Surg 2013;48(1):178–83.

53. Chase J, Robertson VJ, Southwell B, et al. Pilot study using transcutaneous electrical stimulation (interferential current) to treat chronic treatment-resistant constipation and soiling in children. J Gastroenterol Hepatol 2005;20(7):1054–61.

54. Clarke MCC, Chase JW, Gibb S, et al. Decreased colonic transit time after transcutaneous interferential electrical stimulation in children with slow transit constipation. J Pediatr Surg 2009;44(2):408–12.

55. Clarke MCC, Catto-Smith AG, King SK, et al. Transabdominal electrical stimulation increases colonic propagating pressure waves in paediatric slow transit constipation. J Pediatr Surg 2012;47(12):2279–84.

56. Yik YI, Clarke MCC, Catto-Smith AG, et al. Slow-transit constipation with concurrent upper gastrointestinal dysmotility and its response to transcutaneous electrical stimulation. Pediatr Surg Int 2011;27(7):705–11.

57. Clarke MCC, Chase JW, Gibb S, et al. Improvement of quality of life in children with slow transit constipation after treatment with transcutaneous electrical stimulation. J Pediatr Surg 2009;44(6):1268–72 [discussion: 1272].

58. Yik YI, Hutson J, Southwell B. Home-based transabdominal interferential electrical stimulation for six months improves paediatric slow transit constipation (STC). Neuromodulation 2017. https://doi.org/10.1111/ner.12734.

59. Lu PL, Koppen IJN, Orsagh-Yentis DK, et al. Sacral nerve stimulation for constipation and fecal incontinence in children: long-term outcomes, patient benefit, and parent satisfaction. Neurogastroenterol Motil 2018;30(2). [Epub ahead of Print].

60. Lu PL, Asti L, Lodwick DL, et al. Sacral nerve stimulation allows for decreased antegrade continence enema use in children with severe constipation. J Pediatr Surg 2017;52:558–62.

61. Sulkowski JP, Nacion KM, Deans KJ, et al. Sacral nerve stimulation: a promising therapy for fecal and urinary incontinence and constipation in children. J Pediatr Surg 2015;50:1644–7.

62. Goulet O, Sauvat F, Jan D. Surgery for pediatric patients with chronic intestinal pseudo-obstruction syndrome. J Pediatr Gastroenterol Nutr 2005;41(Suppl 1): S66–8.

63. Minneci PC. Intestinal transplantation: an overview. Pathophysiology 2014;21: 119–22.

64. Ganousse-Mazeron S, Lacaille F, Colomb-Jung V, et al. Assessment and outcome of children with intestinal failure referred for intestinal transplantation. Clin Nutr 2015;34:428–35.

65. Millar AJ, Gupte G, Sharif K. Intestinal transplantation for motility disorders. Semin Pediatr Surg 2009;18:258–62.

66. Abu-Elmagd KM, Kosmach-Park B, Costa G, et al. Long-term survival, nutritional autonomy, and quality of life after intestinal and multivisceral transplantation. Ann Surg 2012;256:494–508.

67. Pakarinen MP, Kurvinen A, Koivusalo AI, et al. Surgical treatment and outcomes of severe pediatric intestinal motility disorders requiring parenteral nutrition. J Pediatr Surg 2013;48:333–8.

68. Anderson RB, Newgreen DF, Young HM. Neural crest and the development of the enteric nervous system. Adv Exp Med Biol 2006;589:181–96.

69. Wallace AS, Burns AJ. Development of the enteric nervous system, smooth muscle and Interstitial cells of Cajal in the human gastrointestinal tract. Cell Tissue Res 2005;319:367–82.

70. Bondurand N, Natarajan D, Thapar N, et al. Neuron and glia generating progenitors of the mammalian enteric nervous system isolated from foetal and postnatal gut cultures. Development 2003;130:6387–400.

71. Cooper JE, Natarajan D, McCann CJ, et al. In vivo transplantation of fetal human gut-derived enteric neural crest cells. Neurogastroenterol Motil 2017;29.

72. Hotta R, Stamp LA, Foong JP, et al. Transplanted progenitors generate functional enteric neurons in the postnatal colon. J Clin Invest 2013;123:1182–91.

73. Metzger M, Bareiss PM, Danker T, et al. Expansion and differentiation of neural progenitors derived from the human adult enteric nervous system. Gastroenterology 2009;137:2063–73.e4.

74. Metzger M, Caldwell C, Barlow AJ, et al. Enteric nervous system stem cells derived from human gut mucosa for the treatment of aganglionic gut disorders. Gastroenterology 2009;136:2214–25.e1-3.

75. McCann CJ, Cooper JE, Natarajan D, et al. Transplantation of enteric nervous system stem cells rescues nitric oxide synthase deficient mouse colon. Nat Commun 2017;8:15937.

76. Burns AJ, Thapar N. Neural stem cell therapies for enteric nervous system disorders. Nat Rev Gastroenterol Hepatol 2014;11:317–28.

77. Sun NF, Zhong WY, Lu SA, et al. Co-expression of recombinant adenovirus carrying GDNF and EDNRB genes in neural stem cells in vitro. Cell Biol Int 2013;37:458–63.

78. Lauro A, De Giorgio R, Pinna AD. Advancement in the clinical management of intestinal pseudo-obstruction. Expert Rev Gastroenterol Hepatol 2015;9(2):197–208.

79. Roland BC, Ciarleglio MM, Clarke JO, et al. Small intestinal transit time is delayed in small intestinal bacterial overgrowth. J Clin Gastroenterol 2015;49(7):571–6.

80. Quigley EMM. Microflora modulation of motility. J Neurogastroenterol Motil 2011;17(2):140–7.

81. Parthasarathy G, Chen J, Chen X, et al. Relationship between microbiota of the colonic mucosa vs feces and symptoms, colonic transit, and methane production in female patients with chronic constipation. Gastroenterology 2016;150(2):367–79.e1.

82. van Nood E, Vrieze A, Nieuwdorp M, et al. Duodenal infusion of donor feces for recurrent Clostridium difficile. N Engl J Med 2013;368(5):407–15.

83. Kassam Z, Lee CH, Yuan Y, et al. Fecal microbiota transplantation for Clostridium difficile infection: systematic review and meta-analysis. Am J Gastroenterol 2013;108(4):500–8.

84. Kelly CR, Kahn S, Kashyap P, et al. Update on fecal microbiota transplantation 2015: indications, methodologies, mechanisms, and outlook. Gastroenterology 2015;149(1):223–37.

85. Gu L, Ding C, Tian H, et al. Serial frozen fecal microbiota transplantation in the treatment of chronic intestinal pseudo-obstruction: a preliminary study. J Neurogastroenterol Motil 2017;23(2):289–97.

86. Tian H, Ge X, Nie Y, et al. Fecal microbiota transplantation in patients with slow-transit constipation: a randomized, clinical trial. PLoS One 2017;12(2):e0171308.

Food Sensitivities
Fact Versus Fiction

Catherine DeGeeter, MD[a], Stefano Guandalini, MD[b],*

KEYWORDS

- Food allergy • Food intolerances • Food sensitivities • Wheat • Gluten

KEY POINTS

- There is an overestimation of food allergies, resulting in parents eliminating unnecessarily foods from their children's diet.
- Not all adverse reactions to foods are allergies; diagnosis of a food allergy must follow well-defined criteria.
- Many tests are available to the public that purport detection of food intolerances, but they have no scientific validation whatsoever and should not be used.
- The term non-celiac gluten sensitivity is a misnomer and should be abandoned in favor of non-celiac wheat intolerance, an entity suffering from lack of biomarkers and still not convincingly described in children.

INTRODUCTION

Adverse reactions to foods are increasing in prevalence and are often attributed to allergy. Up to one-third of parents report 1 or more food reactions in their children that they may interpret as allergies.[1] However, not all of these are true intolerances and may result in avoidance of foods that could otherwise be reintroduced into the diet. It must be stressed that food-related disorders can lead to a spectrum of clinical manifestations and degrees of severity, but only some of them are related to allergy. In fact, a true food allergy is defined as an "adverse *immune* response that occurs reproducibly on exposure to a given food and is distinct from other adverse responses to food."[2] Other conditions causing adverse food reactions include congenital or acquired disorders of digestive-absorptive processes, such as lactose intolerance, toxic or pharmacologic reactions, and autoimmune reactions, such as celiac disease (CD). Thus, the noncommitting term "food intolerance" should be used to include all forms

[a] Division of Gastroenterology, Hepatology, Pancreatology, and Nutrition, Stead Family Department of Pediatrics, University of Iowa Health Care, 200 Hawkins Drive, Iowa City, IA, 52242, USA; [b] Section of Pediatric Gastroenterology, Hepatology and Nutrition, University of Chicago, 5721 S. Maryland Avenue, Chicago, IL 60637, USA
* Corresponding author. 2702 Brassie Avenue, Flossmoor, IL 60422.
E-mail address: sguandalini@peds.bsd.uchicago.edu

Gastroenterol Clin N Am 47 (2018) 895–908
https://doi.org/10.1016/j.gtc.2018.07.012
0889-8553/18/© 2018 Elsevier Inc. All rights reserved.

Abbreviations	
AAP	American Academy of Pediatrics
ATI	Amylase-trypsin inhibitors
CD	Celiac disease
EPIT	Epicutaneous
FODMAP	Fermentable oligosaccharides, disaccharides, monosaccharides and polyols
FPIES	Food protein-induced enterocolitis syndrome
IBS	Irritable bowel syndrome
NAS	National Academies of Sciences, Engineering, and Medicine
NCGS	Non-celiac gluten sensitivity
NCWI	Non-celiac wheat intolerance
NIAID	National Institute of Allergy and Infectious Disease
OFC	Oral food challenge
SPT	Skin prick testing
VAS	Visual analog score

of adverse reactions due to ingested foods until an adverse reaction is proven to be due to an immune-mediated process (**Table 1**).

The National Institute of Allergy and Infectious Disease (NIAID) published guidelines for the diagnosis and management of food allergies in 2010 and has been a mainstay in the clinician's approach to food allergies and intolerances.[2] A more recent report published in 2017 by the National Academies of Sciences, Engineering, and Medicine (NAS), entitled "Finding a Path to Safety in Food Allergy: Assessment of the Global Burden, Causes, Prevention, Management, and Public Policy," provides further guidance for the diagnosis, treatment, and prevention of food allergies. The report is based on a study performed by 15 international experts with evidence base including

Table 1
Classification of food intolerances with gastrointestinal manifestations

Type	Pathogenesis	Main Clinical Entities
Immune-mediated (food allergy)	Immunoglobulin (Ig)E mediated	Immediate gastrointestinal hypersensitivity
	Non–IgE mediated	Oral allergy syndrome Food protein–induced Proctocolitis Enterocolitis (FPIES) Enteropathy
	Occasionally IgE mediated	Eosinophilic esophagitis Eosinophilic gastroenteropathy
Unknown, likely mixed, pathogenesis		Non-celiac gluten sensitivity
Autoimmune	Innate as well as adaptive immunity	Celiac disease
Nonimmune mediated	Disorders of digestive-absorptive processes	Glucose-galactose malabsorption Lactase deficiency Sucrase-isomaltase deficiency Enterokinase deficiency
	Toxic or pharmacologic reactions	Food poisoning Tyramine (aged cheeses) Histamine (strawberries, caffeine) Theobromine (chocolate, tea)
	Idiosyncratic reactions	Food additive Food colorants

literature reviews and assessment of published guidelines and practice parameters.[3] Both of these documents provide fundamental points that are discussed throughout this article.

FOOD ALLERGY
Prevalence

The true prevalence of food allergies is difficult to define for several reasons, including that most studies focus on only the most common foods, although more than 170 foods have been identified in causing IgE-mediated reactions.[2] The definition of food allergy often varies in prevalence studies, as well as whether the diagnosis was self-reported versus identified by testing. These, among many other factors, limit the reliability of prevalence estimates and the recent report from the NAS could not give definitive prevalence data for the United States. However, a review published in the *Journal of the American Medical Association* in 2010 estimated that food allergy affects more than 1% to 2% and less than 10% of the US population,[4] and a study published in *Pediatrics* determined 8% of children have food allergy as identified by parental report.[5] It is known that self-reported allergies likely overestimate prevalence,[6] thus it is imperative to use the gold standard oral food challenge (OFC), which has not been used in US studies since the 1980s.[7] A study using skin prick testing (SPT) followed by OFC in Melbourne, Australia, identified the prevalence of food allergies at age 1 year to be 11% and at age 4 to be 3.8%.[8]

IMMUNOGLOBULIN E–MEDIATED FOOD ALLERGY
Myth: "The Immunoglobulin E Allergy Testing Was Positive for Wheat, Eggs, Milk, and Corn, Therefore the Patient Is Allergic to These Foods"

A positive immunoglobulin (Ig)E test shows sensitivity to that allergen, but does not imply clinical relevance. The most common food allergens in the United States include cow's milk, egg, peanut, tree nuts, wheat, shellfish, and soy. Cow's milk proteins followed by soybean proteins are the most common cause of food allergy during infancy, whereas egg protein allergy is most common in school-aged children.[9] Most food allergies have a high rate of resolution. For example, more than 50% of children with a milk allergy will have resolution by ages 5 to 10 years.[10] Egg, wheat, and soy allergies all have nearly 50% resolution by age 9.[10] Allergies to peanuts and tree nuts are less likely to resolve, with only 20% resolution by age 4 for peanuts and only 10% resolution of tree nut allergies.[10] Allergy to seeds, fish, and shellfish are also considered persistent. Achieving tolerance to allergens is likely associated with an increased amount of T regulatory cells and reduction of allergen-specific IgE.[11] A family history of atopy and atopic dermatitis are well-known risk factors for the development of IgE-mediated food allergies. Other risk factors include male sex, race/ethnicity (increased in Asian and black children compared with white children), and genetics.[12] Numerous theories regarding environmental risk factors for food allergy have been proposed, such as the hygiene hypothesis, the allergen avoidance hypothesis, dual allergen exposure hypothesis, and nutritional immunomodulation hypothesis with variable levels of evidence.[12] Other speculations for allergy risk factors that lack firm data include obesity, processed foods, food additives, and genetically modified foods.[3]

Clinical Presentation

IgE-mediated reactions typically have a rapid onset within minutes to hours of ingestion of the offending agent. Numerous organ systems can be involved, including the gastrointestinal tract, skin, lungs, and heart. Gastrointestinal manifestations, such as abdominal pain, nausea, vomiting, and diarrhea are the most common presentation in children (50% to 80%). Skin involvement, such as erythema, itching, and urticaria, is the second most common presentation in children (20% to 40%) followed by respiratory symptoms of cough, wheezing, and rhinorrhea (4% to 25%).[13]

Food allergy should be suspected when symptoms occur within minutes to hours of ingestion of a specific food, especially if it occurs on more than one occasion.[2] Allergy testing also should be considered for infants and children with severe atopic dermatitis, allergic proctocolitis, enterocolitis, enteropathy, and eosinophilic esophagitis. Food allergy is not a typical trigger of chronic asthma or chronic rhinitis so this should not prompt allergy testing.[7]

Diagnosis

The medical history is key to diagnosis and can help identify the likelihood of a food allergy, hone pertinent test selection, and suggest alternative etiologies for symptomatology. The diagnosis of food allergies is challenging, as there is not a uniform set of criteria to follow.[4] In addition to the clinical history, laboratory studies and an OFC are often necessary to confirm a diagnosis. The NIAID guidelines recommend SPTs and serum IgE (sIgE) testing to assist in identifying IgE-mediated food reactions. These tests typically have high sensitivity but poor specificity, thus they should be used in the context of the clinical history and possible food challenge, as positive tests alone are not diagnostic.[14,15] This is demonstrated in a study of 44 children avoiding foods because of positive allergy test results. After 111 OFCs, 93% were found to be tolerant to the avoided foods.[16] Nearly 40% of primary care physicians incorrectly interpreted positive sIgE blood tests or SPTs as sufficient for diagnosis of allergy.[17] With this in mind, physicians should be discouraged from ordering "panels" of food tests without the appropriate rationale. Component testing, which measures sIgE to specific proteins in foods, can improve the specificity of testing. For example, a protein in peanuts called Ara h 2 is associated with clinical reactions and is a more specific identifier of true peanut allergy.[18] A recent systematic review[19] concluded that selected components of cow's milk, hen's egg, peanut, hazelnut, and shrimp allergen showed high specificity, but lower sensitivity. However, few studies exist for each component, and studies vary widely regarding the cutoff values used, making it challenging to synthesize findings across studies.

The gold standard for allergy diagnosis is a double-blind placebo-controlled food challenge; however, due to expense and lengthy time requirements, it is rarely used in clinical practice.[20] More typically, unmasked OFCs are performed in the clinical setting. Both the NAS report and NIAID guidelines advise against the use of many nonvalidated tests that have, however, gained some popularity. These include food allergy patch testing (atopy patch test), measurement of total IgE, and the basophil activation test. Other tests not recommended and considered "unproven and nonstandardized" for diagnosing food allergy are listed in **Box 1**.

Treatment

The mainstay of treatment for IgE-mediated food allergies remains avoidance of the causing allergen. This must occur in numerous settings including home, school, restaurants, and travel, and families should have a written allergy and anaphylaxis emergency plan.[21] Intramuscular epinephrine should be administered as a first line for emergent treatment for food allergy anaphylaxis.[3,22] Antihistamines and steroids also may be used in the case of inadvertent ingestion of allergens. Two additional topics were outlined in the recent NAS report pertinent to the pediatric population: the need for

Box 1
Tests not recommended in the diagnosis of food allergy

- Allergen-specific immunoglobulin (Ig)A, IgG, or IgG4
- Provocation neutralization
- Immune complexes
- Human leukocyte antigen screening
- Lymphocyte stimulation
- Facial thermography
- Gastric juice analysis
- Endoscopic allergen provocation
- Hair analysis
- Applied kinesiology
- Cytotoxic assays
- Electrodermal testing
- Mediator release assays
- Bioresonance
- Iridology

Data from Sicherer SH, Allen K, Lack G, et al. Critical issues in food allergy: a National Academies consensus report. Pediatrics 2017;140(2):3. with permission.

nutritional monitoring for children avoiding foods due to allergy, and attention to psychosocial aspects of food allergy management, including the increased risk of bullying.[7] Immunotherapy is not currently recommended by any of the major allergy guidelines; however, it continues to be aggressively explored. Immunotherapy involves giving gradually increasing doses of specific allergens to induce desensitization and ultimately tolerance.[23] This can be accomplished via oral (OIT), sublingual (SLIT), or epicutaneous (EPIT) routes. OIT appears to be more effective than SLIT and EPIT but with more side effects, including allergic reactions and increased risk of eosinophilic esophagitis. Although there are no currently approved therapies for food allergies, 2 commercial products are in the third phase of clinical trials.[23]

Prevention of Food Allergy

Recommendations for the prevention of food allergy have changed in the past few decades. Previously allergen avoidance during pregnancy, breastfeeding, and infancy was encouraged; however, these myths have been dispelled. There are now numerous studies suggesting early oral exposure may result in the induction of tolerance.

Maternal dietary restriction and breastfeeding
The American Academy of Pediatrics (AAP), NAS, and NIAID all discourage eliminating allergenic food from the diet of pregnant or lactating women, as there is no supportive evidence that this is beneficial in preventing food allergy even in at-risk infants.[2,3,24] There is also no significant evidence for a protective effect of breastfeeding for at-risk infants. However, all 3 entities in addition to the World Health Organization promote nursing of all infants through the first 6 months of life.[2,3,24]

Timing and introduction of complementary foods

There is evidence that very early (during the first 2–3 months of life) introduction of potential allergens put infants at an increased risk for allergy formation; however, there are no convincing data that delaying introduction of solid foods beyond 4 to 6 months of age has any protective effect on the development of food allergy. In the Learning Early About Peanut (LEAP) trial, infants at high risk of peanut allergy (severe eczema or egg allergy) were randomized to receive or avoid peanut to the age of 5 years. The children sensitized to peanut had a peanut allergy rate of 10.6% compared with those in the avoidance group who had peanut allergy rate of 35.3% (*P* = .004; relative risk reduction 70%).[25] The AAP, NAS, and NIAID guidelines all recommend early introduction of peanuts in infants at high risk. Delaying the introduction of egg, cow milk, and wheat seems to have no benefits, so it is suggested that there is a potential benefit for introducing these foods in the first year of life when developmentally ready.[3] Although delaying introduction of these other allergens is not necessary, it is still unclear if early introduction (4–6 months of age) to at-risk infants is beneficial. Two recent randomized control trials investigating egg introduction to at-risk infants had differing outcomes: one study showed a reduced sensitization at 1 year to those exposed early and the other study showed no change in the risk of future egg allergy.[26,27]

Hydrolyzed formulas

There are conflicting studies and recommendations regarding the benefits of using partially and extensively hydrolyzed formulas in lieu of cow milk in the first 4 to 6 months in infants with high risk of developing atopic disease. A recent systemic review and meta-analysis failed to find a beneficial effect of these formulas on allergy.[28] There is no evidence of preventive effects in low-risk children.[29] The NAS committee concluded that there is not enough current evidence to recommend these formulas, which is contrary to the previous AAP Clinical Report in 2008, which suggested there may be a modest benefit in prevention of atopy.[3,24] The Australian Consensus on Infant Feeding Guidelines to Prevent Food Allergy also clearly recommends *against* hydrolyzed (partially or extensively) infant formula for the prevention of allergic disease.[30] The European Academy of Allergy and Clinical Immunology (EAACI) guidelines recommend only hypoallergenic formulas with a documented preventive effect for high-risk children in the first 4 months of life only.[31] Overall, it is evident that more research in this area is necessary to draw firm conclusions.

IMMUNE, non–IgE-MEDIATED FOOD ALLERGY

The non–IgE-mediated food allergies more commonly present with gastrointestinal symptoms and are typically subacute or chronic in nature. This category of food allergy encompasses the following disorders: food protein–induced proctitis and proctocolitis, food protein–induced enterocolitis syndrome (FPIES), and food protein–induced enteropathy.

Food Protein–Induced Proctocolitis

Myth: "A child with milk protein–induced proctocolitis as an infant should continue to avoid milk indefinitely"

Food protein–induced proctocolitis is a cell-mediated reaction that tends to occur in exclusively breastfed infants. Food allergens ingested by the mother then appear in the breast milk to produce the reaction. The most typical food implicated is cow's milk (76%); however, it may be caused by egg (16%), soy (6%), or corn (2%) or multiple foods.[32] Infants often present in the first month of life with low-grade rectal bleeding. This condition is benign, although may be alarming to new parents. Blood loss is minimal and typically does not cause anemia. Diagnosis is made clinically, and flexible sigmoidoscopy may be performed for tissue diagnosis for patients with atypical symptoms or who do not respond to treatment. Treatment is avoidance of the provoking allergen. *If left untreated, this condition will resolve spontaneously.* The offending antigen may be reintroduced as early as 6 months of age with 50% of infants tolerating the antigen and 95% tolerating by 9 months of age.[33]

Food Protein–Induced Enterocolitis Syndrome

Myth: "If skin and IgE blood tests are negative, there is no allergy"

FPIES is an allergic syndrome that also presents in infants; however, they are generally much sicker than those with proctocolitis. Whereas proctocolitis is common in exclusively breastfed infants, FPIES is uncommon in this population and more typically presents in infants who are formula fed. The mechanism of action is unclear but postulated to be due to ingested food antigens causing local T-cell–mediated inflammation that leads to increased intestinal permeability and fluid shifts.[34] The humoral immune response also may be involved. The typical offending agent is cow's milk and, to a lesser extent, soy. Rice, Oats, and poultry have also been implicated.[35] Infants will present in the first month of life with profuse vomiting, diarrhea, and melena or hematochezia. Lethargy, pallor, dehydration, and hypotension are also common. *The diagnosis is made based on the clinical presentation and requires meeting the major criterion of vomiting within 1 to 4 hours after ingestion of the suspect food and the absence of classic IgE-mediated allergic skin or respiratory symptoms in addition to 3 minor criteria.* The minor criteria include additional vomiting, extreme lethargy, marked pallor, need for emergency room visit, need for intravenous fluid, diarrhea, hypotension, and hypothermia.[36] A food challenge also may be performed, especially in the setting of a single episode, as viral gastroenteritis is also common at this age. Treatment is based on eliminating the offending food. Most children presenting with cow's milk and soy FPIES normally become tolerant to the offending food by the age of 3; however, solid food FPIES may have a longer course.

Food Protein–Induced Enteropathy

Food protein–induced enteropathy presents in infants and young children and is the result of a cell-mediated reaction to cow's milk and soy protein. It is most likely to occur in infants younger than 9 months who have been fed regular cow's milk instead of formula. The presentation includes a chronic osmotic diarrhea and failure to thrive and can be very similar to CD. Diagnosis is based on clinical features and confirmed with endoscopy and duodenal biopsy, which will reveal distortion of villous architecture that is indistinguishable from CD. The differentiation from CD is based on negative serologies, including anti–tissue transglutaminase and deamidated gliadin peptides. Treatment is avoidance of the allergen and it typically resolves after 2 years of age.[37]

EOSINOPHILIC GASTROINTESTINAL DISEASE: EOSINOPHILIC ESOPHAGITIS, GASTROENTEROPATHY

Myth: "Food-Specific IgE Testing Determines the Causative Foods for Eosinophilic Gastroenteropathies"

Eosinophilic gastrointestinal disorders (EGIDs) are characterized by eosinophilic infiltration of segments of the intestinal tract in the absence of known causes for eosinophilia.[38] Although EGIDs are typically listed under non-IgE food reactions, they have properties of both IgE-mediated food allergy and cellular-mediated hypersensitivity disorders.[39] These disorders present with a variety of symptoms depending on the location and extent of involvement in the gastrointestinal tract and may include difficulty or pain with swallowing, abdominal pain, nausea, vomiting, and weight loss. *Food-specific IgE tests and SPTs may be used to identify foods associated with EGIDs, but alone are not sufficient to make the diagnosis and if negative do not rule out the possibility of eosinophilic gastroenteropathies.*[2,40] Upper and/or lower endoscopy with mucosal biopsies are necessary for diagnosis in conjunction with the clinical presentation.

Dietary therapy options include elemental diet, which is strict use of amino acid–based formula, targeted diet based on allergy testing, or empiric elimination of the most likely food antigens.[41] Pharmacologic therapy includes topical steroids for both initial and maintenance therapy. Cromolyn, leukotriene receptor antagonists, and immunosuppressive agents are not recommended for treatment.[40]

UNCLEAR, LIKELY MIXED, PATHOGENESIS: NON-CELIAC GLUTEN SENSITIVITY
Myths: "There Is a Test for Gluten Sensitivity; Non-Celiac Gluten Sensitivity Has Been Well Documented in Children Too"

Gluten consumption has been linked to a wide range of disorders, including CD, wheat allergy, dermatitis herpetiformis, gluten ataxia, peripheral neuropathy, and possibly this relatively new entity called "non-celiac gluten sensitivity" (NCGS).

These patients by definition do not meet the criteria for CD or wheat allergy, but report experiencing a number of intestinal and/or extra-intestinal symptoms after consuming gluten-containing foods.[42] They present neither the autoantibodies nor the enteropathy characteristic of CD. In NCGS, symptoms typically occur soon after ingestion of gluten-containing foods and disappear quickly after elimination of wheat-related foods. On reintroduction of wheat, rapid relapse typically occurs. The clinical manifestations are mostly, but not exclusively, gastrointestinal, and are similar to those of irritable bowel syndrome. In 2015, one of us proposed that "NCGS is a misnomer and probably an umbrella term including various clinical entities."[43] With time, it has become even more clear that indeed this entity encompasses various, distinct populations: whereas a small minority may indeed react to gluten itself, most appear to react to FODMAPs (fermentable oligosaccharides, disaccharides, monosaccharides, and polyols), and among them especially fructans, as elegantly demonstrated by Skodje and colleagues[44] in 2017 (**Fig. 1**). But these patients may also react to a series of proteins found in wheat grouped under the name of ATI (Amylase-Trypsin Inhibitors)[45]; or to wheat with non–IgE-mediated mechanisms[46]; or indeed may simply respond to the placebo/nocebo effect.[47]

It is also important to notice that in spite of numerous reports in the adult literature, this entity has not been adequately demonstrated in children. In fact, after a first report that was an open-label, pilot study likely to be biased,[48] very recently the same group published a multicenter double-blind, placebo-controlled trial in children[49]: after screening more than 1000 patients and eventually enrolling only 28 eligible children, the investigators found 4 of them to respond to gluten with a VAS (visual analog score) significantly higher after gluten than after placebo. However (**Fig. 2**), also 4 of these children responded to *placebo* with a VAS significantly higher than after gluten, thus making the interpretation quite doubtful at best.

In conclusion on NCGS:

- Because gluten is responsible at best for a small fraction of these patients, the term NCGS is a misnomer and should be abandoned to the less committing "non-celiac wheat intolerance" (NCWI).

Gastrointestinal symptoms

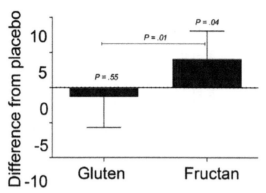

Fig. 1. Mean difference in gluten and fructan response from placebo (95% confidence intervals) for overall Gastrointestinal Symptom Rating Scale-Irritable Bowel Syndrome (GSRS-IBS). (*From* Skodje GI, Sarna VK, Minelle IH, et al. Fructan, rather than gluten, induces symptoms in patients with self-reported non-celiac gluten sensitivity. Gastroenterology 2018;154(3):534; with permission.)

- It cannot be overemphasized how important it is to first rule out the existence of CD or wheat allergy before considering NCWI.
- To this day, there is no convincing documentation of the existence of NCWI in children.

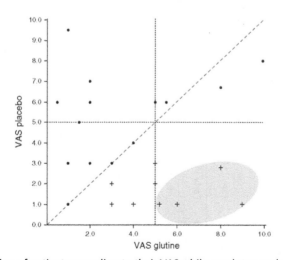

Fig. 2. Distribution of patients according to their VAS while on gluten and placebo; patients on the diagonal line have an equal response to gluten and placebo, children in the lower left quadrant experience a mild degree of overall response (<5) to either gluten or placebo. (*Reprinted by permission from* Springer Nature: Francavilla R, Cristofori F, Verzillo L, et al. Randomized Double-Blind Placebo-Controlled Crossover Trial for the Diagnosis of Non-Celiac Gluten Sensitivity in Children. Am J Gastroenterol 2018;113(3):428.)

Table 2
Diagnostic approach for food intolerances

Condition Suspected	Clinical	Food(s) Involved	Diagnostic Approach
Immediate GI hypersensitivity	Usually infancy to childhood: reactions to offending food within minutes: vomiting, diarrhea, nausea, pain; also rhinoconjunctivitis, skin rash, angioedema	Cow's milk, soy, eggs, peanuts, wheat, shellfish	History, +SPT and/or sIgE
Food protein–induced proctocolitis	Early infancy: streaks of blood and mucus in stools in breastfed, typically healthy infants	Cow's milk, eggs, soy, corn (in mother's diet)	Clinical diagnosis supported by food elimination in mother's diet
Food protein–induced enterocolitis syndrome	Early infancy: vomiting, diarrhea, colitis	Rice, soy, cow's milk, vegetables, fruits, oats, meat, fish	Clinical criteria ± food challenge
Food protein–induced enteropathy	Infants and toddlers: malabsorption syndrome similar to early-onset celiac disease, hypoalbuminemia	Cow's milk, occasionally soy or egg	Clinical diagnosis supported by duodenal biopsies with patchy villous atrophy
Eosinophilic esophagitis	All ages: asymptomatic, refluxlike symptoms, dysphagia	Cow's milk, soy, eggs, peanuts, wheat, shellfish	Endoscopy with biopsies showing typical changes; SPT, sIgE sometimes useful
Eosinophilic gastroenteropathy	Highly variable symptoms depending on localization and extension of eosinophilic infiltrates	Cow's milk, soy, eggs, peanuts, wheat, shellfish	Endoscopy with biopsies
Gluten sensitivity	Adults with IBS-like symptoms	Fructans; wheat components such as ATI; gluten in a minority	Clinical only: no diagnostic marker available
Celiac disease	All ages. Strictly limited to HLA-DQ2 and/or DQ8 positive subjects. GI and extra-GI symptoms	Gluten	Specific serology+, diagnostic features of duodenal biopsies
Lactose intolerance	Increases with age: abdominal pain, bloating, flatulence, diarrhea	Lactose	Clinical, breath hydrogen testing, rarely duodenal biopsy

Abbreviations: ATI, amylase-trypsin inhibitors; GI, gastrointestinal; IBS, irritable bowel syndrome; sIgE, serum immunoglobulin E; SPT, skin prick testing.

AUTOIMMUNE FOOD INTOLERANCE: CELIAC DISEASE
Myth: "Asymptomatic Patients with Celiac Disease Do Not Need a Gluten-Free Diet"

CD is the most common genetically induced food intolerance and is an autoimmune disorder affecting 1% of the population and occurs in individuals of all ages who express the HLA-Class II haplotypes DQ2 and/or DQ8. Ingestion of gluten and related proteins found in wheat, barley, and rye trigger CD in genetically susceptible individuals. It is characterized by an inflammatory enteropathy that leads to flattening of the small intestinal mucosa through a combined adaptive and innate immune response.[50,51] There are variable degrees of severity and clinical manifestations. Gastrointestinal symptoms are prominent, especially in younger children, and include abdominal pain, distention, diarrhea, constipation, and rarely in the present day, malnutrition and failure to thrive. Extra-intestinal manifestations include short stature, iron-deficiency anemia, female infertility, and the typical skin finding of dermatitis herpetiformis. Diagnosis of CD involves serologic screening with autoantibodies that are very sensitive and specific: anti–tissue transglutaminase antibodies (tTG), anti-endomysium antibodies (EMA) and deamidated gliadin peptides.[42] The diagnosis is then typically confirmed by upper endoscopy and obtaining duodenal biopsies, which will show typical histologic changes in the mucosa. *CD is treated by prompt and strict adherence to a life-long gluten-free diet regardless of presenting symptoms.*

NONIMMUNE MEDIATED
Disaccharide Deficiencies: Lactose Intolerance

Myth: "lactose intolerance is the same as a milk allergy"
Among the disaccharidase deficiencies, lactase deficiency is by far the most common, although the exact prevalence is unknown.[52] Intolerance to lactose (one of the FODMAP carbohydrates) is a clinical syndrome in which ingestion of lactose causes symptoms of abdominal pain, bloating, gassiness, and diarrhea. Ingested lactose from dairy-containing foods is broken down by the enzyme lactase on the microvilli surface of the small intestine. *In acquired lactase deficiency, the lactase enzyme is deficient and lactose not absorbed by the small bowel, passing rapidly into the colon. There the lactose is converted to short-chain fatty acids by intestinal bacteria producing fermentation products (including gases such as hydrogen), which cause the typical symptoms.*[52] *There is no immune reaction, as seen with a milk allergy.* Diagnosis primarily can be made clinically with confirmation by resolution of symptoms after avoiding lactose-containing foods for 5 to 7 days. A lactose breath hydrogen test also may be used to confirm the diagnosis, and in rare cases a small bowel biopsy to determine lactase enzyme activity may be used. Treatment includes dietary lactose restriction or enzyme replacement, which is available over the counter.

SUMMARY

Not all adverse reactions are due to food allergy, and an excellent history is the essential first step in making the proper diagnosis. The clinical history will guide appropriate testing selection, and **Table 2** is a suggested diagnostic approach to food intolerances. A positive sIgE or SPT alone is not sufficient to make a diagnosis: testing indicates sensitization but not necessarily clinical allergy. Finally, it is imperative to keep in mind that patient-reported and parental-reported food allergies are often not substantiated by allergy testing and may prompt investigation of other nonallergy causes of food intolerance.

REFERENCES

1. Pyrhonen K, Nayha S, Kaila M, et al. Occurrence of parent-reported food hypersensitivities and food allergies among children aged 1-4 yr. Pediatr Allergy Immunol 2009;20(4):328–38.
2. Boyce JA, Assa'ad A, Burks AW, et al. Guidelines for the diagnosis and management of food allergy in the United States: summary of the NIAID-sponsored expert panel report. J Allergy Clin Immunol 2010;126(6):1105–18.
3. National Academies of Sciences Engineering and Medicine (U.S.). Committee on Food Allergies: global burden causes treatment prevention and public policy. In: Stallings VA, Oria M, National Academies of Sciences, Engineering, and Medicine (U.S.), editors. Finding a path to safety in food allergy: assessment of the global burden, causes, prevention, management, and public policy. Washington, DC: The National Academies Press; 2017. p. 204–10.
4. Chafen JJ, Newberry SJ, Riedl MA, et al. Diagnosing and managing common food allergies: a systematic review. JAMA 2010;303(18):1848–56.
5. Gupta RS, Springston EE, Warrier MR, et al. The prevalence, severity, and distribution of childhood food allergy in the United States. Pediatrics 2011;128(1): e9–17.
6. Rona RJ, Keil T, Summers C, et al. The prevalence of food allergy: a meta-analysis. J Allergy Clin Immunol 2007;120(3):638–46.
7. Sicherer SH, Allen K, Lack G, et al. Critical issues in food allergy: a National Academies consensus report. Pediatrics 2017;140(2):5–6.
8. Peters RL, Koplin JJ, Gurrin LC, et al. The prevalence of food allergy and other allergic diseases in early childhood in a population-based study: HealthNuts age 4-year follow-up. J Allergy Clin Immunol 2017;140(1):145–53.e8.
9. Sicherer SH, Munoz-Furlong A, Godbold JH, et al. US prevalence of self-reported peanut, tree nut, and sesame allergy: 11-year follow-up. J Allergy Clin Immunol 2010;125(6):1322–6.
10. Savage J, Sicherer S, Wood R. The natural history of food allergy. J Allergy Clin Immunol Pract 2016;4(2):196–203 [quiz: 204].
11. Berin MC, Mayer L. Can we produce true tolerance in patients with food allergy? J Allergy Clin Immunol 2013;131(1):14–22.
12. Sicherer SH, Sampson HA. Food allergy: a review and update on epidemiology, pathogenesis, diagnosis, prevention, and management. J Allergy Clin Immunol 2018;141(1):41–58.
13. Sicherer SH, Sampson HA. Food allergy. J Allergy Clin Immunol 2010;125(2 Suppl 2):S116–25.
14. Sampson HA, Ho DG. Relationship between food-specific IgE concentrations and the risk of positive food challenges in children and adolescents. J Allergy Clin Immunol 1997;100(4):444–51.
15. Sampson HA. Utility of food-specific IgE concentrations in predicting symptomatic food allergy. J Allergy Clin Immunol 2001;107(5):891–6.
16. Fleischer DM, Bock SA, Spears GC, et al. Oral food challenges in children with a diagnosis of food allergy. J Pediatr 2011;158(4):578–83.e1.
17. Gupta RS, Springston EE, Kim JS, et al. Food allergy knowledge, attitudes, and beliefs of primary care physicians. Pediatrics 2010;125(1):126–32.
18. Klemans RJ, van Os-Medendorp H, Blankestijn M, et al. Diagnostic accuracy of specific IgE to components in diagnosing peanut allergy: a systematic review. Clin Exp Allergy 2015;45(4):720–30.

19. Flores Kim J, McCleary N, Nwaru BI, et al. Diagnostic accuracy, risk assessment, and cost-effectiveness of component-resolved diagnostics for food allergy: a systematic review. Allergy 2018;73(8):1609–21.

20. Sampson HA, Gerth van Wijk R, Bindslev-Jensen C, et al. Standardizing double-blind, placebo-controlled oral food challenges: American Academy of Allergy, Asthma & Immunology-European Academy of Allergy and Clinical Immunology PRACTALL consensus report. J Allergy Clin Immunol 2012;130(6):1260–74.

21. Wang J, Sicherer SH, Section on A, et al. Guidance on completing a written allergy and anaphylaxis emergency plan. Pediatrics 2017;139(3) [pii:e20164005].

22. Sicherer SH, Simons FER, Section On A, et al. Epinephrine for first-aid management of anaphylaxis. Pediatrics 2017;139(3) [pii:e20164006].

23. Gernez Y, Nowak-Wegrzyn A. Immunotherapy for food allergy: are we there yet? J Allergy Clin Immunol Pract 2017;5(2):250–72.

24. Greer FR, Sicherer SH, Burks AW, American Academy of Pediatrics Committee on Nutrition, American Academy of Pediatrics Section on Allergy and Immunology. Effects of early nutritional interventions on the development of atopic disease in infants and children: the role of maternal dietary restriction, breastfeeding, timing of introduction of complementary foods, and hydrolyzed formulas. Pediatrics 2008;121(1):183–91.

25. Du Toit G, Roberts G, Sayre PH, et al. Randomized trial of peanut consumption in infants at risk for peanut allergy. N Engl J Med 2015;372(9):803–13.

26. Wei-Liang Tan J, Valerio C, Barnes EH, et al. A randomized trial of egg introduction from 4 months of age in infants at risk for egg allergy. J Allergy Clin Immunol 2017;139(5):1621–8.e8.

27. Palmer DJ, Sullivan TR, Gold MS, et al. Randomized controlled trial of early regular egg intake to prevent egg allergy. J Allergy Clin Immunol 2017;139(5):1600–7.e2.

28. Boyle RJ, Ierodiakonou D, Khan T, et al. Hydrolysed formula and risk of allergic or autoimmune disease: systematic review and meta-analysis. BMJ 2016;352:i974.

29. Grimshaw K, Logan K, O'Donovan S, et al. Modifying the infant's diet to prevent food allergy. Arch Dis Child 2017;102(2):179–86.

30. Netting MJ, Campbell DE, Koplin JJ, et al. An Australian consensus on infant feeding guidelines to prevent food allergy: outcomes from the Australian infant feeding summit. J Allergy Clin Immunol Pract 2017;5(6):1617–24.

31. Muraro A, Werfel T, Hoffmann-Sommergruber K, et al. EAACI food allergy and anaphylaxis guidelines: diagnosis and management of food allergy. Allergy 2014;69(8):1008–25.

32. Lake AM. Food-induced eosinophilic proctocolitis. J Pediatr Gastroenterol Nutr 2000;30(Suppl):S58–60.

33. American Academy of Pediatrics. Committee on Nutrition. Hypoallergenic infant formulas. Pediatrics 2000;106(2 Pt 1):346–9.

34. Caubet JC, Nowak-Wegrzyn A. Current understanding of the immune mechanisms of food protein-induced enterocolitis syndrome. Expert Rev Clin Immunol 2011;7(3):317–27.

35. Nowak-Wegrzyn A, Sampson HA, Wood RA, et al. Food protein-induced enterocolitis syndrome caused by solid food proteins. Pediatrics 2003;111(4 Pt 1):829–35.

36. Nowak-Wegrzyn A, Chehade M, Groetch ME, et al. International consensus guidelines for the diagnosis and management of food protein-induced enterocolitis syndrome: executive summary-workgroup report of the adverse reactions to

foods committee, American Academy of Allergy, Asthma & Immunology. J Allergy Clin Immunol 2017;139(4):1111–26.e4.

37. Walker-Smith JA. Cow milk-sensitive enteropathy: predisposing factors and treatment. J Pediatr 1992;121(5 Pt 2):S111–5.

38. Rothenberg ME. Eosinophilic gastrointestinal disorders (EGID). J Allergy Clin Immunol 2004;113(1):11–28 [quiz: 29].

39. Sampson HA. Food allergy. Part 1: immunopathogenesis and clinical disorders. J Allergy Clin Immunol 1999;103(5 Pt 1):717–28.

40. Liacouras CA, Furuta GT, Hirano I, et al. Eosinophilic esophagitis: updated consensus recommendations for children and adults. J Allergy Clin Immunol 2011;128(1):3–20.e6 [quiz: 21–2].

41. Groetch M, Venter C, Skypala I, et al. Dietary therapy and nutrition management of eosinophilic esophagitis: a work group report of the American Academy of Allergy, Asthma, and Immunology. J Allergy Clin Immunol Pract 2017;5(2):312–324 e329.

42. Hill ID, Fasano A, Guandalini S, et al. NASPGHAN clinical report on the diagnosis and treatment of gluten-related disorders. J Pediatr Gastroenterol Nutr 2016; 63(1):156–65.

43. Guandalini S, Polanco I. Nonceliac gluten sensitivity or wheat intolerance syndrome? J Pediatr 2015;166(4):805–11.

44. Skodje GI, Sarna VK, Minelle IH, et al. Fructan, rather than gluten, induces symptoms in patients with self-reported non-celiac gluten sensitivity. Gastroenterology 2018;154(3):529–39.e2.

45. Zevallos VF, Raker V, Tenzer S, et al. Nutritional wheat amylase-trypsin inhibitors promote intestinal inflammation via activation of myeloid cells. Gastroenterology 2017;152(5):1100–13.e2.

46. Carroccio A, Mansueto P, D'Alcamo A, et al. Non-celiac wheat sensitivity as an allergic condition: personal experience and narrative review. Am J Gastroenterol 2013;108(12):1845–52 [quiz: 1853].

47. Molina-Infante J, Carroccio A. Suspected nonceliac gluten sensitivity confirmed in few patients after gluten challenge in double-blind, placebo-controlled trials. Clin Gastroenterol Hepatol 2017;15(3):339–48.

48. Francavilla R, Cristofori F, Castellaneta S, et al. Clinical, serologic, and histologic features of gluten sensitivity in children. J Pediatr 2014;164(3):463–467 e461.

49. Francavilla R, Cristofori F, Verzillo L, et al. Randomized double-blind placebo-controlled crossover trial for the diagnosis of non-celiac gluten sensitivity in children. Am J Gastroenterol 2018;113(3):421–30.

50. Abadie V, Sollid LM, Barreiro LB, et al. Integration of genetic and immunological insights into a model of celiac disease pathogenesis. Annu Rev Immunol 2011; 29:493–525.

51. Husby S, Koletzko S, Korponay-Szabo IR, et al. European Society for Pediatric Gastroenterology, Hepatology, and Nutrition guidelines for the diagnosis of coeliac disease. J Pediatr Gastroenterol Nutr 2012;54(1):136–60.

52. Suchy FJ, Brannon PM, Carpenter TO, et al. National Institutes of Health Consensus Development Conference: lactose intolerance and health. Ann Intern Med 2010;152(12):792–6.

Improving Care in Pediatric Inflammatory Bowel Disease

Matthew D. Egberg, MD, MPH, MMSc[a],*, Michael D. Kappelman, MD, MPH[a,b],
Ajay S. Gulati, MD[c,d]

KEYWORDS

- Crohn disease • Ulcerative colitis • Quality improvement • ImproveCareNow
- Inflammatory bowel disease

KEY POINTS

- Quality improvement (QI) initiatives have been present in health care for more than a century; however, today's care continues to demonstrate gaps in quality, particularly in the care of the inflammatory bowel diseases (IBDs).
- The limited amount of evidence-based care guidelines in pediatric IBD jeopardizes patient outcomes.
- Current IBD QI initiatives, such as ImproveCareNow, are demonstrating the utility and success of collaborative care networks and standardized care stemming from learning health systems.
- Moving forward, efforts in pediatric IBD QI need to center on meaningful outcome measures, utilization of health technology platforms, and creating structured care environments that anticipate the biopsychosocial spectrum of IBD for both patients and families.

INTRODUCTION

The inflammatory bowel diseases (IBDs) are chronic, immune-mediated disorders typically classified as Crohn disease (CD), ulcerative colitis, and IBD-undefined (IBD-U). IBD often presents with intestinal symptoms, including abdominal pain, blood loss, and diarrhea, but can also be associated with systemic symptoms of weight loss, joint and skin changes, and psychological comorbidities, including depression and anxiety.[1]

Disclosure Statement: There are no commercial or financial conflicts of interest to report for any of the listed authors.
[a] Department of Pediatrics, University of North Carolina at Chapel Hill, 130 Mason Farm Road, Bioinformatics Building, CB# 7229, Chapel Hill, NC 27599, USA; [b] Department of Epidemiology, University of North Carolina at Chapel Hill, 130 Mason Farm Road, Bioinformatics Building, CB# 7229, Chapel Hill, NC 27599, USA; [c] Department of Pediatrics, University of North Carolina at Chapel Hill, 230 MacNider, CB# 7229, Chapel Hill, NC 27599, USA; [d] Department of Pathology, University of North Carolina at Chapel Hill, 230 MacNider, CB# 7229, Chapel Hill, NC 27599, USA
* Corresponding author. Division of Pediatric Gastroenterology, Hepatology, and Nutrition, University of North Carolina, Chapel Hill, Center for Gastrointestinal Biology and Disease, 130 Mason Farm Road, Bioinformatics Building, Office# 4101, CB# 7229, Chapel Hill, NC 27599.
E-mail address: Matthew.egberg@med.unc.edu

Gastroenterol Clin N Am 47 (2018) 909–919
https://doi.org/10.1016/j.gtc.2018.07.013
0889-8553/18/© 2018 Elsevier Inc. All rights reserved.

Abbreviations	
AGA	American Gastroenterological Association
CD	Crohn's disease
EHR	Electronic health record
HIT	Health information technology
IBD	Inflammatory bowel diseases
IBD-U	Inflammatory bowel diseases-undefined
ICN	Improve care now
IHI	Institute for Healthcare Improvement
IOM	Institute of Medicine, now the National Academy of Medicine
PM	Population management
PVP	Pre-visit planning; SMS self-management support
QI	Quality improvement
STEEEP	Safe, timely, equitable, efficient, effective, and patient centered
TB	Tuberculosis
TPS	Toyota production system

Although the past several years have brought significant advances in the medical and surgical treatment of IBD, the burden of illness remains substantial. At the individual level, many patients continue to face decreased quality of life, missed days of school, and reduced participation in extracurricular activities.[2] At the societal level, the health care costs of IBD remain staggering, now estimated between $14 and $30 billion.[3] Therefore, additional strategies are needed to promote durable remission, prevent disease and therapy-related complications, and optimize long-term health maintenance.

A focus on quality improvement (QI) to address known gaps in pediatric IBD care can complement the discovery of new treatments and diagnostic tests and accelerate improvement in patient outcomes. QI requires focused effort to address the challenges presented by an evolving disease process, patient population, and health care system. Understanding and appreciating current QI initiatives will position providers and health system leaders to work together to achieve higher quality and more reliable IBD care in the pediatric population. As such, the aims of this article were to (1) briefly review the history of health care QI, (2) highlight gaps in IBD care and the ongoing challenges specific to the field of QI work in IBD, (3) review several pediatric and adult IBD improvement initiatives, and (4) propose directions for future pediatric IBD QI.

BRIEF HISTORY OF HEALTH CARE IMPROVEMENT

In the early 2000s, the Institute of Medicine (IOM, now the National Academy of Medicine) published 2 landmark articles: *To Err is Human: Building a Safer Health System,*[4] and *Crossing the Quality Chasm: A New Healthcare System for the 21st Century.*[5] Both articles challenged the health care field to close the chasm between "the health care we have and the health care we could have."[4] Quality was defined by the IOM as "the degree to which health services for individuals and populations increase the likelihood of desired health outcomes and are consistent with current professional knowledge."[4] To create high-quality and reliable care, the IOM defined 6 key dimensions. These included care that is safe, timely, equitable, efficient, effective, and patient centered (STEEEP). Using the 6 dimensions, health care systems would be better positioned to provide higher quality care to patients.

Although the IOM articles were major milestones in the QI timeline, efforts to improve health care outcomes were in place long before these publications. Ernest

Codman, a Boston surgeon, first described a framework for outcomes measurement in health care using his "end result system" in 1910.[6] Around that time in Japan, Sakichi Toyoda started a textile manufacturing business that would later give rise to the Toyota Motor Company and Toyota Production System (TPS).[7–9] Better known today as Lean Management, the TPS system was founded on production principles that include waste reduction through efficient manufacturing.[8] Moreover, one of its main tenants, *Kaizan*, or "continuous improvement," has taken hold in the health care industry and is used by several large health care organizations to improve care.

In addition to Lean Management, the Model for Improvement is another popular framework for development and implementation of QI initiatives in health care.[7] The model is the result of work in the 1950s by W. Edwards Deming, Walter Shewhart, and Joseph Juran, who popularized the concepts of measuring process variation (heterogeneity in output performance) and methods to increase efficient production (reduction of variability). The Model for Improvement and Lean Management play an important role in today's health care QI environment.

Equally as important as the approaches to improvement science are the organizations working alongside health care systems to facilitate this improvement. The Institute for Healthcare Improvement (IHI) is an independent not-for-profit organization committed to a culturally sensitive and tailored approach to health system improvement rooted in the tenants of improvement science. The IHI seeks to improve the experience of care, improve population health, and reduce per capita health care cost. These goals have become known as the Triple Aim.[10] A fourth dimension, joy in work, has been added to the mission to address the concerns of increasing provider burnout rates, an additional threat to health care quality.[11,12] Although organizations such as the IHI and frameworks like Lean Management and the Model for Improvement have helped the health care industry produce better health care, disparities persist. The health care industry, along with patients and families, need to be mindful of these persistent gaps and work together to eliminate them.

GAPS IN INFLAMMATORY BOWEL DISEASE CARE

Recognizing and addressing care gaps plays a critical role in optimizing disease outcomes in pediatric IBD. Notable care deficiencies include medical knowledge deficits, lack of timely care, and variation in diagnostic and therapeutic strategies. These domains impact all fields of health care, including pediatric IBD.

Deficiencies in Medical Knowledge

As highlighted by the IOM, patient care should keep pace with expanding medical knowledge; however, in reality, research demonstrates many deficits in this area. For example, a recent study demonstrated that nearly 30% of adult gastroenterologists were unaware of recommendations for thrombotic prophylaxis in hospitalized patients with IBD.[13] A second study involving both dermatologists and gastroenterologists showed that only 46% of providers were aware of the association between non-melanoma skin cancer and immunosuppressive medications azathioprine and 6-mercaptopurine.[14] Knowledge gaps like these contribute to outcome heterogeneity and reduce the quality of patient care.

Lack of Timely Care

In addition to knowledge gaps, deficits in the delivery of timely IBD care exist as well. In a study examining clinic attendance of pediatric patients with IBD with active disease, 78% failed to be seen within 2 months of their latest disease flare.[15] Lack of timely patient assessment increases risk for complications due to the disease process, therapy, or both. In addition, poor care coordination reduces patient and family engagement, threatening health outcomes.

Variation in Care

Studies in pediatric CD have highlighted persistent gaps between recommended and actual care.[16] A study of more than 200 pediatric patients diagnosed with CD at 80 sites identified significant heterogeneity in diagnostic practice, including reduced rates of small bowel imaging, stool pathogen testing, documentation of tuberculosis (TB) testing before infliximab initiation, and thiopurine methyltransferase testing before initiation of thiopurine treatment.[16,17] These and other inconsistencies in care delivery negatively impact the reliability of health care provided.

CURRENT CHALLENGES IN INFLAMMATORY BOWEL DISEASE CARE

Gaps in IBD care have significant impact on both the health care system and patient outcomes. Disparities between the care intended and the care delivered are driven by a multitude of challenges. Chief among them are (1) the lack of high-quality clinical and comparative effectiveness data to guide evidence-based decision making, and (2) a system failure to meet the complex needs of the pediatric IBD population via a tailored, multidisciplinary approach. Understanding these driving factors will improve the capability of providers to close current care gaps and expand the quality of care in pediatric IBD.

Lack of Evidence-Based Decision Making

Variation in health care practice is a clear driver of low-quality care[18–20] and may stem from specific patient needs or preferences, the lack of provider adherence to best practices, or paucity of data-driven clinical practice guidelines. Although the introduction of learning health systems has led to significant progress in standardizing care through data generation and outcome measurement in several areas of medicine, this concept remains in its infancy. Improving outcomes in pediatric IBD will require ongoing integration of comparative effectiveness research, guideline development, and continuous QI.

Inadequate Systems to Provide Complex, Chronic Care

IBD is a complex, multifaceted disease that impacts the entire patient and his or her family. Effective treatment requires a thoughtful, multidisciplinary approach focusing on the biopsychosocial spectrum of disease. The *Chronic Illness Care Model* is a co-ordinated multidisciplinary approach to chronic care emphasizing collaboration between engaged and knowledgeable patients and prepared, proactive providers.[21] The model has been successfully applied in pediatric chronic diseases, such as cystic fibrosis and type 1 diabetes[22,23] and in a few pediatric IBD centers. However, widespread use in pediatric IBD remains limited,[24] creating challenges to the provision of patient and family-centered care.

CURRENT INFLAMMATORY BOWEL DISEASE IMPROVEMENT INITIATIVES

Over the past decade, a number of hospitals and practices have successfully implemented QI initiatives targeting key aspects of pediatric IBD care. For example, single-center initiatives have reported increased influenza vaccination rates,[25] adoption of exclusive enteral nutrition protocols,[26] and more efficient transitioning of adolescent patients with IBD to adult providers.[27]

In addition to these single-center initiatives, ImproveCareNow (ICN) is a large, multi-center pediatric IBD QI network. Established in 2007, the purpose of ICN is to transform the health, care, and cost for all children and adolescents with IBD through the development of a sustainable collaborative chronic care network. Over the past decade, ICN has grown into an international consortium composed of 107 pediatric gastrointestinal centers, including 95 in the United States, 2 in England, 1 in Qatar, and 9 in Belgium. Currently, 32,000 patients are registered in the network, and data from 215,000 visits have been collected and analyzed. The network has worked to align the goals of multiple stakeholders: patients, families, clinicians, hospitals, researchers, funding agencies, foundations, and industry. In doing so, ICN has become an important vehicle for overcoming the challenges described previously and will be a critical driver for continuous improvement in the future.

Fig. 1 shows the key driver diagram for ICN. The primary outcome is remission rate, defined by a physician global assessment of disease activity. The remission rate target for the network is currently set at 83%, but each center can define its own goals. The 7 key drivers for improving remission rates are (1) optimal access to care, (2) a prepared

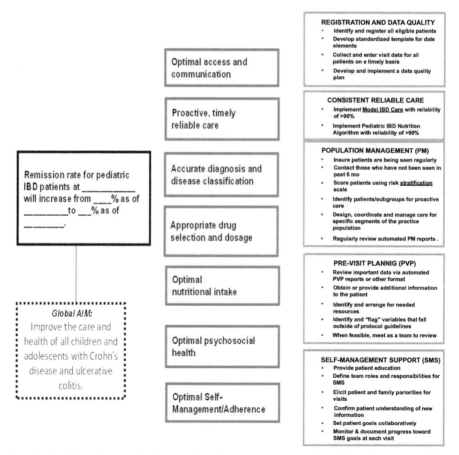

Fig. 1. Key driver diagram for ImproveCareNow demonstrating the global aims of the initiative and areas of focus by which to achieve them. (*Courtesy of* ImproveCareNow Network. Available at: https://www.improvecarenow.org/; with permission.)

and proactive practice team, (3) accurate diagnosis and disease classification, (4) appropriate drug selection and dosage, (5) optimal growth and development, (6) optimal psychosocial health, and (7) informed patients and families who can engage in self-management. The 5 major interventions to support these key drivers are (1) registration and data quality, (2) consistent reliable care, (3) population management (PM), (4) pre-visit planning (PVP), and (5) self-management support.

The ICN Registry provides the foundation for QI work within the network. During each patient encounter, standardized data are collected about the patient, the patient's disease status, and the care provided at the visit. After the visit, these data are entered into the ICN database using a combination of electronic health record (EHR) data extraction and Web-based data entry via a secure server. These data are aggregated, analyzed, and made available to each practice center in real-time as a series of reports and QI tools including (1) QI reports of key clinical measures of process and outcomes; (2) a PM report providing summary, practice-level data; (3) a PVP report providing more detailed, patient-level data; and (4) a data quality report. QI reports contain information about the performance of the individual center, as well as aggregate, network-level data.

In addition to the data collection and analysis infrastructure, the ICN consortium has spent considerable effort defining Model IBD Care Guidelines to provide consistent and reliable care. These were first developed and implemented in 2009, based on evidence from the literature and consensus expert opinion. A Clinical Practice Committee was established in 2013, which supports updating of these guidelines on a regular basis. Targeted didactic sessions at biannual ICN meetings, and open group discussions with clinicians from consortium centers ensure that appropriate diagnostic and therapeutic interventions are consistently updated and recommended for most children and adolescents with IBD.

The cornerstones of data collection and standardized practice guidelines established by the ICN network allow for broadly reaching QI initiatives, including PM and PVP. PM uses large data sets to coordinate health care interventions for specific subsets of patients. Approaching patients in this manner allows for a shift from an episodic care system (in which providers *react* to patients' problems at clinic visits) to a population-based system (in which high-risk patients are managed more *proactively*). ICN has developed a Web-based PM tool that facilitates the rapid identification of high-risk patients. These patients can then be discussed at regular QI meetings to ensure they have timely follow-up in place, optimized drug dosing, and involvement of necessary multidisciplinary care. Such efforts are complemented by PVP tools to assist the clinician in preparing for upcoming patient visits. Patient-specific data can be pulled directly from the database allowing providers to (1) review important clinical data, (2) identify variables that fall outside of protocol guidelines (such as drug dosages and growth parameters), and (3) prearrange needed resources at the upcoming visit (eg, dietitian, psychologist, social worker). The combination of PM and PVP helps ensure centers coordinate and proactively manage both higher-risk and routine patients.

Self-management support (SMS) has been an additional focus of improvement within ICN. Optimal SMS involves providing patient education, eliciting patient and family priorities for visits, confirming patient understanding of new information, setting patient goals collaboratively, and monitoring progress toward these goals at each visit. ICN has implemented a systematic program to develop tools for SMS, which are routinely shared with all participating centers, enabling everyone to benefit from the work of others. This is facilitated through the ICN Web resource center, a listserv, monthly live webinars, and semiannual learning sessions in which teams gather for learning and sharing.

Over the past decade, demonstrable improvements in outcomes have been observed for patients within the ICN network. Remission rates have increased from 52% to 81% with prednisone-free remission rates improving from 49% to 80%. Ninety-three percent of patients now have a satisfactory growth status, and 90% have a satisfactory nutritional status (up from 86% and 85%, respectively). Although the drivers of these improvements are multifactorial (eg, new therapies, monitoring guidelines), ICN is clearly enhancing the care of pediatric patients with IBD.

QI work internationally has also made an impact on IBD quality. In the United Kingdom, a 2006 audit of IBD services revealed large variations in the standard of care. In response, the Crohn's & Colitis UK partnered with the British Society of Gastroenterology and several other organizations to create the "IBD Standards." This published work defines high-quality IBD care and provides benchmarks for health care professionals.[28] In response, there have been clear improvements to the care of patients with IBD, including an increased number of children seen by professionals with appropriate pediatric training in age-appropriate settings.[29] In Australia, similar development of a dedicated IBD service reduced the rates of IBD hospitalization, polypharmacy, and steroid and opiate use.[30] These examples of successful international QI initiatives help guide current and future QI work here in the United States and abroad.

QI work in IBD is not limited to the pediatric population. For example, the American Gastroenterological Association (AGA) has invested in improving several aspects of adult IBD care. Important contributions include the development and implementation of physician performance measurement sets.[31] In addition, the AGA has created several Clinical Care Pathways and Treatment Algorithms.[32–36] Developed through a multi-stakeholder process, these pathways and algorithms incorporate expert consensus and meta-analytic methodology to produce clinical guidance rooted in evidence-based medicine. The Crohn's & Colitis Foundation also supports IBD QI through innovative research, partnership with ICN, and establishment of a multi-stakeholder process to prioritize process and outcome measures.[37] Recently, it has launched IBD Qorus, a collaborative, chronic care network of adult IBD practices that, similar to ICN, empowers health care providers to standardize care, measure and track quality metrics in real time, engage patients, and share QI experience across sites. Currently there are 30 participating sites in the network.[38]

These small and large-scale QI initiatives are important for improving the quality of care provided to patients and families impacted by IBD. As the IBD population grows and the health care system evolves, so too should the approach to QI.

ADVANCING PEDIATRIC INFLAMMATORY BOWEL DISEASE CARE QUALITY FORWARD

Sustaining and accelerating pediatric IBD QI in the future will require a greater focus on measuring and achieving clinical and patient-centered outcomes and continued effort to improve care reliability. Key improvement strategies must include establishing meaningful outcomes, leveraging health technology platforms, and aligning system and provider efforts.

Establishing Meaningful Outcome Measures

Improving health care quality in pediatric IBD begins with measurement of meaningful patient outcomes. The heterogeneous nature of IBD, growing complexity of the health care system, and paucity of research-driven practice guidelines have led to difficulties reaching consensus regarding measures of overall health and patient well-being.[39] Previous research has categorized health care measures using 3 practical domains for QI work.[40] These 3 domains include structural measures (health care system capacity, system architecture, and service organization), process measures (services provided by the health care system to maintain or improve health), and outcome measures (patient-level health care service or interventions that directly affect the health status of the patient).[41] Traditionally, process measures, such as flu vaccination and TB testing, have been the target for health care improvement in pediatric IBD due to their ease of service accounting and subsequent benefits in the pay-for-performance health care structure.[42] However, to continue improving IBD care, a new emphasis on meaningful outcome measures must occur. This will require additional practice algorithms focused on maintaining remission, enhancing recovery from disease flares, and reducing preventable complications. Measures need to be patient/family-centered, scenario-specific (inpatient vs outpatient, emergency room, flare vs remission), and data-driven. Emphasizing meaningful outcome measures in current and future IBD QI work will provide new opportunities for creating better care.

Leveraging Health Technology Platforms

Health information technology (HIT) platforms are important tools for facilitating the collection and measurement of data, as well as the implementation of new knowledge into practice. Platforms like ICN and Qorus directly improve care through embedding data collection directly into the process of clinical practice. HIT platforms can facilitate near real-time data analysis, which accelerates clinical effectiveness research, the dissemination and implementation of findings, and QI. Examples of innovative HIT include EHR-based decision support tools and the use of telehealth to improve access to subspecialty care in resources-poor areas. Gaining popularity are mobile (phone or tablet) applications ("apps") for IBD using Android and iOS operating systems. However, despite their accessibility, research demonstrates limited professional medical involvement and implementation of consensus statements in the development of such apps, thereby limiting their benefit.[43] Increasing access to the current EHR-based platforms while expanding the breadth and professional medical involvement of mobile apps will be important HIT aspects for improving pediatric IBD care moving forward.

System and Provider Alignment

Implementing resources such as HIT and clinical practice guidelines to curtail practice variation and spread best practices in pediatric IBD requires a uniform vision between care team (microsystem) and health system leadership (macrosystem). Lack of this alignment leads to a series of workarounds that fuel variation and ultimately cause deficits in care quality.[44–46] To facilitate vision alignment, both a top-down (leadership) and bottom-up (care team) approach to care quality is needed to support the spread of quality throughout the health care culture. One example of this collaborative approach is a 2010 clinical QI initiative launched by the University of Pittsburgh Medical Center health system in which both microsystems and macrosystems worked together toward a vision for safe and reliable use of intravenous (IV) infusion pumps. In response to the combined effort, development and implementation of Smart pumps enhanced the safety of medication administration for hospitalized patients.[47] Although not strictly an IBD intervention, safer use of IV medication administration will directly impact the quality and reliability of care administered to pediatric patients with IBD.

SUMMARY

QI efforts in health care date back more than a century ago, but despite their recent reinvigoration, gaps persist in the delivery of reliable, high-quality care consistent with cutting-edge scientific knowledge. This is particularly true in the field of pediatric IBD. Initiatives such as ICN have advanced the leading edge of pediatric IBD care quality; however, this expansion is challenged by persistent obstacles, including practice variation and disease complexity. Meeting these challenges will require data-driven practice standardization focused on establishing meaningful outcome measures that are disseminated through a learning health system. This will be facilitated by an increasingly capable HIT system, used by multidisciplinary care teams who interact with engaged and knowledgeable patients in environments aligned toward care excellence and reliability. Prioritizing these aspects of QI as pediatric IBD care moves forward will address not just the health of the pediatric IBD population, but the health of the care system as well.

REFERENCES

1. Keethy D, Mrakotsky C, Szigethy E. Pediatric inflammatory bowel disease and depression: treatment implications. Curr Opin Pediatr 2014;26:561–7.
2. Griffiths AM, Nicholas D, Smith C, et al. Development of a quality-of-life index for pediatric inflammatory bowel disease: dealing with differences related to age and IBD type. J Pediatr Gastroenterol Nutr 1999;28:S46–52.
3. Mehta F. Report: economic implications of inflammatory bowel disease and its management. Am J Manag Care 2016;22:s51–60.
4. Donaldson MS, Corrigan JM, Kohn LT. To err is human: building a safer health system. Washington, DC: National Academies Press; 2000.
5. Institute of Medicine. Crossing the quality chasm: a new health system for the 21st century. Washington, DC: National Academies Press; 2001.
6. Donabedian A. The end results of health care: Ernest Codman's contribution to quality assessment and beyond. Milbank Q 1989;67:233–56.
7. Scoville R. Comparing lean and quality improvement. Cambridge (MA): Institute for Healthcare Improvement; 2014.
8. Mass W. From textiles to automobiles: mechanical and organizational innovation in the Toyoda Enterprises, 1895-1933. Business Econ Hist 1996;25:1–37.
9. Ohno T. Taiichi Ohno's workplace management. New York: McGraw Hill; 2013.
10. Stiefel M. A guide to measuring the triple aim: population health, experience of care, and per capita cost. Cambridge (MA): Institute for Healthcare Improvement; 2012.
11. Bodenheimer T, Sinsky C. From triple to quadruple aim: care of the patient requires care of the provider. Ann Fam Med 2014;12:573–6.
12. Perlo J. IHI framework for improving joy in work. Cambridge (MA): Institute for Healthcare Improvement; 2017.
13. Tinsley A, Naymagon S, Trindade AJ, et al. A survey of current practice of venous thromboembolism prophylaxis in hospitalized inflammatory bowel disease patients in the United States. J Clin Gastroenterol 2013;47:e1–6.
14. De Luca JF, Severino R, Lee YS, et al. Dermatologist and gastroenterologist awareness of the potential of immunosuppressants used to treat inflammatory bowel disease to cause non-melanoma skin cancer. Int J Dermatol 2013;52:955–9.
15. Dykes D, Williams E, Margolis P, et al. Improving pediatric inflammatory bowel disease (IBD) follow-up. BMJ Qual Improv Rep 2016;5 [pii:u208961.w3675].

16. Colletti RB, Baldassano RN, Milov DE, et al. Variation in care in pediatric Crohn disease. J Pediatr Gastroenterol Nutr 2009;49:297–303.

17. Kappelman MD, Bousvaros A, Hyams J, et al. Intercenter variation in initial management of children with Crohn's disease. Inflamm Bowel Dis 2007;13:890–5.

18. Ahmed S, Siegel CA, Melmed GY. Implementing quality measures for inflammatory bowel disease. Curr Gastroenterol Rep 2015;17:14.

19. Adler J, Sandberg KC, Shpeen BH, et al. Variation in infliximab administration practices in the treatment of pediatric inflammatory bowel disease. J Pediatr Gastroenterol Nutr 2013;57:35–8.

20. Reddy S, Friedman S, Telford J, et al. Are patients with inflammatory bowel disease receiving optimal care? Am J Gastroenterol 2005;100:1357–61.

21. Wagner EH, Austin BT, Davis C, et al. Improving chronic illness care: translating evidence into action. Health Aff (Millwood) 2001;20:64–78.

22. Bodenheimer T, Wagner EH, Grumbach K. Improving primary care for patients with chronic illness: the chronic care model, Part 2. JAMA 2002;288:1909–14.

23. Lozano P, Finkelstein JA, Carey VJ, et al. A multisite randomized trial of the effects of physician education and organizational change in chronic-asthma care. Arch Pediatr Adolesc Med 2004;158:875–83.

24. Pearson ML, Wu S, Schaefer J, et al. Assessing the implementation of the chronic care model in quality improvement collaboratives. Health Serv Res 2005;40: 978–96.

25. Keith C, Kuo H-C, Knight T, et al. Use of quality improvement process to increase influenza vaccination in pediatric inflammatory bowel disease patients. Gastroenterology 2018;154:S65.

26. Mansoor S, Costantino J, Molle-Rios Z. Development of care pathway for initiation of enteral nutrition therapy for pediatric Crohn's disease—single center quality improvement initiative. Inflamm Bowel Dis 2017;23:S74–5.

27. Schaefer M, Tung J, Maddux M, et al. Implementing transition of care and transfer of care systems in pediatric IBD. Inflamm Bowel Dis 2017;23:S73.

28. IBD Standards Group. Standards for the healthcare of people who have inflammatory bowel disease (IBD); Update. 2013. Available at: http://s3-eu-west-1. amazonaws.com/files.crohnsandcolitis.org.uk/Publications/PPR/ibd_standards_ 13.pdf. Accessed January 3, 2018.

29. Fitzgerald MP, Mitton SG, Protheroe A, et al. The organisation and structure of inflammatory bowel disease services for children and young people in the UK in 2010: significant progress but still room for improvement. Frontline Gastroenterol 2013;4:25–31.

30. Phan VH, van Langenberg DR, Grafton R, et al. A dedicated inflammatory bowel disease service quantitatively and qualitatively improves outcomes in less than 18 months: a prospective cohort study in a large metropolitan centre. Frontline Gastroenterol 2012;3:137–42.

31. American Gastroenterological Association. Adult inflammatory bowel disease physician performance measures set. 2011. Available at: http://www.gastro.org/ practice/quality-initiatives/IBD_Measures.pdf. Accessed January 3, 2018.

32. Nguyen GC, Loftus EV Jr, Hirano I, et al. American Gastroenterological Association Institute Guideline on the management of Crohn's disease after surgical resection. Gastroenterology 2017;152:271–5.

33. Terdiman JP, Gruss CB, Heidelbaugh JJ, et al. American Gastroenterological Association Institute guideline on the use of thiopurines, methotrexate, and anti-TNF-alpha biologic drugs for the induction and maintenance of remission in inflammatory Crohn's disease. Gastroenterology 2013;145:1459–63.

34. Feuerstein JD, Nguyen GC, Kupfer SS, et al. American Gastroenterological Association Institute guideline on therapeutic drug monitoring in inflammatory bowel disease. Gastroenterology 2017;153:827–34.

35. Vande Casteele N, Herfarth H, Katz J, et al. American Gastroenterological Association Institute technical review on the role of therapeutic drug monitoring in the management of inflammatory bowel diseases. Gastroenterology 2017;153: 835–57.e6.

36. Dassopoulos T, Sultan S, Falck-Ytter YT, et al. American Gastroenterological Association Institute technical review on the use of thiopurines, methotrexate, and anti-TNF-alpha biologic drugs for the induction and maintenance of remission in inflammatory Crohn's disease. Gastroenterology 2013;145:1464–78.e1-5.

37. Melmed GY, Siegel CA, Spiegel BM, et al. Quality indicators for inflammatory bowel disease: development of process and outcome measures. Inflamm Bowel Dis 2013;19:662–8.

38. Crohns and Colitis Foundation. QORUS improvement project. 2017. Available at: http://www.crohnscolitisfoundation.org/science-and-professionals/ibdqorus/. Accessed January 3, 2018.

39. Martin L, Nelson E, Rakover J, et al. Whole system measures 2.0: a compass for health system leaders. Cambridge (MA): Institute for Healthcare Improvement; 2016.

40. Donabedian A. The role of outcomes in quality assessment and assurance. QRB Qual Rev Bull 1992;18:356–60.

41. Agency for Healthcare Research and Quality/National Quality Measures Clearinghouse. Selecting process measures for clinical quality measurement. 2017. Available at: https://www.qualitymeasures.ahrq.gov/help-and-about/quality-measure-tutorials/selecting-process-measures. Accessed January 3, 2018.

42. Werner RM, Kolstad JT, Stuart EA, et al. The effect of pay-for-performance in hospitals: lessons for quality improvement. Health Aff (Millwood) 2011;30:690–8.

43. Con D, De Cruz P. Mobile phone apps for inflammatory bowel disease self-management: a systematic assessment of content and tools. JMIR Mhealth Uhealth 2016;4:e13.

44. Halbesleben JR, Savage GT, Wakefield DS, et al. Rework and workarounds in nurse medication administration process: implications for work processes and patient safety. Health Care Manage Rev 2010;35:124–33.

45. Spear SJ, Schmidhofer M. Ambiguity and workarounds as contributors to medical error. Ann Intern Med 2005;142:627–30.

46. Debono DS, Greenfield D, Travaglia JF, et al. Nurses' workarounds in acute healthcare settings: a scoping review. BMC Health Serv Res 2013;13:175.

47. Skledar SJ, Niccolai CS, Schilling D, et al. Quality-improvement analytics for intravenous infusion pumps. Am J Health Syst Pharm 2013;70:680–6.

Molecular Mechanisms in Pediatric Cholestasis

James E. Squires, MD, MS*, Patrick McKiernan, MD

KEYWORDS

- Jaundice • Children • Pediatric • Genetic causes of cholestasis • Bile acids

KEY POINTS

- Pediatric cholestasis is a common manifestation with wide-ranging etiologies.
- Advances in genetic and molecular understandings of bile formation, processing, and flow have enabled improved diagnostic capabilities.
- A systematic diagnostic approach to the jaundiced child can be beneficial in identifying the etiology.
- Management of cholestasis with genetic causes is generally supportive; however, identifying the underlying etiology and implementing appropriate treatment may be life-saving in some.

INTRODUCTION

Cholestasis often results from mechanical obstruction of the biliary tract or a genetic defect with subsequent absent or dysfunctional protein critical to the process of forming, processing, or excreting bile. The phenotypic homogeneity, commonly manifesting as jaundice, should not distract from the etiologic heterogeneity that is reflected in the large and growing number of identified disorders affecting infants and children. Importantly, isolated jaundice in the neonatal period is often the product of normal physiologic adaption and results in transient elevation of the unconjugated bilirubin fraction. Conversely, jaundice associated with conjugated hyperbilirubinemia and serum bile acid elevation is never physiologic, reflecting an underlying pathology within the hepatobiliary system. Several frameworks have been used to classify cholestatic diseases, including anatomic (intrahepatic or extrahepatic), pathophysiologic (eg, infection, inflammatory, metabolic, toxin/drug), and age-based (neonatal-, childhood-, adolescent-onset). Although overlap may exist as it relates to various demographic and clinical features, common to all is the expansion in understanding of how malfunctions within pathways regulating bile production and flow drive the development of cholestasis in children. The goal of this article was to present a practical review of pediatric cholestatic syndromes, with a focus on those with known molecular mechanisms of disease.

Conflicts of Interest and Source of Funding: The authors report no conflicts of interest and no external sources of funding were used for the purposes of the information presented.
Division of Gastroenterology, Hepatology and Nutrition, Children's Hospital of Pittsburgh, One Children's Hospital Drive, 6th Floor FP, 4401 Penn Avenue, Pittsburgh, PA 15224, USA
* Corresponding author.
E-mail address: James.Squires2@chp.edu

Gastroenterol Clin N Am 47 (2018) 921–937
https://doi.org/10.1016/j.gtc.2018.07.014
0889-8553/18/© 2018 Elsevier Inc. All rights reserved.

Abbreviations	
AGS	Alagille syndrome
CFTR	Cystic fibrosis transmembrane conductance regulator
DCDC2	Doublecortin domain containing protein 2
MRP2	Multidrug resistance–associated protein 2
NISCH	Neonatal ichthyosis and sclerosing cholangitis syndrome
PFIC	Progressive familial intrahepatic cholestasis
Pi	Protease inhibitor
UDCA	Ursodeoxycholic acid
UGT	Uridine diphosphate-glucuronyl transferase

GENERAL MANAGEMENT OF CHILDREN WITH CHOLESTASIS

Critical to management of all children with cholestasis, particularly with conjugated bilirubin elevations, is the early recognition and implementation of appropriate interventions that can dramatically impact outcomes. Vital factors, such as the age of presentation, clinical and family histories, extrahepatic symptoms, comorbidities, and exposure history, will help form the differential diagnosis and guide initial investigations. Importantly, there is often an acute focus on the infant with cholestasis, as specific, timely interventions can dramatically decrease morbidity in this population. This has resulted in specific guidelines that are available.[1] A general approach to the cholestatic child is presented in **Table 1**.

Table 1
General diagnostic approach to cholestasis in children

Clinical history	• Symptoms of non-hepatic disease
	  ○ Infection/Sepsis
	  ○ Panhypopituitarism
	• Drug/Toxin exposure
	  ○ Comprehensive medication history
	• Family history
	  ○ + consanguinity = ↑ risk of recessive conditions
	  ○ + history of neonatal cholestasis = ↑ suspicion for genetic condition (eg, AGS, PFIC, A1AT, CF)
	• Prenatal history
	  ○ Prenatal ultrasound for structural abnormalities
	  ○ + cholestasis of pregnancy: suspect PFIC
	  ○ + acute fatty liver of pregnancy: suspect LCHAD
	  ○ + maternal infection: suspect TORCH

Physical examination	• Assess for overall ill appearance, palpate for HSM
	• Visualization of stool. + acholic – suspect BA, obstruction
	• Assess for findings of chronic liver disease:
	  ○ Ascites
	  ○ Prominent, superficial abdominal vessels
	  ○ Palmar erythema
	  ○ Spider nevi
	  ○ Digital clubbing
	  ○ Pruritic excoriations
	• Syndromic features:
	  ○ + facial features: suspect AGS
	  ○ Skeletal/bone malformations: suspect ARC
	• Cardiac defects: suspect AGS, BA
	• Laterality defects: suspect BA
	• Pulmonary symptoms: suspect CF, TJP2 deficiency

(continued on next page)

Table 1 (continued)		

Laboratory tests	• First-line testing:
	  ○ Blood: CBC, culture, PT/INR, AST, ALT, ALP, GGT, TB, DB, albumin. Glucose, TSH, T4, review NBS, A1AT levels and phenotype
	  ○ Urine: urinalysis, culture, reducing substances
		• Second-line considerations:
		  ○ General: serum and urinary bile acids, cortisol
		  ○ Metabolic: NH$_3$, lactate, cholesterol, RBC galactose-1-phosphate, urine SA and OA, ceruloplasmin, 24-h urine copper
		  ○ Infectious: HAV, HBV, HCV, EBV, HSV, enterovirus
		  ○ Sweat chloride testing
		  ○ Autoimmune markers: ANA, Anti-Sm, LKM Ab, IgG
		  ○ Genetic testing

Radiographic tests	• Abdominal/Liver ultrasound (to include Doppler and spleen examination) • CXR (to assess heart and vertebral bodies) • Echocardiogram • HIDA scan/Cholangiogram (if suspect BA)	
Additional considerations	• Liver biopsy when BA is suspected • Comprehensive/Targeted genetic testing	

Abbreviations: A1AT, Alpha-1 antitrypsin; AGS, Alagille syndrome; ALP, alkaline phosphatase; ALT, alanine aminotransferase; ANA, antinuclear antibodies; Anti-SM, Anti-Smooth Muscle; ARC, arthrogryposis-renal dysfunction-cholestasis; AST, aspartate aminotransferase; BA, biliary atresia; CBC, complete blood count; CF, cystic fibrosis; CXR, chest X-ray; DB, Direct bilirubin; EBV, Epstein-Barr virus; HAV, hepatitis A virus; HBV, hepatitis B virus; HCV, hepatitis C virus; HIDA, hepatobiliary; HSM, hepatosplenomegaly; HSV, herpes simplex virus; GGT, gamma glutamyl transferase; Ig, immunoglobulin; LCHAD, L-3 hydroxyacyl-CoA dehydrogenase deficiency; LKM, Liver Kidney Microsomal Antibody; NBS, newborn screen; OA, organic acids; PFIC, progressive familial intrahepatic cholestasis; PT/INR, prothrombin time/international normalized ratio; RBC, red blood cell; SA, succinylacetone; TB, total bilirubin; TJP2, tight-junction protein 2; TORCH, toxoplasmosis, other, rubella, cytomegalovirus, herpes; TSH, thyroid-stimulating hormone; ↑, increased; ↓, decreased.

Although targeted therapies may be available to only a minority of children once a diagnosis is established, those who are found to have chronic or progressive disease processes will benefit from intensive nutritional management and support with secondary benefits on development and growth.[2]

ETIOLOGY, MECHANISM OF INJURY, CLINICAL CHARACTERISTICS, AND TREATMENT
Progressive Familial Intrahepatic Cholestasis

Progressive familial intrahepatic cholestasis (PFIC) refers to a group of disorders that cause hepatocellular cholestasis secondary to the disruption of bile formation. Specific genetic defects have been identified that are associated with defective bile acid transport[3–8] **(Table 2)**. Several of these diseases have been discriminated due to recent advancements in next-generation sequencing technologies and it is likely that additional causative defects will be identified in the future. Collectively, these efforts to expand the understanding of the genetic basis of cholestatic disease in the neonate has enabled the identification of an expanded role for mutations in these genes in the development of phenotypic manifestations in older individuals, such as recurrent cholestasis, cryptogenic cirrhosis, and intrahepatic cholestasis of pregnancy.[9]

Symptomatic improvement in pruritus, optimization of nutritional status, and management of complications of chronic liver disease constitute the main medical avenues of treatment for patients with disorders of bile acid transport.[10] Supportive treatment requires aggressive supplementation of fat-soluble vitamins (A, D, E, and K) and administration of medium-chain triglycerides, which are absorbed

Table 2
Defects in bile acid or phospholipid transport

Etiology	Genetic Defect	Histology	Mechanism of Disease	Clinical Characteristics	Treatment
FIC1 Deficiency (PFIC1, Byler syndrome)[8]	ATP8B1	• Bland cholestasis, mild lobular fibrosis, varying degrees of hepatocellular ballooning and giant cell transformation	• Uncertain ○ Possibly involved in maintenance of canalicular membrane integrity ○ Possible effect on FXR with resultant BSEP downregulation	• ↑ AST/ALT/bilirubin. ↓/normal GGTP • + extrahepatic symptoms: diarrhea/malabsorption • Symptom onset in infancy with progression over first decade	• Supportive care • Biliary diversion • Liver transplantation ○ Diarrhea may worsen after transplant ○ Allograft steatohepatitis can occur
BSEP deficiency (PFIC2)[8]	ABCB11	• Nonspecific giant cell hepatitis, IHC staining for BSEP available	• Dysfunctional secretion of bile acids from hepatocyte into canalicular space	• ↑ AST/ALT/bilirubin. ↓/normal GGTP • Symptom onset in infancy with rapid progression over first few years of life • High risk of development of hepatocellular malignancy	• Supportive care • Biliary diversion • Liver transplantation ○ Antibody-mediated recurrent disease can occur
MDR3 deficiency (PFIC3)[8]	ABCB4	• Ductular proliferation	• Decreased excretion of cytoprotective biliary phospholipids with resultant bile duct damage from the detergent activity of bile acids	• ↑ AST/ALT/bilirubin. ↑↑ GGTP • Symptom onset ranges from late infancy to early adulthood with more gradual disease course	• Supportive care • Biliary diversion • Liver transplantation
TJP2 deficiency[6]	TJP2	• Giant cell transformation, micronodular cirrhosis • Absent expression of TJP2 with IHC	• Impairment of hepatocyte tight junctions with resultant leakage of biliary components into liver parenchyma	• ↑ AST/ALT/bilirubin. ↓/normal GGTP • Liver disease if often refractory, requiring liver transplantation	• Supportive care • Liver transplantation

Disease	Gene	Histology	Mechanism	Clinical Features	Treatment
FXR[3]	NR1H4	• Ductular reaction, giant cell transformation and ballooning • Intralobular cholestasis • Absent BSEP expression	• Loss of FXR function results in decreased BSEP promoter activation and absent BSEP expression in the canaliculus	• ↑ AST/ALT/bilirubin. ↓/normal GGTP • Neonatal onset with rapid progression to ESLD • Coagulopathy is common • ↑↑ AFP	• Supportive care • Liver transplantation
Myosin VB[4,5]	MYO5B	• Giant cell transformation, intralobular cholestasis • Abnormal BSEP distribution, coarse granular dislocation of MYO5B	• Impaired targeting of BSEP to the canalicular membrane with decreased bile acid excretion	• ↑ AST/ALT/bilirubin. ↓/normal GGTP • Presentation in the first months of life • Liver disease has been reported to be transient, recurrent, and/or progressive	• Supportive care
Arthrogryposis, renal dysfunction and cholestasis (ARC)[15]	VPS33B (75%) or VIPAR	• Bland cholestasis and ductopenia • Abnormal BSEP distribution	• Missorting of canalicular proteins involved in bile secretion	• ↑AST/ALT/bilirubin. ↓/normal GGTP • Poor growth • Polyuria and proteinuria • Usually fatal in the first year of life but occasional long-term survivors	• Supportive care

Abbreviations: AFP, alpha fetoprotein; ALT, alanine aminotransferase; AST, aspartate aminotransferase; BSEP, bile salt exporter pump; ESLD, End-stage liver disease; FIC, familial intrahepatic cholestasis; FXR, Farnesoid X receptor; GGTP, gamma-glutamyl transpeptidase; IHC, immunohistochemistry; TJP2, tight-junction protein 2; ↑, increased; ↓, decreased.

independently of bile acids. Antipruritic agents, such as ursodeoxycholic acid, rifaximin, hydroxyzine, cholestyramine, naloxone, and sertraline have demonstrated varying degrees of success.[11] Surgical interruption of the enterohepatic circulation through approaches such as ileal exclusion and partial biliary diversion has been shown to be well tolerated, and generally, although not uniformly, results in improvement of pruritus and cholestasis.[12] However, the presence of cirrhosis at the time of diversion has been associated with poor outcomes, and recurrent, self-limited cholestasis episodes can occur.[10] If all else fails, liver transplantation can lead to good overall outcomes, with normalization of bile acid synthesis and growth, even in patients who receive a live-donor organ from a potentially heterozygous parent.[8] However, extrahepatic manifestations of FIC1 deficiency, such as diarrhea, can worsen after transplantation. The development of fatty infiltration of the graft liver is concerning, as this can progress to the development of cirrhosis and require re-transplantation. In these rare cases, internal and external biliary diversions have demonstrated some success in ameliorating the disease process.[13] Additionally, de novo blocking anti-BSEP (bile salt export pump) antibody may cause phenotypic BSEP deficiency following transplant for BSEP disease, particularly in patients with severe truncating or early deleterious mutations.[14]

Disorders of Development

An improved understanding of genes associated with normal hepatobiliary development has led to the identification of several disease processes whereby defects in these genes result in cholestasis (**Table 3**).

The autosomal dominant Alagille syndrome (AGS) is perhaps the most well recognized of these diseases. Disordered cell fate signaling during development can result in bile duct paucity on liver biopsy with cholestasis. The hepatic phenotype in AGS is variable, and although the overall prognosis is relatively good, long-term outcomes are directly linked to the severity of liver or cardiac involvement with approximately one-third of patients requiring a liver transplant.[20]

Neonatal sclerosing cholangitis, with and without ichthyosis, are severe cholangiopathies of neonates. The neonatal ichthyosis and sclerosing cholangitis syndrome (NISCH) is a rare autosomal recessive disorder of sclerosing cholangitis accompanied by scalp hypertrichosis, alopecia, and ichthyosis.[19] In confirmed cases of NISCH, the hepatic phenotype is variable and progression unpredictable. Ursodeoxycholic acid (UDCA) therapy may have some benefit in slowing disease progression, and liver transplantation should be reserved for those with severe disease, as most extrahepatic manifestations persist following surgery.[21] The application of whole-exome sequencing to individuals with the sclerosing cholangitis phenotype, but without ichthyosis revealed novel doublecortin domain containing protein 2 (DCDC2) mutations, expanding not only the molecular spectrum of neonatal sclerosing cholangitis, but also the clinical spectrum of DCDC2 mutations, which had previously been reported in dyslexia, deafness, and nephronpothisis.[18] The resultant ciliopathy in DCDC2-associated sclerosing cholangitis is unlikely to fully explain the severe hepatobiliary phenotype. This is supported by the disparity between the cholestasis and duct destruction seen in DCDC2 disease and other ciliopathies that can involve the liver, such as autosomal recessive polycystic kidney disease (PKHD1 mutations) and autosomal dominant polycystic liver disease (PRKCSH mutations). Subsequently, it has been proposed that the absence of DCDC2 may enable the formation of "cytotoxic" bile or dysregulated cholangiocyte homeostasis, which contributes to the more severe phenotype.[22]

Table 3
Disorders of development

Etiology	Genetic Defect	Histology	Mechanism of Disease	Clinical Characteristics	Treatment

Alagille syndrome (AGS)[16]	JAG1 (>90%) or NOTCH2	• Bile duct paucity (may not be present during infancy)[17]	• Disruption of Notch signaling pathway, which is involved in regulating cell fate during embryogenesis	• Cholestasis, ↑↑ GGTP
				• Hypercholesterolemia with cutaneous xanthomas
				• Cardiovascular malformation
				  ○ Peripheral pulmonic stenosis
				  ○ Tetralogy of Fallot
				• Posterior embryotoxon
				• Unique facial features
				• Vertebral arch defects (butterfly vertebrae)
				• Cerebrovascular anomalies (Moyamoya)
					• Supportive care
					• Antipruritics
					• Biliary diversion
					• Liver transplant

Neonatal sclerosing cholangitis[18]	DCDC2	• Fibrosis, cirrhosis, tortuous bile ducts inserted into the fibrosis • Electron microscopy may show cholangiocytes without cilia	• Normal DCDC2 is part of the microtubule structure involved in ciliary function • DCDC2 mutations lead to failure of primary cilia development • How loss of cilia leads to inflammation and cholestasis is not clear, as it is not typical of hepatorenal ciliopathies	• Neonatal cholestasis • Variable manifestations including pale stools, hepatosplenomegaly, coagulopathy, ascites • ↑ALT, GGTP • Extrahepatic renal disease	• Supportive care • Liver transplantation
Neonatal ichthyosis-sclerosing cholangitis (NISCH)[19]	CLDN1	• Hepatocellular cholestasis, canalicular bile plugs. • Portal fibrosis, steatosis, ductular proliferations and ductopenia have been reported • Absent Claudin-1 expression	• Defect in the tight-junction protein Claudin-1 • Results in increased paracellular permeability and subsequent paracellular bile leakage	• Neonatal cholestasis • ↑ALT, GGTP • Ichthyosis • Alopecia • Portal hypertension	• Supportive care • Ursodeoxycholic acid (UDCA) • Liver transplant (has shown to improve skin lesions in some cases, but most extrahepatic manifestations do not improve)

Abbreviations: ALT, alanine aminotransferase; GGTP, gamma-glutamyl transpeptidase; ↑, increased.

Disorders of Bile Acid Synthesis

Bile acids are the natural detergents made by the liver, which promote bile-induced bile flow and enable fat and fat-soluble vitamin absorption. The primary bile acids, cholic acid and chenodeoxycholic acid, are synthesized by the liver from cholesterol through a series of 17 enzymatic steps. There are 2 principal causes of morbidity in disorders of bile acid synthesis: (1) the failure to make "normal" bile acids results in impaired bile flow with attendant reduction of biliary excretion of individual components, including cholesterol and other fats, proteins, drugs, and environmental toxins out of the liver; and (2) the production and accumulation of "toxic" intermediary metabolites produced because of the block in the bile acid production. Because each of the enzymes in the pathway is regulated by a gene, it is believed that abnormalities in any of the steps of the pathway can be inherited. The clinical phenotype of these disorders are variable with hyperbilirubinemia, liver transaminase elevations, and hepatosplenomegaly being common in individuals with defects in the enzymes responsible for catalyzing reactions in the steroid nucleus.[23] Mild liver disease is seen in those with defects that involve modifications to the cholesterol side with phenotypic manifestations dominated by fat-soluble vitamin malabsorption and/or neurologic disease[23] (**Table 4**). Diagnosis of these disorders is often made with liquid secondary ionization mass spectrometry, formerly known as fast atom bombardment mass spectrometry, or genetic-based testing.

Disorders of Bilirubin Metabolism and Transport

Bilirubin is formed by the breakdown of heme, most notably from red blood cells into carbon monoxide and biliverdin. Biliverdin is then metabolized to bilirubin by the enzyme biliverdin reductase. Most bilirubin is bound to albumin and transported to the liver where it is taken up by hepatic cells for secretion into the biliary ductal system via the multidrug resistance–associated protein 2 (MRP2) after undergoing conjugation via the enzyme uridine diphosphate-glucuronyl transferase (UGT). Defects of this process at various steps can lead to the clinical manifestation of jaundice with a wide spectrum of morbidity and mortality (**Table 5**).

Metabolic Disorders

Several inherited metabolic liver diseases present with cholestasis as major clinical manifestation. Although the phenotype of chronic intrahepatic cholestasis may be shared by these syndromes, the molecular basis for the disease processes as well as prognosis and treatment courses vary (**Table 6**).

Defective cystic fibrosis transmembrane conductance regulator (CFTR) in the cholangiocytes results in a varied spectrum of hepatobiliary manifestations collectively referred to cystic fibrosis associated liver disease (CFLD). A joint National Institutes of Health and Cystic Fibrosis Foundation Clinical Research Workshop on CFLD suggested criteria to diagnose progressive liver disease in patients with cystic fibrosis (CF)[44] (**Box 1**).

CFLD constitutes a significant disease burden, reflective in the fact that it is the third leading cause of mortality in CF.[44] The manifestations of CFLD most commonly become apparent in early childhood; however, cholestasis associated with CF has been reported to be causative in 2% of neonates with jaundice.[45]

Nutritional support and liver health optimization constitute the major management strategies for individuals with CFLD. UDCA therapy is commonly prescribed; however, few trials have assessed its effectiveness and evidence to justify its routine use in CF is insufficient.[46] Monitoring and mitigating the complications of portal hypertension is crucial. Synthetic liver function often remains intact; thus, liver transplantation is often

Table 4
Disorders of bile acid synthesis in children

Etiology	Genetic Defect	Histology	Mechanism of Disease	Clinical Characteristics	Treatment
3β-HSD deficiency[24]	HSD3B7	• Giant cell hepatitis • Can have chronic hepatitis	• Failure to convert 7α-hydroxycholesterol is to 7α-hydroxy-4-cholesten-3-one	• Most common defect • Presents in infancy or later childhood • Neonatal jaundice, poor growth, +HSM • ↑AST/ALT, low/normal GGTP • Fat-soluble vitamin deficiency • Clinical features like PFIC (↑ CB), but usually low serum bile acids and without pruritic	• Oral cholic acid[25]
Δ4-3-oxosteroid 5β-reductase deficiency[24]	AKR1D1	• Lobular disarray with giant cell and pseudoacinar transformation of hepatocytes • Bile stasis • Extramedullary hematopoiesis	• Failure to convert the intermediates 7α-hydroxy-4-cholesten-3-one and 7α,12α-dihydroxy-4-cholesten-3-one to the corresponding 3-oxo-5β(H) intermediates	• Neonatal jaundice, poor growth, +HSM • Fat-soluble vitamin deficiency • Clinical features similar to PFIC (↑ CB), but usually without pruritic and low serum bile acids • ↑AST/ALT, and GGTP	• Oral cholic acid[25]
Oxysterol 7α-hydroxylase deficiency[24]	CYP7B1	• Cholestasis • Bridging fibrosis • Giant cell transformation • Proliferating ductules	• Accumulation of high concentrations of hepato-toxic monohydroxy bile acids with the 3b-hydroxy-D5 structure	• Progressive cholestasis • ↑AST/ALT, low/normal GGTP, +HSM • Synthetic liver dysfunction	• Supportive care • Cholic acid ineffective but chenodeoxycholic may be effective[26] • Liver transplant
27-hydroxylase deficiency (aka CTX)[27]	CYP27A1	• Lobular disarray • Giant cell transformation • Portal tract fibrosis • Ductular reaction	• Reduced synthesis of the primary bile acids leads classically to accumulation of C27 sterol intermediates	• + neurologic dysfunction • Neonatal cholestasis[27] • Diarrhea	• Liver transplant for those with severe neonatal disease • Oral cholic acid[25]

(continued on next page)

Table 4
(continued)

Etiology	Genetic Defect	Histology	Mechanism of Disease	Clinical Characteristics	Treatment
2-methylacyl-CoA racemase deficiency[24]	AMCAR	• Cholestasis • Giant cell transformation • Modest inflammation	• Defects have profound effects on both the bile acid and the fatty acid pathways	• Neonatal cholestasis and fat-soluble vitamin deficiency • Adult presentation with sensory motor neuropathy	• Oral cholic acid[25]
Amidation defects[28]	BAAT	• Bile plugs and lobular cholestasis • Giant cell transformation • Periportal fibrosis	• Defect in the final step in bile acid synthesis, which normally results in glycine and taurine conjugates • Without conjugation, bile acids are less efficient at absorbing fats	• Neonatal cholestasis • Fat-soluble vitamin deficiency • Growth failure • Hepatomegaly can occur • Liver failure has been reported • AST/ALT can be elevated or normal	• Glycocholic acid[29] • Liver transplant in severe cases
Zellweger spectrum disorder[30]	PEX genes	• Nonspecific changes of hepatocyte degeneration • EM with lack of peroxisomes	• Impaired peroxisomal assembly	• Multiorgan dysfunction + neurologic dysfunction • Hepatomegaly • Cholestasis • Abnormal VLCFA • ↑Phytanic and/or pristanic acids	• Supportive care • Multidisciplinary approach to extrahepatic manifestations • Oral cholic acid (no effect on extrahepatic manifestations)[25]

Abbreviations: 3β HSD, 3β-Hydroxy-C27-steroid oxidoreductase; ALT, alanine aminotransferase; AST, aspartate aminotransferase; CTX, cerebrotendinous xanthomatosis; CYP7A1, cholesterol 7α-hydroxylase; CB, conjugated bilirubin; EM, electron microscopy; GGTP, gamma-glutamyl transpeptidase; HSM, hepatosplenomegaly; PFIC, progressive familial intrahepatic cholestasis; VLCFA, very-long-chain fatty acids; ↑, increased.

Table 5
Disorders of bilirubin metabolism and transport

Etiology	Genetic Defect	Histology	Mechanism of Disease	Clinical Characteristics	Treatment

Crigler-Najjar[31]	UGT1A1	• Classically described as normal
		• Fibrosis can be seen, generally in older individuals[32]
			• Severely dysfunctional or deficient UGT1A1 results in pathologic elevation in unconjugated bilirubin (UB)	• 2 described phenotypes
				  ○ Type I: severe congenital nonhemolytic jaundice (UB level >20 mg/dL) with kernicterus
				  ○ Type II: less severe than type I (UB level 10–20 mg/dL), kernicterus is less common
					• Intensive phototherapy
					• Avoidance of medications that displace bilirubin
					• Phenobarbital for Type II
					• Plasmapheresis
					• Albumin infusions
					• Liver transplant is curative

Gilbert syndrome[31]	UGT1A1 (often in the TATA promoter region)	• Normal	• Promoter region mutations result in reduced expression, but normal function, of UGT1A1 • Other exonal mutations have been described with resultant mild effects on protein function	• Mild UB elevation (usually UB level <3 mg/dL) without bilirubinuria or hemolysis • Often with mild scleral icterus	• No specific therapy needed • Avoidance of unnecessary testing
Rotor syndrome[33]	SLCO1B1 and SLCO1B3	• Normal	• Dysfunctional organic anion transporting polypeptides (OATP) 1B1 and 1B3, which act to normally reuptake bilirubin conjugates	• Mild conjugated and unconjugated hyperbilirubinemia (total bilirubin levels 2–5 mg/dL) • Scleral icterus • Normal AST/ALT • Increased urine coproporphyrin	• No specific therapy needed • Avoidance of unnecessary testing
Dubin-Johnson[34,35]	ABCC2	• Accumulation of dark melaninlike pigment in lysosomes • Pigment may be absent in infants • Normal hepatic architecture	• Absent or dysfunctional multidrug resistance–associated protein 2 (MRP2) • Abnormal excretion of conjugated bilirubin across the canalicular membrane	• Usually presents in young adulthood with elevated conjugated bilirubin • Can present in neonatal period	• No specific therapy needed • Avoidance of unnecessary testing

Abbreviations: ALT, alanine aminotransferase; AST, aspartate aminotransferase.

Table 6
Metabolic disorders

Etiology	Genetic Defect	Histology	Mechanism of Disease	Clinical Characteristics	Treatment

CFLD[36]	CFTR	• Pathognomonic focal biliary cirrhosis
		• May progress to multilobular biliary cirrhosis
		• 50% may have steatosis
			• Complex; thought to result from defective CFTR protein with resulting small duct obstruction, inflammation, bile duct proliferation, and portal fibrosis	• Variable phenotype that can include
				  ○ ↑AST/ALT, rare to have synthetic dysfunction
				  ○ Neonatal cholestasis
				  ○ Portal hypertension (d/t biliary cirrhosis)
					• Supportive care
					• Surgical porto-systemic shunt placement
					• Liver transplantation

A1AT[37]	SERPINA1	• Can change with age
		• In infancy: paucity or proliferation, intracellular cholestasis, inflammation, giant cell transformation
		• Characteristic periodic acid-Schiff (PAS)-positive, diastase resistant globules
			• Misfolded A1AT Z protein is retained in hepatocyte
			• Gain-of-function defect with several proposed mechanisms:
			  ○ Impaired endoplasmic reticulum-associated degradation
			  ○ Abnormal unfolded protein response (UPR) activation
			  ○ Decreased autophagy
				• Wide variability
				• ↑ AST/ALT/GGTP in minority (~20%) of PiZZ individuals
				• Sever phenotype is possible with neonatal cholestasis and liver disease progression
				• Hepatocellular carcinoma can occur
					• Supportive care
					• No disease-specific therapy
					• Future targets:
					  ○ Autophagy enhancers
					  ○ Decreasing Z protein production
					• Liver transplantation

Wilson disease[38]	ATP7B	• Wide range of patterns
		• Most show steatosis, portal and lobular inflammation, and fibrosis
		• Elevated hepatic copper content
			• Due to abnormal copper transport
			• Normal biliary copper excretion is reduced and copper accumulates in the liver
				• Degree of liver disease and timing on symptom onset is variable due to:
				  ○ Difference in dietary copper
				  ○ Genetic susceptibility
				  ○ Comorbidities
				• Extrahepatic copper deposition occurs: CNS/symptoms, K-F rings
				• ↓ Ceruloplasmin
				• Anemia is common
				• ↑ Hepatic copper content
				• ↑ Urinary copper
				• ALF can be initial presentation
					• Chelation therapy (D-penicillamine or trientine) +/− zinc
					• Guidelines are available[39]
					• Low-copper diet
					• Management of disease complications such as portal hypertension and CNS symptoms

Disease	Gene	Histology	Molecular mechanism	Clinical features	Management

Niemann-Pick type C[40]	NPC1	• Giant cell transformation
		• Neonatal hepatitis
		• Storage material and fibrosis is prominent in more progressive disease
		• EM with whorled and irregular lamellar inclusions[41]
			• Abnormal endosomal-lysosomal trafficking results in accumulation of multiple lipids in lysosomes	• Age-based presentation:
				  ○ Pre-perinatal (<2 mo)
				  ○ Early infantile (2 mo to <2 y)
				  ○ Late infantile (2–6 y)
				  ○ Juvenile (6–15 y)
				  ○ Adult (>15 y)
				• Cholestasis associated with perinatal and early infantile forms:
				  ○ Prolonged jaundice
				  ○ Mild HSM
				  ○ Neurologic morbidity is severe
				• ALF can be manifestation
					• Mainstay of therapy is symptom management, often with multidisciplinary team
					• Miglustat may slow neurologic deterioration.
					• Clinical guidelines are available[40]

NICCD[42]	SLC25A13	• Classic "tetralogy" of steatosis, necrotic inflammation, cholestasis, and fibrosis[43]	• Citrin is a mitochondrial solute carrier protein • Functions as Ca^{2+}-binding aspartate-glutamate carrier • Involved in glycolysis, gluconeogenesis, and urea cycle functions	• Neonatal intrahepatic cholestasis • Variable liver dysfunction • Hepatomegaly • ↑ NH_3, hypoglycemia • Most cases resolve by 12 mo • Minority of disease progresses to liver failure	• Supportive care • Liver transplant in severe, progressive cases

Abbreviations: A1AT, Alpha-1 antitrypsin; ALF, Acute Liver Failure; ALT, alanine aminotransferase; AST, aspartate aminotransferase; CFLD, cystic fibrosis associated liver disease; CFTR, Cystic fibrosis transmembrane conductance regulator; CNS, central nervous system; EM, electron microscopy; GGTP, gamma-glutamyl transpeptidase; HSM, hepatosplenomegaly; K-F, Kayser-Fleischer rings; ↑, increased; ↓, decreased.

Box 1
Diagnostic criteria for cystic fibrosis associated liver disease (CFLD)

Requires ≥2 of the following:

- Hepatomegaly (eg, liver edge palpable >2 cm below the costal margin) and/or splenomegaly, confirmed by ultrasonography.
- Abnormalities of alanine aminotransferase, aspartate aminotransferase, and gamma-glutamyl transpeptidase above the laboratory upper limits of normal for more than 6 months, after excluding other causes of liver disease.
- Ultrasonographic evidence of coarseness, nodularity, increased echogenicity, or portal hypertension.
- Liver biopsy showing focal biliary cirrhosis or multilobular cirrhosis (if performed).

---

reserved for those with severe complications related to their portal hypertension. A portosystemic shunt can be an effective treatment in select patients with variceal bleeding; long-term outcomes are comparable to those for patients who undergo liver transplantation.[47]

A1AT liver disease is the most frequent genetic cause of liver disease in children and the most common indication for liver transplantation.[48] The A1AT protein is a protease inhibitor (Pi) that is produced in the liver and primarily acts in the lung to degrade neutrophil elastase and regulate inflammation. Thus, in deficiency states, A1AT disease can cause unmitigated inflammation in the airway with resultant emphysema. Unlike this *loss of function* mechanism driving lung pathology, the liver disease is a *gain-of-function* process in which abnormal protein folding results in aberrant retention in the hepatocyte and subsequent cirrhosis.[49,50] More than 100 variants of the Pi protein have been identified, with PiMM representing the normal phenotype. Most of the disease burden is manifest in PiZZ individuals; however, other rarer variants have been associated with morbidity. There is a wide spectrum of liver disease among patients with the classic form of A1AT (PiZZ) deficiency and very little is known about what predisposes those affected to a severe, progressive decline in hepatic function.[51] There are no current disease-specific therapies for the hepatic manifestations in A1AT deficiency and the initial treatment remains symptomatic care. The importance of providing fat-soluble vitamins when indicated, adequate nutrition, and counseling to avoid obesity, alcohol, smoking, and second-hand smoke cannot be overemphasized. However, as the pathophysiology is increasingly elucidated, more and more therapeutic targets are being identified.[37]

Wilson disease is due to defective copper transport and can result in excessive hepatic copper accumulation and subsequent damage.[38] The cholestasis associated with Wilson disease is often the result of substantial liver damage, and can be severe in those who develop acute liver failure. Importantly, other cholestatic liver disease, especially sclerosing cholangitis, can have evidence of systemic copper overload and laboratory abnormalities indicating dysfunctional copper metabolism.[52,53] Low ceruloplasmin, high 24-hour urinary copper, and D-penicillamine challenge have been shown to be specific for Wilson.[53,54] Treatment strategies in Wilson disease are aimed at chelation and/or preventing copper absorption with zinc. Symptomatic patients are recommended to receive higher dosages of medications to stabilize and then reverse hepatic damage, whereas asymptomatic patients are dosed lower with the goal to prevent additional copper accumulation and damage. A low-copper diet, as well as the management of portal hypertension and neurologic morbidity, are important considerations.[38]

SUMMARY

Cholestasis in children, while the result of disparate etiologies, is increasingly being recognized to result from specific defects in many of the processes that regulate the normal formation and flow of bile. Identification of the causative molecular abnormality can prove highly beneficial for those individuals in whom precise, disease-altering therapies or interventions can be implemented. Furthermore, the recognition of specific abnormality may enable future efforts aimed at gene replacement or protein augmentation therapies. Finally, an understanding of the genetic and molecular basis for disease may be beneficial as it relates to prognosis and family planning.

REFERENCES

1. Fawaz R, Baumann U, Ekong U, et al. Guideline for the evaluation of cholestatic jaundice in infants: joint recommendations of the North American Society for Pediatric Gastroenterology, Hepatology, and Nutrition and the European Society for Pediatric Gastroenterology, Hepatology, and Nutrition. J Pediatr Gastroenterol Nutr 2017;64(1):154–68.
2. Nightingale S, Ng VL. Optimizing nutritional management in children with chronic liver disease. Pediatr Clin North Am 2009;56(5):1161–83.
3. Gomez-Ospina N, Potter CJ, Xiao R, et al. Mutations in the nuclear bile acid receptor FXR cause progressive familial intrahepatic cholestasis. Nat Commun 2016;7:10713.
4. Gonzales E, Taylor SA, Davit-Spraul A, et al. MYO5B mutations cause cholestasis with normal serum gamma-glutamyl transferase activity in children without microvillous inclusion disease. Hepatology 2017;65(1):164–73.
5. Qiu YL, Gong JY, Feng JY, et al. Defects in myosin VB are associated with a spectrum of previously undiagnosed low gamma-glutamyltransferase cholestasis. Hepatology 2017;65(5):1655–69.
6. Sambrotta M, Strautnieks S, Papouli E, et al. Mutations in TJP2 cause progressive cholestatic liver disease. Nat Genet 2014;46(4):326–8.
7. Sambrotta M, Thompson RJ. Mutations in TJP2, encoding zona occludens 2, and liver disease. Tissue Barriers 2015;3(3):e1026537.
8. Srivastava A. Progressive familial intrahepatic cholestasis. J Clin Exp Hepatol 2014;4(1):25–36.
9. Vitale G, Gitto S, Raimondi F, et al. Cryptogenic cholestasis in young and adults: ATP8B1, ABCB11, ABCB4, and TJP2 gene variants analysis by high-throughput sequencing. J Gastroenterol 2018;53(8):945–58.
10. Squires JE, Celik N, Morris A, et al. Clinical variability after partial external biliary diversion in familial intrahepatic cholestasis 1 deficiency. J Pediatr Gastroenterol Nutr 2017;64(3):425–30.
11. Thebaut A, Habes D, Gottrand F, et al. Sertraline as an additional treatment for cholestatic pruritus in children. J Pediatr Gastroenterol Nutr 2017;64(3):431–5.
12. Wang KS, Tiao G, Bass LM, et al. Analysis of surgical interruption of the enterohepatic circulation as a treatment for pediatric cholestasis. Hepatology 2017;65(5):1645–54.
13. Usui M, Isaji S, Das BC, et al. Liver retransplantation with external biliary diversion for progressive familial intrahepatic cholestasis type 1: a case report. Pediatr Transplant 2009;13(5):611–4.
14. Siebold L, Dick AA, Thompson R, et al. Recurrent low gamma-glutamyl transpeptidase cholestasis following liver transplantation for bile salt export pump (BSEP) disease (posttransplant recurrent BSEP disease). Liver Transpl 2010;16(7):856–63.

15. Gissen P, Tee L, Johnson CA, et al. Clinical and molecular genetic features of ARC syndrome. Hum Genet 2006;120(3):396–409.

16. Saleh M, Kamath BM, Chitayat D. Alagille syndrome: clinical perspectives. Appl Clin Genet 2016;9:75–82.

17. Clouston AD. Pathologic features of hereditary cholestatic diseases. Surg Pathol Clin 2018;11(2):313–27.

18. Girard M, Bizet AA, Lachaux A, et al. DCDC2 mutations cause neonatal sclerosing cholangitis. Hum Mutat 2016;37(10):1025–9.

19. Grosse B, Cassio D, Yousef N, et al. Claudin-1 involved in neonatal ichthyosis sclerosing cholangitis syndrome regulates hepatic paracellular permeability. Hepatology 2012;55(4):1249–59.

20. Kamath BM, Baker A, Houwen R, et al. Systematic review: the epidemiology, natural history, and burden of Alagille syndrome. J Pediatr Gastroenterol Nutr 2018; 67(2):148–56.

21. Paganelli M, Stephenne X, Gilis A, et al. Neonatal ichthyosis and sclerosing cholangitis syndrome: extremely variable liver disease severity from claudin-1 deficiency. J Pediatr Gastroenterol Nutr 2011;53(3):350–4.

22. Grammatikopoulos T, Sambrotta M, Strautnieks S, et al. Mutations in DCDC2 (doublecortin domain containing protein 2) in neonatal sclerosing cholangitis. J Hepatol 2016;65(6):1179–87.

23. Setchell KD, Heubi JE. Defects in bile acid biosynthesis—diagnosis and treatment. J Pediatr Gastroenterol Nutr 2006;43(Suppl 1):S17–22.

24. Heubi JE, Setchell KD, Bove KE. Inborn errors of bile acid metabolism. Semin Liver Dis 2007;27(3):282–94.

25. Heubi JE, Bove KE, Setchell KDR. Oral cholic acid is efficacious and well tolerated in patients with bile acid synthesis and Zellweger spectrum disorders. J Pediatr Gastroenterol Nutr 2017;65(3):321–6.

26. Dai D, Mills PB, Footitt E, et al. Liver disease in infancy caused by oxysterol 7 alpha-hydroxylase deficiency: successful treatment with chenodeoxycholic acid. J Inherit Metab Dis 2014;37(5):851–61.

27. Gong JY, Setchell KDR, Zhao J, et al. Severe neonatal cholestasis in cerebrotendinous xanthomatosis: genetics, immunostaining, mass spectrometry. J Pediatr Gastroenterol Nutr 2017;65(5):561–8.

28. Setchell KD, Heubi JE, Shah S, et al. Genetic defects in bile acid conjugation cause fat-soluble vitamin deficiency. Gastroenterology 2013;144(5):945–55.e946 [quiz: e914–5].

29. Heubi JE, Setchell KD, Jha P, et al. Treatment of bile acid amidation defects with glycocholic acid. Hepatology 2015;61(1):268–74.

30. Steinberg SJ, Raymond GV, Braverman NE, et al. Zellweger spectrum disorder. In: Adam MP, Ardinger HH, Pagon RA, et al, editors. Seattle (WA: GeneReviews((R)); 1993.

31. Sampietro M, Iolascon A. Molecular pathology of Crigler-Najjar type I and II and Gilbert's syndromes. Haematologica 1999;84(2):150–7.

32. Mitchell E, Ranganathan S, McKiernan P, et al. Hepatic parenchymal injury in Crigler-Najjar type I. J Pediatr Gastroenterol Nutr 2018;66(4):588–94.

33. Jirsa M, Knisely AS, Schinkel A, et al. Rotor syndrome. In: Adam MP, Ardinger HH, Pagon RA, et al, editors. Seattle (WA: GeneReviews((R)); 1993.

34. Memon N, Weinberger BI, Hegyi T, et al. Inherited disorders of bilirubin clearance. Pediatr Res 2016;79(3):378–86.

35. Togawa T, Mizuochi T, Sugiura T, et al. Clinical, pathologic, and genetic features of neonatal Dubin-Johnson syndrome: a multicenter study in Japan. J Pediatr 2018;196:161–7.e1.
36. Kamal N, Surana P, Koh C. Liver disease in patients with cystic fibrosis. Curr Opin Gastroenterol 2018;34(3):146–51.
37. Lomas DA, Hurst JR, Gooptu B. Update on alpha-1 antitrypsin deficiency: new therapies. J Hepatol 2016;65(2):413–24.
38. Schilsky ML. Wilson disease: diagnosis, treatment, and follow-up. Clin Liver Dis 2017;21(4):755–67.
39. Roberts EA, Schilsky ML, American Association for Study of Liver Diseases (AASLD). Diagnosis and treatment of Wilson disease: an update. Hepatology 2008;47(6):2089–111.
40. Geberhiwot T, Moro A, Dardis A, et al. Consensus clinical management guidelines for Niemann-Pick disease type C. Orphanet J Rare Dis 2018;13(1):50.
41. Jevon GP, Dimmick JE. Histopathologic approach to metabolic liver disease: part 1. Pediatr Dev Pathol 1998;1(3):179–99.
42. Chen ST, Su YN, Ni YH, et al. Diagnosis of neonatal intrahepatic cholestasis caused by citrin deficiency using high-resolution melting analysis and a clinical scoring system. J Pediatr 2012;161(4):626–631 e622.
43. Jiang GY, Cheng ZM, Liu KS. Neonatal intrahepatic cholestasis caused by citrin deficiency: a histopathologic study of 10 cases. Zhonghua Bing Li Xue Za Zhi 2012;41(7):452–5 [in Chinese].
44. Leung DH, Narkewicz MR. Cystic fibrosis-related cirrhosis. J Cyst Fibros 2017; 16(Suppl 2):S50–61.
45. Stonebraker JR, Ooi CY, Pace RG, et al. Features of severe liver disease with portal hypertension in patients with cystic fibrosis. Clin Gastroenterol Hepatol 2016; 14(8):1207–15.e3.
46. Cheng K, Ashby D, Smyth RL. Ursodeoxycholic acid for cystic fibrosis-related liver disease. Cochrane Database Syst Rev 2017;(9):CD000222.
47. Gooding I, Dondos V, Gyi KM, et al. Variceal hemorrhage and cystic fibrosis: outcomes and implications for liver transplantation. Liver Transpl 2005;11(12): 1522–6.
48. Silverman GA, Pak SC, Perlmutter DH. Disorders of protein misfolding: alpha-1-antitrypsin deficiency as prototype. J Pediatr 2013;163(2):320–6.
49. Gooptu B, Dickens JA, Lomas DA. The molecular and cellular pathology of alpha(1)-antitrypsin deficiency. Trends Mol Med 2014;20(2):116–27.
50. Joly P, Vignaud H, Di Martino J, et al. ERAD defects and the HFE-H63D variant are associated with increased risk of liver damages in Alpha 1-antitrypsin deficiency. PLoS One 2017;12(6):e0179369.
51. Perlmutter DH. Alpha-1-antitrypsin deficiency: importance of proteasomal and autophagic degradative pathways in disposal of liver disease-associated protein aggregates. Annu Rev Med 2011;62:333–45.
52. Gross JB Jr, Ludwig J, Wiesner RH, et al. Abnormalities in tests of copper metabolism in primary sclerosing cholangitis. Gastroenterology 1985;89(2):272–8.
53. Martins da Costa C, Baldwin D, Portmann B, et al. Value of urinary copper excretion after penicillamine challenge in the diagnosis of Wilson's disease. Hepatology 1992;15(4):609–15.
54. Sood V, Rawat D, Khanna R, et al. Cholestatic liver disease masquerading as Wilson disease. Indian J Gastroenterol 2015;34(2):174–7.

Assessment and Treatment of Nonadherence in Transplant Recipients

Caitlin Shneider, BA[a], Claire Dunphy, MA[b], Eyal Shemesh, MD[c],*,
Rachel A. Annunziato, PhD[d]

KEYWORDS

- Transplant • Adherence • MLVI • CoV • Intervention

KEY POINTS

- Despite potentially severe consequences of nonadherence to immunosuppressant medications after organ transplantation, no "gold standard" exists to routinely and objectively measure adherence.
- There are 2 types of adherence measurement methods: direct measurements, which includes medication level variation, and indirect measurements, which include self-reports and electronic monitoring.
- Although several clinical interventions have sought to improve adherence, no conclusive evidence exists to support the use of any specific intervention strategy to date.
- Clinicians may consider routinely monitoring medication blood levels to identify nonadherence and evaluate psychosocial risks to tailor specific intervention efforts.

The number of solid organ transplant operations is increasing; in 2016, more than 33,000 transplant operations were performed, marking an almost 20% increase from 2012.[1,2] Adherence to immunosuppressant drug regimens after transplantation is a critical aspect of the success of organ transplantation.[3] And yet, nonadherence to immunosuppressant regimen remains the leading cause of preventable graft failure and is a significant cause of morbidity and mortality.[4–11] Therefore, it is essential to examine behavioral and psychological aspects of organ transplantation and the

Disclosure Statement: Supported by NIH/NIDDK award #U34 DK112661 (E. Shemesh). The funders had no role in data accumulation, interpretation, or publication efforts.
[a] Center for Translational Science, Children's National Medical Center, 111 Michigan Avenue Northwest, 5th Floor Main, Suite 5500, Office 5533, Washington, DC 20010, USA; [b] Clinical Psychology, Department of Psychology, Fordham University, 441 East Fordham Road, Dealy Hall, Bronx, NY 10458, USA; [c] Division of Behavioral and Developmental Health, The Department of Pediatrics, Kravis Children's Hospital, Icahn School of Medicine at Mount Sinai, Box 1198, 1 Gustave L Levy Place, New York, NY 10029, USA; [d] Psychology, Fordham College at Rose Hill, Fordham University, 441 East Fordham Road, Dealy Hall, Bronx, NY 10458, USA
* Corresponding author.
E-mail address: eyal.shemesh@mssm.edu

Gastroenterol Clin N Am 47 (2018) 939–948
https://doi.org/10.1016/j.gtc.2018.07.015
0889-8553/18/© 2018 Elsevier Inc. All rights reserved.

Abbreviations

CoV	Coefficient of variability
MALT	Medication Adherence in Children Who Had a Liver Transplant
MLVI	Medication level variability index
RCT	Randomized controlled trials
WRBL	Within-range blood levels

---

posttransplantation period, in an effort to identify patients at risk of nonadherence, bolster support to encourage adherence, and prolong organ (and patient) survival.

Despite the clinical relevance of nonadherence, to date, there has not been an accepted "gold standard" approach to measure adherence, let alone to target and improve nonadherence.[12] In this article, we attempt to summarize evidence related to assessment, monitoring, and treatment of nonadherence, and review the potential clinical relevance of this information.

DEFINING "ADHERENCE"

The term "nonadherence" is used to describe general behaviors that deviate from a prescribed health regimen,[13] in cases in which the patient (or, parent, guardian, caretaker) has agreed to follow the regimen.[14] This can include improper medication ingestion, failure to attend follow-up clinic visits, failure to comply with recommendations from physicians, as well as others. In the World Health Organization (WHO) framework, nonadherence does not include cases in which the patient/caretaker overtly disagrees with treatment recommendations. In this article, we focus on nonadherence to immunosuppressant medications (and not other aspects of the regimen), given its direct impact on organ rejection and graft loss, and given that most of the data pertain to medication adherence, not other types of adherence. Even though the WHO definition makes a distinction between cases in which patients agree with the prescribed regimen or not, this issue has not been systematically examined in the transplant setting: it is presumably highly unusual that patients or caretakers overtly disagree with the recommendation to take immunosuppressants.

DIRECT AND INDIRECT MEASUREMENTS OF ADHERENCE

To date, there is no agreed "gold standard" method to measure adherence, and no threshold has been defined and widely accepted for the determination that a patient is "nonadherent." The issue of threshold is important: most, if not all, patients sometimes miss a dose. If we do not know at what point "missing some doses" starts to predict poor transplant outcomes, we will not know which patients or families to target for intervention. This fact has led to interventions that do not predefine a certain degree of nonadherence as an entry criterion, resulting in an inability to show an effect on transplant outcomes, because most patients in intervention studies are sufficiently adherent at entry anyway.[15] Nevertheless, various assessment methods have been used, and those have been classified as either direct or indirect. A direct measurement includes a direct observed therapy, measurement of the level of a drug or metabolite in blood or urine, and detection or measurement of a biological marker added to the drug formulation.[16] These direct methodologies are recognized as more accurate but are frequently more expensive. Examples of direct measures include direct observation of medication intake,[17,18] the Proteus Chip,[19] and medication blood levels. Such measures are less subject to bias but sometimes require significant resources to implement.[16] The transplant field is particularly fortunate in this regard because medication blood-level assessments are a part of standard care and therefore do not require additional resources to obtain. Indirect measures include patient report of such ingestion, medication refill rates, or electronic pill-box monitoring devices (none of which directly measure actual ingestion, although they may be related to it).[15]

Direct observation of medication-taking is costly, time-consuming, and largely impractical, except in specific settings such as inpatient units or jails. The Proteus Chip is a technology innovation that detects ingestion by adding an inert component to a capsule; an extracorporeal sensor detects the presence of that component once the medication is digested, and sends the information in real-time to a prespecified recipient (eg, the patient, physician). The chip is costly and currently unavailable in transplant settings. Even if it were available, it is not clear that truly nonadherent patients would be able or willing to use it. Therefore, in practice, direct measurement of nonadherence to immunosuppressant medications after transplantation has been largely focused on medication blood levels, which are obtained routinely in clinical practice. Those include 2 methods evaluating the degree of fluctuation between individual levels: the medication level variability index (MLVI) and the Coefficient of Variability (CoV), as well as an evaluation of within-range blood levels (WRBLs). MLVI, which is the most extensively studied construct, is calculated as the standard deviation of a set of at least 3 tacrolimus trough blood levels.[20] A high MLVI denotes erratic medication blood levels. A threshold of 2.0 to 2.5 MLVI has been consistently found to be indicative of future risk in children and adult liver transplant recipients,[20-22] as well as other organ transplant groups.[23] The CoV approach builds on the MLVI calculation by dividing it by the patient average. The result is a number that expresses variability as a fraction or percentage that is "adjusted" to the mean. This approach is advantageous in cases in which means are substantially different between examined cohorts and therefore allows for comparisons between populations that have different target levels. This approach has frequently been used in kidney transplant recipients, where the primary immunosuppressant is cyclosporine. In this group, immunosuppressant levels are higher and more variable, which is favorable for this construct.[24,25] However, several limitations exist. CoV is not as good a measure of variance when the dataset's mean is close to zero. Similarly, CoV is limited when the data are "constrained" in one direction and not in the other.[26] A final direct measurement of nonadherence, WRBL, is a classification of the amount of medication in the blood as either within or out of a predefined target range.[27-31] This measurement approach is subject to "white-coat adherence" bias (a situation in which patients take the medication only or primarily before a blood-level draw), and has not been robustly correlated with outcomes.

Objective but indirect measurements of nonadherence to immunosuppressant medications include electronic monitoring,[5,32-41] tracking pill counts,[27,42,43] and determining medication refill rates.[27,44,45] Electronic monitoring typically involves a microchip in the cap of a pill bottle that records the date and time that the container was opened. This method provides information about the frequency and timing of the pill bottle opening. Of course, opening a pill bottle is not the same as ingestion of a medication. In addition, electronic monitoring is relatively cumbersome (some patients will simply not use it) and expensive.[46] Therefore, the most nonadherent patients are less likely to use it, making this method largely unsuited for screening efforts. We found that when electronic measurement of adherence was used in intervention studies, the studies failed to show an effect on transplant outcomes even though they largely did find an improvement in adherence, as measured by the electronic device. This suggests that electronic monitoring is not a suitable way to measure adherence in intervention studies or perhaps clinical care in transplant settings.[15] Pill count estimate (the number of pills ingested by counting the remaining the pills in the bottles), and refill rates (or, medication possession ratio) similarly extrapolate the number of pills consumed by quantifying the number of pills left in the bottle or the number of refill prescription refills. These methods do not directly measure whether the patient actually ingested the medication but are less expensive and cumbersome than electronic monitors. Obtaining accurate refill information requires the provider to know which pharmacy the patient gets the medications from, and a pharmacy's agreement to provide this information must be secured (both of which may sometimes be hard to accomplish in the United States). In addition, refill rates cannot be used to measure patient adherence in situations in which automatic refills are used, an increasingly prevalent practice.

Other indirect measurement methods include patient self-report or parent-proxy report[27,47–57] and clinic attendance rates.[56,58] Self-report has been collected through questionnaire completion or clinician-conducted interviews. Although self-report can be a clinically useful tool to help patients and families reflect on their perception of adherence, a more rigorous methodology is needed for objective assessment and ongoing monitoring, as patient self-report that a medication was taken is not synonymous with actually taking the medication.[12]

TREATMENT OF NONADHERENCE

Nonadherence to immunosuppressant medication has been firmly established as a key risk factor for adverse outcomes among transplant recipients.[59] Therefore, implementation of empirically supported methods to address it has been labeled a priority for research and practice in the field.[60] Because the reasons for nonadherence are many and vary widely, a number of intervention strategies have been investigated (eg, patient education techniques, cognitive behavioral approaches, behavioral interventions) across pediatric, adolescent, and adult patient groups and within different transplant groups.

Several challenges to studying adherence interventions have been described previously.[15] These include the prevalence of single-center studies with small sample sizes, selection bias (nonadherent patients are less likely to attend clinic appointments and participate in research studies, and therefore many studies may not be capturing the truly nonadherent population), selection of inappropriate outcome variables (notably, behavioral outcomes, such as medication-taking, are often used in place of objective indicators of adherence or medical outcomes), and failure to target only those patients who are nonadherent (improvement in adherence for patients who are already quite adherent does not translate to improvement in adherence for nonadherent patients).[15]

With these caveats in mind, a substantial body of literature has accumulated dedicated to the investigation of such interventions, yet a successful approach for the management of medication nonadherence has yet to be identified. As highlighted by a recent systematic review of studies in transplant medicine,[12] only a small minority of studies has shown statistically significant improvement in transplant outcomes.[29,61,62] Notably, all of these studies were conducted using nonrandomized research designs and with small sample sizes. None of the randomized-controlled trials (RCTs) published thus far have demonstrated any improvement in transplant outcomes.[31,33–41,45,51–55,57,63–66] As no RCTs, and few studies overall, have shown improvement in outcomes, such as rejection, organ loss, and other objective measures of graft function, the search for an effective way to treat nonadherence remains elusive.

A related consideration is timing of intervention, as previous studies have suggested that adherence is variable, not stable, over time.[67–69] As observed in the Medication

Adherence in Children Who Had a Liver Transplant (MALT) cohort, which included a nationally representative sample of 400 pediatric liver transplant recipients, patients who are adherent to medication do not necessarily continue to be adherent.[70] Unfortunately, MALT also reported that nonadherence appears to persist among a majority of patients once it is present, with the risk of poor clinical outcomes increasing with time of nonadherence. In the MALT study, nearly 60% of patients who were nonadherent during the first year of the study were also nonadherent during the second year.

NONADHERENCE DURING THE TRANSITION TO ADULTHOOD

The period of time during which transplant recipients transition from pediatric to adult health care settings, where the burden of self-management rests more fully with the patient, has been identified as a period of increased risk for patients. The transition process has been characterized by an increase in rates of nonadherence to medications as well as likelihood for poor clinical outcomes, including rejection.[20,71–73] This transitional time is a potentially promising area for intervention,[74] and a specific area of interest for intervention focus is the acquisition of self-management skills. One approach to this issue has been to advocate for increasing patients' degree of self-management during the transition process, but findings suggest that during this transitional period, greater self-management actually may be associated with worse adherence.[58,75] Similar results were reported in MALT, in which a higher level of patient-reported self-management at baseline was associated with worse adherence and, furthermore, emerged as a predictor of graft rejection during a 2-year follow-up period.[76] Although the achievement of self-management is an important part of the transition process, increasing the degree of self-management may actually lead to worse outcomes. Given these findings, it seems likely that more consideration should be given to an individual patient's level of readiness for this responsibility. More individualized, developmentally sensitive interventions, rather than more generalized interventions applied on the basis of age alone, are likely to be more appropriate for this time period.

SUMMARY

From this constellation of findings, it follows that changes should be made in the way interventions are studied and implemented. For example, recruitment strategies are important considerations, and must include specific efforts to prevent selection bias.[77] To account for variability in adherence, interventions should use longer-term surveillance of adherence, even for patients who appear to display good adherence at any given time. Additionally, interventions should use objective measures of adherence shown to be related to clinical outcomes, such as the MLVI, rather than indirect indicators, which may provide a poor representation of adherence. Successful interventions should result in better clinical outcomes (eg, rejection rates), and therefore these outcomes must be measured for intervention programs to be appropriately evaluated.

CLINICAL IMPLICATIONS

Although measures such as the MLVI can be used to monitor adherence in posttransplant care, to date, it has not yet been convincingly shown that such monitoring, or any monitoring of adherence, results in improvements in transplant outcomes. Much more work is needed to determine how we can help patients to improve their adherence once we determine that adherence is not optimal in a specific case. High-risk periods, such as adolescence, in which transition to adulthood happens, should be a specific focus of attention, but again rigorous intervention studies are needed to move the field forward. In the absence of robust evidence to support any particular intervention strategy, we believe that clinicians should consider monitoring adherence as a part of routine clinical practice and adding psychosocial assessments as needed to help focus intervention efforts.[78] We cannot recommend a specific standard approach to improving adherence at this point, but we definitely do recommend a multipronged clinical approach that tailors interventions to specific patient needs.

REFERENCES

1. Scutti S. US organ transplants increased nearly 20% in five years. In: CNN. 2017. Available at: https://www.cnn.com/2017/01/09/health/organ-donation-2016/index.html. Accessed on December 12, 2017.
2. Organs & tissues for transplant. In: LifeCenter Northwest. Available at: http://www.lcnw.org/donation/organs-tissues-for-transplant/. Accessed December 28, 2017.
3. Colaneri J. An overview of transplant immunosuppression–history, principles, and current practices in kidney transplantation. Nephrol Nurs J 2014;41(6):549–60.
4. Cromer BA, Tarnowski KJ. Noncompliance in adolescents: a review. J Dev Behav Pediatr 1989;10:207–15.
5. De Geest S, Schafer-Keller P, Denhaerynck K, et al. Supporting medication adherence in renal transplantation (SMART): a pilot RCT to improve adherence to immunosuppressive regimens. Clin Transplant 2006;20:359–68.
6. Dew MA, Kormos RL, Roth LH, et al. Early post-transplant medical compliance and mental health predict physical morbidity and mortality one to three years after heart transplantation. J Heart Lung Transplant 1999;18:549–62.
7. Didlake RH, Dreyfus K, Kerman RH, et al. Patient noncompliance: a major cause of late graft failure in cyclosporine-treated renal transplants. Transplant Proc 1988;20:63–9.
8. McDermott MM, Schmitt B, Wallner E. Impact of medication nonadherence on coronary heart disease outcomes. A critical review. Arch Intern Med 1997;157:1921–9.
9. Milgrom H, Bender B. Nonadherence to asthma treatment and failure of therapy. Curr Opin Pediatr 1997;9:590–5.
10. Murri R, Ammassari A, De Luca A, et al. Self-reported nonadherence with antiretroviral drugs predicts persistent condition. HIV Clin Trials 2001;2:323–9.
11. Chisholm-Burns MA, Spivey CA. The 'cost' of medication nonadherence: consequences we cannot afford to accept. J Am Pharm Assoc 2003;52(6):823–6.
12. Duncan S, Annunziato RA, Dunphy C, et al. A systematic review of immunosuppressant adherence interventions in transplant recipients: decoding the streetlight effect. Pediatr Transplant 2017;22(1):1–12.
13. Fine RN, Becker Y, De Geest S, et al. Nonadherence consensus conference summary report. Am J Transplant 2009;9(1):35–41.
14. Adherence to long-term therapies: evidence for action. World Health Organization, 2003. p.9–21. ISBN 9241545992. Available at: http://www.who.int/chp/knowledge/publications/adherence_report/en/. Accessed January 10, 2018.
15. Lieber SR, Helcer J, Shemesh E. Monitoring drug adherence. Transplant Rev (Orlando) 2015;29(2):73–7.
16. Lam WY, Fresco P. Medication adherence measures: an overview. Biomed Res Int 2015;2015:217047.

17. Hoffman JA, Cunningham JR, Suleh AJ, et al. A technical feasibility pilot using mobile phones in Nairobi, Kenya. Am J Prev Med 2010;39(1):78–80.
18. Weis SE, Slocum PC, Blais FX, et al. The effect of directly observed therapy on the rates of drug resistance and relapse in tuberculosis. N Engl J Med 1994; 330(17):1179–84.
19. U.S. FDA accepts first digital medicine new drug application for Otsuka and Proteus digital health. In: press releases. 2015. Available at: https://www.proteus.com/press-releases/u-s-fda-accepts-first-digital-medicine-new-drug-application-for-otsuka-and-proteus-digital-health/. Accessed December 28, 2017.
20. Shemesh E, Bucuvalas JC, Anand R, et al. The Medication Level Variability Index (MLVI) predicts poor liver transplant outcomes: a prospective multi-site study. Am J Transplant 2017;17(10):2668–78.
21. Shemesh E, Shneider BL, Savitzky JK, et al. Medication adherence in pediatric and adolescent liver transplant recipients. Pediatrics 2004;113(4):825–32.
22. Supelana C, Annunziato RA, Schiano T, et al. The medication level variability index (MLVI) predicts rejection, possibly due to nonadherence, in adult liver transplant recipients. Liver Transpl 2014;20(10):1168–77.
23. Pollock-Barziv SM, Finkelstein Y, Manlhiot C, et al. Variability in tacrolimus blood levels increases the risk of late rejection and graft loss after solid organ transplantation in older children. Pediatr Transplant 2010;14(8):968–75.
24. Kreuzer M, Prufe J, Oldhafer M, et al. Transitional care and adherence of adolescents and young adults after kidney transplantation in Germany and Austria: a binational observatory census within the TRANSNephro trial. Medicine 2015; 94(48):e2196.
25. Eid L, Tuchman S, Moudgil A. Late acute rejection: incidence, risk factors, and effect on graft survival and function. Pediatr Transplant 2014;18(2):155–62.
26. Golay P, Fagot D, Lecerf T. Against coefficient of variation for estimation of intra-individual variability with accuracy measures. Tutor Quant Methods Psychol 2013;9(1):6–14.
27. Rianthavorn P, Ettenger RB. Medication non-adherence in the adolescent renal transplant recipient: a clinician's viewpoint. Pediatr Transplant 2005;9(3): 398–407.
28. Shaw RJ, Palmer L, Blasey C, et al. A typology of non-adherence in pediatric renal transplant recipients. Pediatr Transplant 2003;7(6):489–93.
29. Chisholm MA, Spivey CA, Mulloy LL. Effects of a medication assistance program with medication therapy management on the health of renal transplant recipients. Am J Health Syst Pharm 2007;64(14):1506–12.
30. Giacoma T, Ingersoll GL, Williams M. Teaching video effect on renal transplant patient outcomes. ANNA J 1999;26:29–33.
31. Suhling H, Rademacher J, Zinowsky I, et al. Conventional vs. tablet computer-based patient education following lung transplantation–a randomized controlled trial. PLoS One 2014;9(6):e90828.
32. Denhaerynck K, Schafer-Keller P, Young J, et al. Examining assumptions regarding valid electronic monitoring of medication therapy: development of validation framework and its application on a European sample of kidney transplant patients. BMC Med Res Methodol 2008;8:5.
33. Kuypers DR, Peeters PC, Sennesael JJ, et al. Improved adherence to tacrolimus once-daily formulation in renal recipients: a randomized controlled trial using electronic monitoring. Transplantation 2013;95(2):333–40.

34. McGillicuddy JW, Gregoski MJ, Weiland AK, et al. Mobile health medication adherence and blood pressure control in renal transplant recipients: a proof-of-concept randomized controlled trial. JMIR Res Protoc 2013;2(2):e32.

35. Russell C, Conn V, Ashbaugh C, et al. Taking immunosuppressive medications effectively (TIMELink): a pilot randomized controlled trial in adult kidney transplant recipients. Clin Transplant 2011;25(6):864–70.

36. Reese PP, Bloom RD, Trofe-Clark J, et al. Automated reminders and physician notification to promote immunosuppression adherence among kidney transplant recipients: a randomized trial. Am J Kidney Dis 2017;69(3):400–9.

37. Hardstaff R, Green K, Talbot D. Measurement of compliance posttransplantation–the results of a 12-month study using electronic monitoring. Transplant Proc 2003; 35(2):796–7.

38. Joost R, Dorje F, Schwitulla J, et al. Intensified pharmaceutical care is improving immunosuppressive medication adherence in kidney transplant recipients during the first post-transplant year: a quasi-experimental study. Nephrol Dial Transplant 2014;29(8):1597–607.

39. Klein A, Otto G, Kramer I. Impact of a pharmaceutical care program on liver transplant patients' compliance with immunosuppressive medication: a prospective, randomized, controlled trial using electronic monitoring. Transplantation 2009;87(6):839–47.

40. Dobbels F, De Bleser L, Berben L, et al. Efficacy of a medication adherence enhancing intervention in transplantation: the MAESTRO-Tx trial. J Heart Lung Transplant 2017;36(5):499–508.

41. Henriksson J, Tyden G, Hoijer J, et al. A prospective randomized trial on the effect of using an electronic monitoring drug dispensing device to improve adherence and compliance. Transplantation 2016;100(1):203–9.

42. Fennell RS, Foulkes LM, Boggs SR. Family-based program to promote medication compliance in renal transplant children. Transplant Proc 1994;26:102–3.

43. Beck DR, Fennell RS, Yost RL, et al. Evaluation of an education program on compliance with medication regimens in pediatric patients with renal transplants. J Pediatr 1980;96(6):1094–7.

44. Chisholm MA, Vollenweider LJ, Mulloy LL, et al. Renal transplant patient compliance with free immunosuppressive medications. Transplantation 2000;23: 745–58.

45. Chisholm MA, Mulloy LL, Jagadeesan M, et al. Impact of clinical pharmacy services on renal transplant patients' compliance with immunosuppressive medications. Clin Transplant 2001;15(5):330–6.

46. Shellmer DA, Zelikovsky N. The challenges of using medication event monitoring technology with pediatric transplant patients. Pediatr Transplant 2007;11(4): 422–8.

47. Dew MA, DiMartini AF, Dabbs ADV, et al. Adherence to the medical regimen during the first two years after lung transplantation. Transplantation 2008;85(2): 193–202.

48. Freier C, Oldhafer M, Offner G, et al. Impact of computer-based patient education on illness-specific knowledge and renal function in adolescents after renal transplantation. Pediatr Transplant 2010;14(5):596–602.

49. Traiger GL, Bui LL. A self-medication administration program for transplant recipients. Crit Care Nurse 1997;17:71–9.

50. Beckebaum S, Iacob S, Sweid D, et al. Efficacy, safety, and immunosuppressant adherence in stable liver transplant patients converted from a twice-daily

tacrolimus-based regimen to once-daily tacrolimus extended-release formulation. Transpl Int 2011;24:666–75.

51. Cukor D, Ver Halen N, Pencille M, et al. A pilot randomized controlled trial to promote immunosuppressant adherence in adult kidney transplant recipients. Nephron 2017;135(1):6–14.

52. DeVito DA, Dew M, Myers B, et al. Evaluation of a hand-held, computer-based intervention to promote early self-care behaviors after lung transplant. Clin Transplant 2009;23:537–45.

53. Garcia MF, Bravin AM, Garcia PD, et al. Behavioral measures to reduce nonadherence in renal transplant recipients: a prospective randomized controlled trial. Int Urol Nephrol 2015;47(11):1899–905.

54. DeVito Dabbs A, Song MK, Myers BA, et al. A randomized controlled trial of a mobile health intervention to promote self-management after lung transplantation. Am J Transplant 2016;16(7):2172–80.

55. Breu-Dejean N, Driot D, Dupouy J, et al. Efficacy of psychoeducational intervention on allograft function in kidney transplant patients: 10-year results of a prospective randomized study. Exp Clin Transplant 2016;14(1):38–44.

56. Fredericks EM, Magee JC, Opipari-Arrigan L, et al. Adherence and health-related quality of life in adolescent liver transplant recipients. Pediatr Transplant 2008; 12(3):289–99.

57. Urstad KH, Oyen O, Andersen MH, et al. The effect of an educational intervention for renal recipients: a randomized controlled trial. Clin Transplant 2012;26(3): E246–53.

58. Fredericks EM, Dore-Stites D, Well A, et al. Assessment of transition readiness skills and adherence in pediatric liver transplant recipients. Pediatr Transplant 2010;14(8):944–53.

59. Shemesh E, Shneider BL, Emre S. Adherence to medical recommendations in pediatric transplant recipients: time for action. Pediatr Transplant 2008;12(3): 281–3.

60. Kelly DA, Bucuvalas JC, Alonso EM, et al. Long-term medical management of the pediatric patient after liver transplantation: 2013 practice guideline by the American Association for the Study of Liver Diseases and the American Society of Transplantation. Liver Transpl 2013;19(8):798–825.

61. Annunziato RA, Emre S, Shneider BL, et al. Transitioning health care responsibility from caregivers to patient: a pilot study aiming to facilitate medication adherence during this process. Pediatr Transpl 2008;12(3):309–15.

62. Miloh T, Annunziato R, Arnon R, et al. Improved adherence and outcomes for pediatric liver transplant recipients by using text messaging. Pediatrics 2009; 124(5):e844–50.

63. Chisholm-Burns MA, Spivey CA, Graff Zivin J, et al. Improving outcomes of renal transplant recipients with behavioral adherence contracts: a randomized controlled trial. Am J Transplant 2013;13(9):2364–73.

64. McGillicuddy JW, Taber DJ, Mueller M, et al. Sustainability of improvements in medication adherence through a mobile health intervention. Prog Transplant 2015;25(3):217–23.

65. Rosenberger EM, DeVito Dabbs AJ, DiMartini AF, et al. Long-term follow-up of a randomized controlled trial evaluating a mobile health intervention for self-management in lung transplant recipients. Am J Transplant 2017;17(5):1286–93.

66. Schmid A, Hils S, Kramer-Zucker A, et al. Telemedically supported case management of living-donor renal transplant recipients to optimize routine evidence-

based aftercare: a single-center randomized controlled trial. Am J Transplant 2017;17(6):1594–605.

67. Loiselle KA, Gutierrez-Colina AM, Eaton CK, et al. Longitudinal stability of medication adherence among adolescent solid organ transplant recipients. Pediatr Transplant 2015;19(4):428–35.

68. Lieber SR, Shemesh E. Longitudinal stability of medication adherence: trying to decipher an important construct. Pediatr Transplant 2015;19(4):348–50.

69. Lee JL, Eaton C, Gutierrez-Colina AM, et al. Longitudinal stability of specific barriers to medication adherence. J Pediatr Psychol 2014;39(7):667–76.

70. Shemesh E, Duncan S, Anand R, et al. Trajectory of adherence behavior in pediatric and adolescent liver transplant recipients—the MALT cohort. Liver Transpl 2018;24(1):80–8.

71. Kahana SY, Frazier TW, Drotar D. Preliminary quantitative investigation of predictors of treatment non-adherence in pediatric transplantation: a brief report. Pediatr Transplant 2008;12(6):656–60.

72. Watson AR. Non-compliance and transfer from paediatric to adult transplant unit. Pediatr Nephrol 2000;14(6):469–72.

73. Annunziato RA, Emre S, Shneider B, et al. Adherence and medical outcomes in pediatric liver transplant recipients who transition to adult services. Pediatr Transplant 2007;11(6):608–14.

74. Annunziato RA, Duncan SE. Closer to fine: a transition success story. Pediatr Transplant 2017;21(1).

75. Bilhartz JL, Lopez MJ, Magee JC, et al. Assessing allocation of responsibility for health management in pediatric liver transplant recipients. Pediatr Transplant 2015;19(5):538–46.

76. Annunziato R, Bucuvalas JC, Wanrong Y, et al. Self-management measurement and prediction of clinical outcomes in pediatric transplant. J Pediatr 2017;193:128–33.e2.

77. Shemesh E, Mitchell J, Neighbors K, et al. Recruiting a representative sample in adherence research-The MALT multisite prospective cohort study experience. Pediatr Transplant 2017;21(8):1–8.

78. Annunziato RA, Fisher M, Jerson B, et al. Psychosocial assessment prior to pediatric transplantation: a review and summary of key considerations. Pediatr Transplant 2010;14(5):565–74.

Advances in Pediatric Fatty Liver Disease

Pathogenesis, Diagnosis, and Treatment

Hayley A. Braun, MPH[a],*, Sarah A. Faasse, MD[a,b],
Miriam B. Vos, MD, MSPH[a,b]

KEYWORDS

- Pediatric NAFLD • Review • Treatment • Type II diabetes • Diagnosis

KEY POINTS

- Pediatric nonalcoholic fatty liver disease (NAFLD) is increasing in prevalence and is a significant public health problem worldwide.
- The natural history is largely unknown but recent data suggest that mortality is increased in young adults with NAFLD and that type II diabetes is a frequent comorbidity.
- Factors implicated in NAFLD include genetic polymorphisms, environmental triggers, and dysregulated lipid metabolism. As advancements have been made in understanding the pathophysiology, there is greater opportunity for developing therapeutics.
- The use of MRI for steatosis measurement has been validated in children and is a useful noninvasive diagnostic, although it remains limited in availability and expensive.
- Therapeutic development is robust in pediatric NAFLD, with many drugs in early-stage trials; however, lifestyle improvements in diet and exercise remain the standard of care.

INTRODUCTION

As nonalcoholic fatty liver disease (NAFLD) has become the leading liver diseases in children, the critical questions surrounding it have grown in importance. These questions include what causes it, who is at risk for progression, whether it is treatable, and whether it is reversible. This article reviews the recent advances in understanding NAFLD as it occurs in children.

Disclosure: S.A. Faasse and H.A. Braun declare that they have no competing interests. M.B. Vos has NAFLD-related research support or in-kind research services from Resonance Health, Nutrition Science Initiative, AMRA, Gemphire, Immuron, Siemens, Shire, Target PharmaSolutions, Labcorp, and Perspectum and serves as an NAFLD consultant for Allergan, AMRA, Boehringer Ingelheim, Bristol-Myers Squibb, Immuron, Intercept, Shire, and Target PharmaSolutions.
[a] Division of Gastroenterology, Hepatology, and Nutrition, Department of Pediatrics, Emory University School of Medicine, 1760 Haygood Drive North East, Atlanta, GA 30322, USA;
[b] Division of Gastroenterology, Hepatology, and Nutrition, Children's Healthcare of Atlanta, 1405 Clifton Road, Atlanta, GA 30329, USA
* Corresponding author. 1760 Haygood Drive North East, Atlanta, GA 30322.
E-mail address: Hayley.Braun@emory.edu

Gastroenterol Clin N Am 47 (2018) 949–968
https://doi.org/10.1016/j.gtc.2018.07.016
0889-8553/18/© 2018 Elsevier Inc. All rights reserved.

Abbreviations	
ARFI	Acoustic radiation force impulse imaging
ALT	Alanine transaminase
ARB	Angiotensin receptor blocker
BMI	Body mass index
CAP	Controlled attenuation parameter
COX-2	Cyclooxygenase-2
CRN	Clinical Research Network
FA	Fatty acid
FGF-19	Fibroblast growth factor 19
FGF-21	Fibroblast growth factor 21
FIB-4	Fibrosis-4
FXR	Farnesoid X receptor
GCKR	Glucokinase regulatory protein
GLP-1	Glucagonlike peptide 1
GLP-1R	Glucagonlike peptide 1 receptor
GLUT1	Glucose transporter 1
GLUT8	Glucose transporter 8
GWAS	Genome-wide association study
HFD	High-fat diet
HOMA-IR	Homeostatic model assessment of insulin resistance
IGWLD	Intragastric weight loss device
LDL	Low-density lipoprotein
LSG	Laparoscopic sleeve gastrectomy
MMP	Matrix metalloproteinase
MR	Magnetic resonance
MRE	Magnetic resonance elastography
MRS	Magnetic resonance spectroscopy
NAFLD	Nonalcoholic fatty liver disease
NAS	NAFLD activity score
NASH	Nonalcoholic steatohepatitis
NSWL	Nonsurgical weight loss
PAI-1	Plasminogen activator inhibitor-1
PDFF	Proton density fat fraction
PPAR	Peroxisome proliferator-activated receptor
PUFA	Polyunsaturated fatty acids
SAF	Steatosis, activity, fibrosis
SNP	Single nucleotide polymorphism
T2DB	Type II diabetes
TG	Triglyceride
TNF-α	Tumor necrosis factor alpha
VAT	Visceral adipose tissue
VLDL	Very-low-density lipoprotein

PREVALENCE OF NONALCOHOLIC FATTY LIVER DISEASE

Over time, NAFLD has increased in prevalence and become the most common liver disease in children worldwide. In a recent review of prevalence across the world, a striking feature was the similarity in the pediatric populations of regions from Asia to Europe to North America: 5.9%, 5.7%, and 6.5% respectively.[1] Although some clinicians have questioned the contribution of increased awareness of NAFLD to these numbers, studies that compare prevalence over time applying a standard definition show that the prevalence of disease has more than doubled.[2] Estimated prevalence in the United States based on suspected NAFLD (defined as overweight; body mass index [BMI] ≥85th percentile) plus increased alanine aminotransferase levels (boys, >25.8 U/L; girls, >22.1 U/L) in 2007 to 2010 was 11% of all children, whereas 48.1% (3.7) of all obese boys and 56.0% (3.5) of obese Mexican American male adolescents had suspected NAFLD.[2] NAFLD risk increases with age, BMI z-score, male sex, and in Mexican American children, and is more common in Mexican American children.[2,3]

DEFINING NONALCOHOLIC FATTY LIVER DISEASE

NAFLD is defined both by the clinical scenario and by pathologic findings within the liver. A diagnosis requires evidence of hepatic steatosis and exclusion of other secondary causes of steatosis, such as viral hepatitis, Wilson disease, alpha-1-antitrypsin deficiency, autoimmune hepatitis, metabolic disease, lysosomal acid lipase deficiency, excess alcohol consumption, hepatotoxic medications, malnutrition, or parenteral nutrition.[4] It is the only liver disease diagnosed through the absence of other conditions, as the non in the name implies.[5] Particularly in pediatrics, the name nonalcoholic is problematic because it is confusing for parents and clinicians less familiar with the disease. The name fatty liver is commonly used in patient education materials and in communicating with patients; however, it is a broader category because fat overload in the liver can be caused by other conditions, as listed earlier. Thus, an appropriate name does not exist at this time. Previous appeals have been made for metabolic syndrome steatohepatitis.[5] Another possibility is fatty liver insulin resistance syndrome because the critical difference between other sources of fatty liver and NAFLD is that the disease includes insulin-glucose dysregulation.

The term NAFLD refers to the full spectrum of disease from steatosis alone to steatohepatitis to cirrhosis. Nonalcoholic steatohepatitis (NASH) is a more severe phenotype, defined by histologic findings including steatosis, inflammation, and hepatocyte ballooning.[6] In 2005, a unique pattern of injury on pediatric biopsies was described, designated as the pediatric pattern (or type 2), consisting of a periportal (zone 1) pattern of inflammation and steatosis that is rarely seen in adults but occurs in children.[7,8] In general, 3 histologic phenotypes of NAFLD in children are delineated:

1. A panacinar (diffuse) macrosteatosis pattern
2. A periportal steatosis
3. A zone 3 pattern similar to that seen in adults[9]

Although the pediatric pattern has generated great interest, with speculation that it might represent a different disease, instead growing evidence suggests that it is an early immature phenotype of the same disease. The pediatric pattern is more common in younger children and in male patients.[7] The National Institutes of Health NASH Clinical Research Network (CRN) recently reported the 2-year natural history of the pediatric pattern and showed that it was not predictive of any specific future clinical or histologic outcome.[10]

There are 2 widely accepted, validated methods for grading and staging the pathologic lesions of NAFLD: the NASH CRN proposed score (NAFLD activity score [NAS][11]) and a score proposed by the European Fatty Liver Inhibition of Progression centers that includes fibrosis (steatosis, activity, fibrosis [SAF][12]).

- NAS is the sum of steatosis (0–3), lobular inflammation (0–3), and hepatocyte ballooning (0–2). This score does not differentiate NASH, which is a separate characterization assigned by pathologists.
- SAF is the sum of steatosis (0–3), activity (0–4: lobular inflammation 0–2 and ballooning 0–2), and fibrosis (0–4).

Both of these are useful because they provide standardized language to semiquantitatively describe the severity of the histologic findings. The primary difference is the inclusion of fibrosis in SAF, which may be a benefit given the importance of fibrosis for prognosis, as supported by adult natural history studies. Both score steatosis as the percentage of hepatocytes involved: less than 5% = 0, 5% to 33% = 1, 34% to 66% = 2, and greater than 66% = 3.[9]

The definition of steatosis or abnormal levels of lipid deposition in hepatocytes has evolved over time. Most clinicians accept steatosis as lipid deposition in greater than 5% of hepatocytes.[13] This definition developed out of the measurement of fat within a healthy liver, which is less than 5% by weight, and levels more than 5% are considered pathologic.[14] However, newer MRI data suggest that the cutoff of normal liver fat by MRI is less than 5%. This change is an example of how the understanding of NAFLD is evolving as newer technologies provide additional data.

Another notable pediatric feature is that hepatocyte ballooning is rarely present. The lack of hepatocyte ballooning has led to a semantic issue because, although severe inflammation and stage 2 and 3 fibrosis are seen in children, they may not meet the definition for NASH because of the lack of hepatocyte ballooning. The term borderline NASH is applied when some, but not all, of the features of NASH are present. In adults, this is typically milder phenotypes (zone 3 borderline NASH); however, it may not be mild in children.

NATURAL HISTORY

The available data for the pediatric natural history of NAFLD are from small case series and a limited number of longitudinal reports. In adults, NAFLD is predictive of earlier mortality[15] and associated with early cardiovascular disease, type II diabetes (T2DB), and hepatocellular carcinoma.[16] It seems that, even in childhood, a diagnosis of NAFLD is associated with increased mortality as a young adult.[17,18] In studies evaluating change by liver biopsy over several years, approximately half of children increase fibrosis and half improve.[10,19] The presence of fibrosis is most predictive of future adverse outcomes for adults, and the rate of fibrosis progression is estimated to be approximately 9 years per stage. Thus, a child diagnosed with NASH and stage 2 fibrosis at age 12 years could progress to cirrhosis by age ~40 years if progression is the same for NASH identified in childhood as that identified in adulthood. In adults, the presence of fibrosis has increasingly been identified as the most reliable marker of future liver-related outcomes such as cirrhosis, portal hypertension, and hepatocellular carcinoma, and fibrosis is associated with mortality when present with steatosis alone or with NASH.[20] However, in pediatrics, there are insufficient data to predict which child will have progressive fibrosis and this remains an area in need of longitudinal investigations.

Growing evidence suggests that one of the earliest comorbidities of pediatric NAFLD is the onset of T2DB. In a placebo-based cohort of children with NAFLD who were receiving lifestyle treatment, 3.5% progressed to T2DB over 1 year.[10] In cross-sectional studies, pediatric NAFLD is strongly associated with prediabetes as well as dyslipidemia and hypertension.[4]

ADVANCES IN UNDERSTANDING FACTORS IMPLICATED IN NONALCOHOLIC FATTY LIVER DISEASE
Genetics

The development of pediatric NAFLD is the result of environmental influences superimposed on genetic variants that predispose the individual to the disease. One of the most well-studied genetic variants implicated in NAFLD is in the PNPLA3 gene, which encodes a protein involved in lipid metabolism called adiponutrin. A 2008 genome-wide association study (GWAS) described 2 important mutations. The first is a single nucleotide polymorphism (SNP) in codon 148 labeled rs738409, which results in the missense mutation of isoleucine to methionine (I148M). This mutation was found more frequently in Hispanic individuals, and a more recent study showed that the mutation has a synergistic effect with adiposity, compounding the risk of NAFLD in susceptible patients.[21,22] In the same GWAS study, the PNPLA3 rs6006460 serine to isoleucine missense SNP (S453I) was found to confer a hepatoprotective effect via lower intrahepatic fat content. Significantly, this SNP was found more commonly in African Americans, who overall have a lower prevalence of NAFLD.[21] Two other SNPs that have been identified as potentially significant in the pathogenesis of NAFLD (glucokinase regulatory protein [GCKR] rs1260326[23] and transmembrane 6 superfamily member 2 rs58542926[24]) seem to have a synergistic effect on determining intrahepatic fat content when combined with PNPLA3 rs6006460.[24]

The SNP rs1260326 found in the GCKR promotes de novo lipogenesis, which, as discussed later, is a major component of the pathophysiology of hepatic steatosis. Importantly, there is a lower incidence of rs1260326 in African Americans than in Hispanics or caucasians, suggesting one reason that NAFLD may be less prevalent in this group.[25]

Prenatal Programming and Epigenetics

Emerging research also indicates that the origins of chronic diseases such as NAFLD may lie in predisposing factors from the prenatal environment. Nonhuman primate studies have implicated prenatal exposure in long-term negative effects on the fetal hepatic immune system and de novo lipogenesis. For instance, a set of experiments by Friedman and colleagues[26,27] showed that when pregnant, insulin-resistant female Japanese macaques were fed a high-fat diet, this was predictive of fatty liver in their infants, regardless of postnatal infant diet. In addition, these primates had abnormally activated macrophage and natural killer cells.[28]

This crucial role of the prenatal environment is supported by imaging studies of infants born to obese mothers with gestational diabetes. At 1 to 3 weeks of age, these infants had, on average, 68% more intrahepatic fat deposition[28] as well as more adipose tissue overall.[29] Another study found that 79% of stillborn infants of mothers with either prepregnancy diabetes or gestational diabetes had hepatic steatosis compared with 17% of stillborn infants born to mothers without diabetes.[30] It may be that maternal obesity is sufficient to program hepatic effects because a longitudinal study of mother-child pairs found an effect of maternal BMI but not gestational diabetes on hepatic fat at age 16 years.[31]

Obesity and Fat Distribution

NAFLD often does not occur in isolation but is present within the spectrum of cardiometabolic disease and insulin resistance. Several available studies support that NAFLD is not only a comorbidity of obesity but an independent risk factor for insulin resistance and metabolic syndrome. In a study of Egyptian overweight and obese children, those with NAFLD were significantly more likely to show insulin resistance than overweight and obese children without NAFLD.[32] Further, a study of obese adolescents showed not only lower insulin sensitivity but poorer efficiency of fat oxidation in patients with NAFLD compared with those without.[33] The difference in children with metabolic syndrome may lie in the predominant type of adiposity that they have. Metabolically unhealthy individuals, in general, not only have increased central adiposity but also have increased visceral adipose tissue (VAT).[34] There is a higher prevalence of NAFLD and metabolic syndrome in individuals with a higher proportion of VAT, which has been shown to be metabolically active.[35] Significantly, intrahepatic fat may be more important than VAT in driving the metabolic dysfunction and insulin resistance present in NAFLD.[36,37] De novo lipogenesis plays a major role in the steatosis of NAFLD, significantly more so than in metabolically healthy individuals,[38] and even more in the setting of weight gain.[39]

Although the emphasis has been on excess fat in the liver and viscera, tissue deficiencies may also play a role. Decreased muscle mass, or sarcopenia, combined with increased visceral fat is also associated with NAFLD[40] and was shown to be predictive of significant liver fibrosis in adults.[41,42] Although children with end-stage liver disease have been found to have sarcopenia,[31] no data are available regarding children with NAFLD. Inadequate expansion of subcutaneous fat has been implicated as a driver of multiple ectopic fats, including hepatic fat, visceral fat, intramuscular fat, and pancreatic fat.[43] One hypothesized mechanism proposes that it is the failure of subcutaneous fat to expand in the setting of increasing calories that drives metabolic disease.[44] Adiponectin is secreted by the subcutaneous adipocytes and it may play a protective role against the development of NASH. In control patients, serum adiponectin levels were significantly increased postprandially, whereas patients with NASH showed decreased levels of adiponectin. These levels were inversely correlated with postprandial lipemia. In addition, low circulating adiponectin levels were significantly associated with steatosis, necroinflammation, and fibrosis.[45] Fat distribution and metabolic activity is a promising area of investigation that needs more attention in pediatric NAFLD, because this may inform prevention and treatment.

There has been significant interest in further defining the actions of fibroblast growth factor 21 (FGF-21), a metabolic regulatory hormone primarily synthesized in and released from the liver. Through its receptor and coreceptor, the hepatic klotho receptor, it increases glucose uptake in adipocytes via the GLUT1 transporter, and it is upregulated by peroxisome proliferator-activated receptor (PPAR) gamma.[46] Significantly, both FGF-19 and FGF-21 were decreased in patients with NAFLD compared with healthy controls; the decrease was even more dramatic in patients with NASH.[47] In a longitudinal study of obese and normal-weight children, FGF-21 was significantly higher in obese children than in normal-weight children but did not correlate with NAFLD,[48] underscoring the concept that NAFLD is part of a dysmetabolic process and is not simply related to patient obesity.

The liver is central in regulating lipids in the human body, and understanding of the alterations found in lipid flux in NAFLD is growing. Triglyceride (TG) metabolism is the most disturbed in NAFLD, although cholesterol alterations have also been described. There are multiple sources contributing to fatty acids (FAs) used for very-low-density lipoprotein (VLDL)–TG synthesis, including dietary FA, FA synthesized de novo from dietary carbohydrates, nonesterified FA from adipose tissue, nonesterified FA from spillover of chylomicron-TG, and FA stored in liver lipid droplets.[49] Normally, there is essentially no storage of TG in the liver and the normal liver is ~5% lipid by weight; this consists of lipid that is in transit through one of these processes and lipids contained within cell membranes and structures. In NAFLD, dietary supply of lipids and precursors for de novo lipogenesis are increased because of hypercaloric diets and excess return of FA from adipose tissue. In direct comparison of individuals with NAFLD and individuals without, the critical difference in NAFLD is an inappropriately increased rate of de novo lipogenesis.[38] Under conditions of weight gain, de novo lipogenesis rate increases further.[39] VLDL secretion is normal and children with NAFLD have large, TG-rich VLDL. Thus, it seems that steatosis in NAFLD results from excess supply of metabolites to de novo lipogenesis, producing excess TG beyond that able to be exported by VLDL.[39]

Dietary Contributors

Diet is one of the major environmental causes of NAFLD in both children and adults. Of dietary causes of NAFLD, fructose and added sugars have growing evidence to support their importance in the disease. In an epidemiologic study, children who consumed an energy-adjusted higher fructose intake had a significantly increased risk of NAFLD within 3 years.[50] Fructose is also implicated in insulin resistance, because it is processed differently by the liver than glucose, and uniquely upregulates lipogenic transcription factors.[51] Compared with glucose, fructose promotes increased de novo lipogenesis, visceral adiposity, and decreased insulin sensitivity.[52] Specifically, the GLUT8 transporter protein mediates hepatic fructose uptake; GLUT8-deficient mice show lower fructose uptake and reduced de novo lipogenesis, showing a protective effect from NAFLD when GLUT8 is deficient.[53]

The mechanisms through which fructose may contribute to NAFLD are likely multiple, including serving as a source of excess calories, direct stimulation of de novo lipogenesis, and modification of the microbiome or its products such as endotoxin. In a series of pediatric cohorts, those with NAFLD had increased endotoxin levels, which correlated to increased insulin resistance and levels of inflammatory cytokines, compared with levels in obese control patients without steatosis. Further, this study found that consistent ingestion of fructose-containing beverages results in persistently increased endotoxin levels 4 weeks after the fructose is removed.[54]

Oxidative stress is well established as a critical mechanism in NAFLD and may be at least partially the result of deficient glutathione. In recent studies, amino acids related to glutathione synthesis have been found to be altered in NAFLD. In particular, glutamate, tyrosine, and a ratio of glutamate, serine, and glycine were correlated with hepatic insulin resistance.[55] In a pediatric study of the metabolome of NAFLD, similar dysfunction was found in amino acid pathways.[56] However, whether these findings are causal or an effect of liver dysfunction remains to be evaluated.

Intestinal Microbiome/Gut-Liver Axis

The intestinal microbiome may also provide proinflammatory signaling mechanisms that are important in the pathogenesis of NAFLD. Evidence suggests a relationship between small intestine bacterial overgrowth, a so-called leaky gut caused by increased intestinal permeability, and NAFLD pathogenesis.[57] In the setting of increased permeability, bacteria, pathogen-associated molecular patterns, and damage-associated molecular patterns pass through the endothelium and into the mesenteric portal bloodstream.[58] Importantly, not only could alterations in the intestinal microbiome in patients with NASH contribute to increased permeability but the by-products of the bacteria may also contribute to the oxidative stress that has been implicated in NAFLD. In a study of 63 children in New York with NASH, obesity without liver disease, and healthy controls, patients with NASH not only had a different microbiome profile but these bacteria produced more ethanol than those in healthy patients. As a result, patients with NASH had higher detectable endogenous ethanol levels, which could contribute to the oxidative stress and injury of hepatocytes.[59] In addition, a recent Italian metagenomics and metabolomics study examined the bacterial profiles and volatile organic compounds present in stool samples from 61 pediatric patients with NAFLD, NASH, or obesity and 54 healthy controls. Subjects with NAFLD had an increase in 26 of 292 known volatile organic compounds and a decrease in 2 compounds. The investigators were able to temporally identify a decrease in *Oscillospira* bacteria to onset of NAFLD and the increase of *Ruminococcus* and *Dorea* to the progression of NAFLD to NASH.[60] These intriguing findings could have major noninvasive diagnostic, and potentially mechanistic and therapeutic, implications.

Bile acids have powerful metabolic actions as regulators of genes important in nutrient absorption and lipid metabolism, and different bile acids have both protective and injurious effects on hepatocytes. Therefore, there has been great interest in analysis of both bile acid levels and profiles in the pathophysiology of NAFLD in recent years, although their exact role in NAFLD is not yet clear. Bile acids and insulin are synergistic ligands for protein kinase B and extracellular signal-regulated kinase 1/2 signaling pathways.[61] In a study of obese adult patients, changes in bile acid ratios were associated with greater insulin resistance, but there was not a significant change in bile acid profiles of patients with NASH compared with those without.[62] These findings emphasize that both the steatosis and fibrosis disease processes, although interrelated, are important in NAFLD and may have different biochemical stimuli. Bile acid levels were higher in patients with NAFLD with fibrosis compared with patients with NAFLD without fibrosis, but both were lower than in control patients, supporting that bile acids may be important in lipid metabolism.[63]

DIAGNOSIS OF NONALCOHOLIC FATTY LIVER DISEASE AND INNOVATION IN DIAGNOSTICS

The typical diagnostic pathway for NAFLD includes establishing the presence of steatosis through either imaging or liver biopsy and ruling out other chronic liver diseases through history and laboratory screening. Although laboratory tests and imaging can provide information on diagnosis and estimations of liver fat content, only histologic assessment can accurately stage NAFLD and distinguish NASH, simple steatosis, and steatosis with fibrosis.[11] Liver biopsies are limited by cost, invasiveness, precision, and issues with the subjective nature of histologic reading. In particular, for repeated measurements, the invasiveness of the procedure makes it problematic.[64] Another issue for liver biopsies is that the distribution of fat may not be consistent throughout the liver, and thus the biopsied section may not be representative in determining liver fat.[65,66] For these reasons, there is great interest in developing accurate noninvasive biomarkers and diagnostic tests for NAFLD, which will be especially beneficial for children.

Histologic Assessment

Histology is useful for ruling out other liver diseases and for grading and staging the disease. A typical clinicopathologic assessment includes a description of the presence of steatosis, the location and type of steatosis, the type and amount of inflammation, the determination of NASH or not, as well as the stage of fibrosis by location. The NASH CRN has proposed an assessment approach that is described in an article by Kleiner and Brunt.[65]

Detection of Steatosis

Ultrasonography and MRI are the two primary noninvasive tools used to detect and measure steatosis. Historically, ultrasonography was the primary method to detect steatosis for NAFLD diagnosis; however, it has fallen out of favor because of the lack of accuracy.[4] Newer magnetic resonance (MR)–based methods have been developed to measure hepatic fat. MR spectroscopy (MRS) is highly precise and is becoming the new gold standard for hepatic fat quantification.[67] MRI–proton density fat fraction (PDFF) is also widely available. In one study, MRI-PDFF and MRS showed a strong correlation and both had a positive correlation with histologically determined steatosis grade.[68] There is strong evidence that quantitative MRI can accurately estimate pediatric liver fat compared with histology. The corresponding MRI-PDFF value for histologic grade 1 steatosis in a cohort of pediatric patients with NAFLD was a mean of 11%, whereas grade 2 and 3 were 18% and 26% respectively.[69] Volumetric liver fat fraction is another MR-based methodology[70] recently validated in children that is useful because of its wide availability and precision.[71]

Controlled attenuation parameter (CAP) measurements have been assessed in 2 studies of pediatric patients.[72,73] CAP is a noninvasive assessment of hepatic fat based on the radiofrequency ultrasonography signal acquired by a transient elastography device. At this time, CAP seems to be most useful to differentiate between marked steatosis and none.

Detection and Staging of Fibrosis

Several noninvasive serologic scores have been developed for NAFLD, most developed using adult cohorts. One of the most frequently used is the Fibrosis-4 (FIB-4) score. However, in a pediatric validation study, FIB-4 was insensitive for pediatric disease.[74] Efforts have been made to develop pediatric-specific scores but again have not been proved to have sufficient sensitivity or specificity to be useful in clinical practice.[74] There is substantial development in detection of fibrosis by imaging. Most technologies are developed first in adults and then applied to children. A note of caution was raised by a study in which healthy adults were compared with children using MR elastography (MRE) to measure liver stiffness.[75] Liver stiffness was significantly lower in children and adolescents compared with adults and increased with age over normal development. This study suggested that direct application of adult values may underestimate severity of disease in children and emphasized the need for pediatric studies of new technologies. Transient elastography has been used extensively in Europe to evaluate liver fibrosis and received US Food and Drug Administration approval in 2013.[76] It has been tested in a pediatric cohort and found to be accurate and reproducible; however, it was most useful in predicting advanced fibrosis, whereas differentiation between no fibrosis and stage 1 or 2 was less accurate.[77] Acoustic radiation force impulse imaging (ARFI), an ultrasonography-based assessment, uses high-intensity acoustic pulses to create shear waves. The wave velocity correlates with liver stiffness.[76] ARFI is commonly available but few validation data exist in pediatrics. A small study of children undergoing liver biopsy and ARFI showed that it was able to detect significant fibrosis; however, more studies are needed.[78]

MRE is an MR-based method of measuring fibrosis that is becoming clinically available at many pediatric facilities. There are several reports of MRE in children[79] and it has been validated against liver biopsy in a study of 114 children.[80] The data from this study show that MRE had an overall accuracy for discriminating between any versus no fibrosis of 72% and 87% to 90% for classifying advanced fibrosis (stage $\geq$3).[80] These data are promising, but further studies in larger cohorts will be helpful to improve the utility for clinical decision making.

In summary, MR-based methods are sufficiently validated for clinical use in children for detecting and quantifying hepatic steatosis. Ultrasonography-based methods are less accurate, although they have the advantage of greater availability. For fibrosis, at this time both ultrasonography-based methods and MR need further study before they can be applied in the clinical pathway of diagnosis.

TREATMENTS AND THERAPEUTIC DEVELOPMENT
Lifestyle Modifications

Lifestyle modification is a commonly prescribed treatment plan for the management of NAFLD. NAFLD pathogenesis is related to obesity and the metabolic syndrome and thus lifestyle modifications may address these disorders. A review of lifestyle interventions including nutrition, exercise, or both assessed the role of lifestyle interventions in the treatment of NAFLD and highlighted the need for large-scale randomized trials to form an evidence base for supporting lifestyle recommendations.[81] When considering dietary modifications, one question that commonly arises concerns which diet works best. In a study of low fat versus low glycemic load, both types of interventions showed significant decrease in hepatic fat fraction (37% and 36% respectively) by MRS, with no difference between groups.[82] Another area of interest is whether different carbohydrates affect the liver differently. One study assessed whether glucose or fructose contributed more to steatosis and liver profiles. Children consumed a 237-mL (8-oz) beverage containing either glucose or fructose 3 times a day for 4 weeks. Although no difference was found in hepatic fat, alanine transaminase (ALT), homeostatic model assessment of insulin resistance (HOMA-IR), or body weight, the glucose group had significantly lower free FAs, adipose insulin resistance, high-sensitivity C-reactive protein, and low-density lipoprotein (LDL) oxidation.[83]

Lifestyle modification interventions also included combined exercise and dietary interventions. One study in children with biopsy-proven NAFLD assessed the impact of a 1-year combined exercise and dietary intervention focused on a balanced, low-calorie diet. Of the 84 initially enrolled patients, 57 completed the study. In the patients not lost to follow-up, significant decreases in BMI, ALT, and HOMA-IR were noted.[84] Another study compared types of lifestyle interventions: inpatient, ambulatory outpatient, and usual care. Over the 6-month follow-up period, liver fat normalized in 43%, 29%, and 22% in the inpatient group, ambulatory, and usual care groups respectively. ALT levels significantly decreased in the inpatient and ambulatory care groups at 6 months, but only the inpatient group remained decreased at 18 months.[85] These consistent findings support the use of lifestyle interventions for the treatment of NAFLD and it remains the standard of care. Other developing areas for treatment relevant to children are discussed later.

Bariatric Surgery

Laparoscopic sleeve gastrectomy (LSG) is a radical but potentially useful procedure in reversing NAFLD or NASH in patients with a BMI greater than or equal to 35 kg/m^2 who have unsuccessfully attempted nonsurgical weight loss options. In a study of older adolescents who received LSG, an intragastric weight loss device (IGWLD), or a nonsurgical weight loss option (NSWL), LSG had a much greater reversal rate of fibrosis among all 3 groups: 90% compared with 40% in the IGWLD group (the NSWL group had <50% retention, so comparisons cannot be made). In addition, the percentage of patients with an NAS of 5 or greater went from 30% to 0% and the number of patients with an NAS of 1 went from 0% to 66.5% in the LSG group, indicating a drastic reversal in histologic features. Patients receiving the IGWLD also showed favorable, although less drastic, decreases in percentage of patients with an NAS of 5, decreasing by 30%, and the number of patients with a score of 1 increasing by 25%. LSG also showed favorable results in improving comorbidities, with significant decreases in percentage of patients with hypertension, obstructive sleep apnea syndrome, dyslipidemia, and impaired glucose tolerance.[86]

Modification of the Gut Microbiota and Endotoxin

There is evidence to suggest that gut microbiota play a role in hepatic fat deposition, and regulation of the gut-liver axis may improve the course of NAFLD. Two potential therapeutic options are probiotics and antilipopolysaccharides. Rat models have shown that high-fat diets increase liver lipid peroxidation, expression of cyclooxygenase-2 (COX-2), increased inflammatory markers such as tumor necrosis factor alpha (TNF-α) and matrix metalloproteinase (MMP), and decreased PPAR-α expression.[87] In contrast, rats fed a high-fat diet in combination with VSL#3, a multi-strain probiotic of *Streptococcus thermophilus* and multiple species of *Lactobacillus* and *Bifidobacterium*, showed significantly lower TNF-α levels, MMP activity, and expression of inducible nitric oxide synthase and COX-2, and PPAR-α levels were significantly higher, suggesting an overall antiinflammatory effect with improved lipid metabolism.[87]

A 2016 meta-analysis of probiotic use in NAFLD reported positive outcomes in patients taking probiotics. The meta-analysis indicated improvement in HOMA-IR, total cholesterol, high-density lipoprotein, LDL, and TNF-α in Italian and Spanish participants taking probiotic regimens, including VSL#3, *Lactobacillus*, *Bifidobacterium*, *Bifidobacterium longum*, fructo-oligosaccharides, *Lactobacillus bulgaricus*, S thermophilus, *Lactobacillus* GG, *Lactobacillus acidophilus*, dung *Enterococcus*, *Bacillus subtilis*, and *Enterococcus* compared with placebo.[88] No difference in BMI, glucose, and insulin in adults with NAFLD was seen. Notable limitations include variations in probiotic regimens, the small sample size of the studies, the lack of studies providing histologic evaluation, and disproportionately fewer studies in children.[88] A study in children did show significantly lower odds of severe versus less severe steatosis by ultrasonography after 4 months of VSL#3 probiotic use.[89] In addition, in patients taking the probiotic, levels of GLP-1 and the activated form (aGLP-1) were significantly increased.

Another focus of gut microbiome–related disorder in NAFLD is the gut endotoxin lipopolysaccharides found on the outer cell wall of gram-negative bacteria.[90] Plasma levels of lipopolysaccharides and inflammatory cytokines interleukin-1beta, interleukin-6, and TNF-α were significantly increased in children with biopsy-proven NAFLD. One hypothesis is that lipopolysaccharides activate a proinflammatory pathway that involves hepatic stellate cell cytokine production through lipopolysaccharide-induced signaling. This hypothesis is supported by lipopolysaccharide-inducible TNF-α factor–dependent transcription of proinflammatory cytokines in hepatic stellate LX-2 cells and subsequent suppression by lipopolysaccharide-inducible TNF-α factor silencing. Further implicating this pathway in the pathogenesis of NASH is that children with NAFLD had significantly higher levels of lipopolysaccharide-induced TNF-α factor, which correlated with the presence of NASH and the NAS.[90]

Farnesoid X Receptor Agonists/Bile Acids

The farnesoid X receptor (FXR) of the nuclear receptor superfamily is another potential therapeutic option. FXRs are highly expressed in the liver, kidney, intestines, and adrenal glands and are regulated by bile acids.[91,92] They are thought to have many roles in metabolism, including bile acid excretion, TG biosynthesis, and glucose homeostasis. FXR agonists improved glucose tolerance and hepatic steatosis in animal models.[91] These results have been supported in adult studies, although side effects such as increased serum cholesterol level and pruritus raised questions about the safety of the drug.[93]

Omega-3 Fatty Acids

Omega-3 polyunsaturated FAs (PUFAs), such as eicosapentaenoic acid and docosahexaenoic acid, have been shown to have both hepatic metabolic effects as well as an antiinflammatory role as a ligand for PPARα.[94] As described earlier, PPARα has an antiinflammatory effect and upregulates fatty acid oxidation. A meta-analysis of omega-3 PUFA supplementation supports these findings and has shown PUFA supplementation to be associated with significantly improved hepatic steatosis grade on ultrasonography.[95] This finding is supported by a study assessing hepatic fat fraction by MRI, which showed significantly decreased hepatic fat levels in children receiving omega-3 PUFAs compared with controls.[96]

Insulin Resistance

Metformin has been suggested as a potential treatment option for NAFLD. The Treatment of NAFLD in Children (TONIC) study in 2011 in children with NAFLD compared 1000 mg of metformin, 800 IU of vitamin E, or placebo for 96 weeks. The primary outcome of sustained reduction in ALT levels was no different than placebo for either the metformin or vitamin E group.[97] Although these results did not seem promising, a commentary published the following year suggested potential limitations of the study. One limitation was that the metformin dosing may have been too small to induce any physiologic changes in NAFLD, because the metformin at this dose was unable to change measures of insulin sensitivity, which is the drug's primary mechanism of action.[98] Although not directly assessing hepatic measures, metformin has been shown to improve insulin sensitivity in adolescents with NAFLD, addressing common NAFLD comorbidities.

Antioxidants

Antioxidants such as vitamin E and cysteamine bitartrate have been researched for their potential in protecting against NASH. Children with NAFLD did not meet the recommended daily allowance of vitamin E and lower median consumption was associated with a higher grade of steatosis.[99] With supplementation, ALT and alkaline phosphatase levels were found to decrease in a small pilot study.[100] However, in the TONIC randomized controlled trial, vitamin E supplementation improved liver histology in NAFLD, with affected hepatocytes showing a lesser degree of ballooning than before treatment.[97] There has been considerable interest in antioxidant therapy for NAFLD in recent years; thus far, the most promising improvements seem to be when coupled with lifestyle changes.[101]

Another antioxidant of interest is cysteamine bitartrate. In the Cysteamine Bitartrate Delayed-Release for the Treatment of NAFLD in Children (CyNCh) trial, which tested the efficacy of cysteamine bitartrate delayed release, there was no change in overall NAS, although children receiving cysteamine bitartrate delayed release had lower serum ALT and aspartate transaminase levels, and a larger proportion had reduced lobular inflammation than children receiving the placebo.[102]

Angiotensin Receptor Blockers

Losartan is an orally administered angiotensin II receptor blocker (ARB) that is currently marketed for hypertension. Losartan also acts to decrease plasminogen activator inhibitor-1 (PAI-1) and to increase insulin sensitivity, properties that may confer protective anti-NAFLD effects. Rat models show that rats fed a high-fat diet (HFD) plus losartan had significantly reduced liver fat compared with HFD rats alone. In addition, PAI-1 levels were significantly reduced in the rats that received losartan.[103] In an adult study of patients with insulin resistance, hypertension, NAFLD, and type II diabetes, losartan did not improve hepatic fat content derived from liver-to-spleen ratio based on computed tomography scan.[104] An attempted study of losartan failed to recruit sufficient participants because of the high rate of patients already taking either ARBs or angiotensin-converting enzyme inhibitors.[105] A pilot study of losartan in children has been reported in abstract form and on clinicaltrials.gov, and larger studies are needed.

Glucagonlike Peptide 1 Receptor Agonist

Glucagonlike peptide 1 (GLP-1) is an intestinal peptide secreted by neuroendocrine cells with a wide range of downstream effects thought to include weight loss; decreased inflammation by immune cells; and decreased hepatic steatosis, inflammation, fibrosis, and hepatocyte injury.[106] A small adult study of liraglutide, a GLP-1 receptor (GLP-1R) agonist, showed resolution in significantly more participants (39%) receiving liraglutide compared with 9% in controls.[107] Because of these positive findings, a large multicentered trial is now being conducted to further investigate these results (Clinicaltrials.gov NCT02970942). As mentioned earlier, probiotics increased expression of GLP-1, suggesting another way to elicit the positive effects of activated GLP-1R in patients with NAFLD.[89]

Current Clinical Trials

At the time of this article, on clinicaltrials.gov (www.clinicaltrials.gov), 14 studies in pediatric NAFLD were listed. Two studies are completed with published results, 4 studies are complete without peer-reviewed published results that the authors were able to obtain, 1 study is active but not recruiting, 1 study was terminated because of poor recruitment, and 2 studies are listed with an unknown status, although on further investigation 1 study has published results.[108] The unpublished studies are on losartan, diet (4), antilipopolysaccharides, supplementations (4), and weight loss surgery. The number of studies and the extensive development in place for pediatric NAFLD treatment bodes well for the future because more effective therapies are an urgent need.

SUMMARY

Pediatric nonalcoholic fatty liver disease is an increasingly prevalent disease, but the pathophysiology is not fully elucidated, diagnosis is expensive and invasive, and therapeutic options are limited (**Table 1**). Recent advancements in understanding the pathophysiology of NAFLD suggest that environmental exposures contributing to NAFLD may begin in the fetal period, that NAFLD is closely tied to the metabolic syndrome and dietary composition, and that the disease process may have a tightly regulated relationship with the gastrointestinal system. New MRI and ultrasonography modalities have advanced the quality of diagnostic information. The understanding of pathophysiology has grown, and new therapeutic options are in development.

Table 1
Pediatric nonalcoholic fatty liver disease overview

	Criteria	Histologic Phenotypes	Grading and Staging Criteria

Pediatric NAFLD	1. Evidence of hepatic steatosis, with lipid deposition in >5% hepatocytes[10]
	2. Exclusion of other secondary causes of steatosis[1]
		1. A panacinar (diffuse) macrosteatosis pattern
		2. A periportal steatosis
		3. A zone 3 pattern similar to that seen in adults[6]
		4. NASH: inflammation ± hepatocyte ballooning
			NAS[8]:
			1. Steatosis (0–3)
			2. Lobular inflammation (0–3)
			3. Hepatocyte ballooning (0–2)
			SAF[9]:
			1. Steatosis (0–3)
			2. Activity (0–4):
			  • Lobular inflammation (0–2)
			  • Ballooning (0–2)
			3. Fibrosis (0–4)

REFERENCES

1. Anderson EL, Howe LD, Jones HE, et al. The prevalence of non-alcoholic fatty liver disease in children and adolescents: a systematic review and meta-analysis. PLoS One 2015;10(10):e0140908.
2. Welsh JA, Karpen S, Vos MB. Increasing prevalence of nonalcoholic fatty liver disease among United States adolescents, 1988-1994 to 2007-2010. J Pediatr 2013;162(3):496–500.
3. Schwimmer JB, Deutsch R, Kahen T, et al. Prevalence of fatty liver in children and adolescents. Pediatrics 2006;118(4):1388–93.
4. Vos MB, Abrams SH, Barlow SE, et al. NASPGHAN clinical practice guideline for the diagnosis and treatment of nonalcoholic fatty liver disease in children: recommendations from the Expert Committee on NAFLD (ECON) and the North American Society of Pediatric Gastroenterology, Hepatology and Nutrition (NASPGHAN). J Pediatr Gastroenterol Nutr 2017;64(2):319–34.
5. Brunt EM. What's in a NAme? Hepatology 2009;50(3):663–7.
6. Brunt E. Nonalcoholic steatohepatitis: definition and pathology. Semin Liver Dis 2001;21(1):3–16.
7. Schwimmer JB, Behling C, Newbury R, et al. Histopathology of pediatric nonalcoholic fatty liver disease. Hepatology 2005;42(3):641–9.
8. Africa JA, Behling CA, Brunt EM, et al. In children with nonalcoholic fatty liver disease, zone 1 steatosis is associated with advanced fibrosis. Clin Gastroenterol Hepatol 2018;16(3):438–46.e1.
9. Brunt EM. Nonalcoholic fatty liver disease and the ongoing role of liver biopsy evaluation. Hepatol Commun 2017;1(5):370–8.
10. Xanthakos SLJ, Yates KP, Schwimmer JB, et al. Natural history of nonalcoholic fatty liver disease (NAFLD) in children receiving standard lifestyle counseling and placebo in NASH Clinical Research Network (CRN) trials. Hepatology 2017;66(Suppl 1):31A.
11. Kleiner DE, Brunt EM, Van Natta M, et al. Design and validation of a histological scoring system for nonalcoholic fatty liver disease. Hepatology 2005;41(6): 1313–21.
12. Bedossa P. Utility and appropriateness of the fatty liver inhibition of progression (FLIP) algorithm and steatosis, activity, and fibrosis (SAF) score in the evaluation of biopsies of nonalcoholic fatty liver disease. Hepatology 2014; 60(2):565–75.
13. Tannapfel A, Denk H, Dienes HP, et al. Histopathological diagnosis of nonalcoholic and alcoholic fatty liver disease. Virchows Arch 2011;458(5):511–23.
14. Jin R, Vos MB. Fructose and liver function–is this behind nonalcoholic liver disease? Curr Opin Clin Nutr Metab Care 2015;18(5):490–5.
15. Haflidadottir S, Jonasson JG, Norland H, et al. Long-term follow-up and liver-related death rate in patients with non-alcoholic and alcoholic related fatty liver disease. BMC Gastroenterol 2014;14:166.
16. Stein E, Bays H, Koren M, et al. Efficacy and safety of gemcabene as add-on to stable statin therapy in hypercholesterolemic patients. J Clin Lipidol 2016;10(5): 1212–22.
17. Cioffi CE, Welsh JA, Cleeton RL, et al. Natural history of NAFLD diagnosed in childhood: a single-center study. Children (Basel) 2017;4(5) [pii:E34].
18. Feldstein AE, Charatcharoenwitthaya P, Treeprasertsuk S, et al. The natural history of non-alcoholic fatty liver disease in children: a follow-up study for up to 20 years. Gut 2009;58(11):1538–44.

19. A-Kader H, Henderson J, Vanhoesen K, et al. Nonalcoholic fatty liver disease in children: a single center experience. Clin Gastroenterol Hepatol 2008;6(7):799–802.

20. Younossi ZM, Stepanova M, Rafiq N, et al. Nonalcoholic steatofibrosis independently predicts mortality in nonalcoholic fatty liver disease. Hepatol Commun 2017;1(5):421–8.

21. Romeo S, Kozlitina J, Xing C, et al. Genetic variation in PNPLA3 confers susceptibility to nonalcoholic fatty liver disease. Nat Genet 2008;40(12):1461–5.

22. Stender S, Kozlitina J, Nordestgaard BG, et al. Adiposity amplifies the genetic risk of fatty liver disease conferred by multiple loci. Nat Genet 2017;49(6):842–7.

23. Santoro N, Zhang CK, Zhao H, et al. Variant in the glucokinase regulatory protein (GCKR) gene is associated with fatty liver in obese children and adolescents. Hepatology 2012;55(3):781–9.

24. Goffredo M, Caprio S, Feldstein AE, et al. Role of TM6SF2 rs58542926 in the pathogenesis of nonalcoholic pediatric fatty liver disease: a multiethnic study. Hepatology 2016;63(1):117–25.

25. Umano GR, Martino M, Santoro N. The association between pediatric NAFLD and common genetic variants. Children (Basel) 2017;4(6) [pii:E49].

26. Thorn SR, Baquero KC, Newsom SA, et al. Early life exposure to maternal insulin resistance has persistent effects on hepatic NAFLD in juvenile nonhuman primates. Diabetes 2014;63(8):2702–13.

27. McCurdy CE, Bishop JM, Williams SM, et al. Maternal high-fat diet triggers lipotoxicity in the fetal livers of nonhuman primates. The Journal of clinical investigation 2009;119(2):323–35.

28. Brumbaugh DE, Tearse P, Cree-Green M, et al. Intrahepatic fat is increased in the neonatal offspring of obese women with gestational diabetes. J Pediatr 2013;162(5):930–6.e1.

29. Modi N, Murgasova D, Ruager-Martin R, et al. The influence of maternal body mass index on infant adiposity and hepatic lipid content. Pediatr Res 2011; 70(3):287–91.

30. Patel KR, White FV, Deutsch GH. Hepatic steatosis is prevalent in stillborns delivered to women with diabetes mellitus. J Pediatr Gastroenterol Nutr 2015; 60(2):152–8.

31. Bellatorre A, Scherzinger A, Stamm E, et al. Fetal overnutrition and adolescent hepatic fat fraction: the exploring perinatal outcomes in children study. J Pediatr 2018;192:165–70.e1.

32. El-Karaksy HM, El-Raziky MS, Fouad HM, et al. The value of different insulin resistance indices in assessment of non-alcoholic fatty liver disease in overweight/obese children. Diabetes Metab Syndr 2015;9(2):114–9.

33. Lee S, Rivera-Vega M, Alsayed HM, et al. Metabolic inflexibility and insulin resistance in obese adolescents with non-alcoholic fatty liver disease. Pediatr Diabetes 2015;16(3):211–8.

34. Neeland IJ, Ayers CR, Rohatgi AK, et al. Associations of visceral and abdominal subcutaneous adipose tissue with markers of cardiac and metabolic risk in obese adults. Obesity (Silver Spring) 2013;21(9):E439–47.

35. Fontana L, Eagon JC, Trujillo ME, et al. Visceral fat adipokine secretion is associated with systemic inflammation in obese humans. Diabetes 2007;56(4): 1010–3.

36. D'Adamo E, Cali AM, Weiss R, et al. Central role of fatty liver in the pathogenesis of insulin resistance in obese adolescents. Diabetes Care 2010;33(8):1817–22.

37. Fabbrini E, Magkos F, Mohammed BS, et al. Intrahepatic fat, not visceral fat, is linked with metabolic complications of obesity. Proc Natl Acad Sci U S A 2009; 106(36):15430–5.

38. Lambert JE, Ramos-Roman MA, Browning JD, et al. Increased de novo lipogenesis is a distinct characteristic of individuals with nonalcoholic fatty liver disease. Gastroenterology 2014;146(3):726–35.

39. Fabbrini E, Tiemann Luecking C, Love-Gregory L, et al. Physiological mechanisms of weight gain-induced steatosis in people with obesity. Gastroenterology 2016;150(1):79–81.e2.

40. Shida T, Akiyama K, Oh S, et al. Skeletal muscle mass to visceral fat area ratio is an important determinant affecting hepatic conditions of non-alcoholic fatty liver disease. J Gastroenterol 2018;53(4):535–47.

41. Lee YH, Kim SU, Song K, et al. Sarcopenia is associated with significant liver fibrosis independently of obesity and insulin resistance in nonalcoholic fatty liver disease: nationwide surveys (KNHANES 2008-2011). Hepatology 2016;63(3): 776–86.

42. Petta S, Ciminnisi S, Di Marco V, et al. Sarcopenia is associated with severe liver fibrosis in patients with non-alcoholic fatty liver disease. Aliment Pharmacol Ther 2017;45(4):510–8.

43. Caprio S, Perry R, Kursawe R. Adolescent obesity and insulin resistance: roles of ectopic fat accumulation and adipose inflammation. Gastroenterology 2017; 152(7):1638–46.

44. Lotta LA, Gulati P, Day FR, et al. Integrative genomic analysis implicates limited peripheral adipose storage capacity in the pathogenesis of human insulin resistance. Nat Genet 2017;49(1):17–26.

45. Musso G, Gambino R, Durazzo M, et al. Adipokines in NASH: postprandial lipid metabolism as a link between adiponectin and liver disease. Hepatology 2005; 42(5):1175–83.

46. Lakhani I, Gong M, Wong WT, et al. Fibroblast growth factor 21 in cardiometabolic disorders: a systematic review and meta-analysis. Metabolism 2018;83:11–7.

47. Alisi A, Ceccarelli S, Panera N, et al. Association between serum atypical fibroblast growth factors 21 and 19 and pediatric nonalcoholic fatty liver disease. PLoS One 2013;8(6):e67160.

48. Reinehr T, Woelfle J, Wunsch R, et al. Fibroblast growth factor 21 (FGF-21) and its relation to obesity, metabolic syndrome, and nonalcoholic fatty liver in children: a longitudinal analysis. J Clin Endocrinol Metab 2012;97(6):2143–50.

49. Jacome-Sosa MM, Parks EJ. Fatty acid sources and their fluxes as they contribute to plasma triglyceride concentrations and fatty liver in humans. Curr Opin Lipidol 2014;25(3):213–20.

50. O'Sullivan TA, Oddy WH, Bremner AP, et al. Lower fructose intake may help protect against development of nonalcoholic fatty liver in adolescents with obesity. J Pediatr Gastroenterol Nutr 2014;58(5):624–31.

51. Softic S, Gupta MK, Wang GX, et al. Divergent effects of glucose and fructose on hepatic lipogenesis and insulin signaling. J Clin Invest 2017;127(11): 4059–74.

52. Stanhope KL, Schwarz JM, Keim NL, et al. Consuming fructose-sweetened, not glucose-sweetened, beverages increases visceral adiposity and lipids and decreases insulin sensitivity in overweight/obese humans. J Clin Invest 2009; 119(5):1322–34.

53. Debosch BJ, Chen Z, Saben JL, et al. Glucose transporter 8 (GLUT8) mediates fructose-induced de novo lipogenesis and macrosteatosis. J Biol Chem 2014; 289(16):10989–98.
54. Jin R, Willment A, Patel SS, et al. Fructose induced endotoxemia in pediatric nonalcoholic fatty liver disease. Int J Hepatol 2014;2014:560620.
55. Gaggini M, Carli F, Rosso C, et al. Altered amino acid concentrations in NAFLD: impact of obesity and insulin resistance. Hepatology 2018;67(1):145–58.
56. Jin R, Banton S, Tran VT, et al. Amino acid metabolism is altered in adolescents with nonalcoholic fatty liver disease-an untargeted, high resolution metabolomics study. J Pediatr 2016;172:14–9.e5.
57. Miele L, Valenza V, La Torre G, et al. Increased intestinal permeability and tight junction alterations in nonalcoholic fatty liver disease. Hepatology 2009;49(6): 1877–87.
58. Paolella G, Mandato C, Pierri L, et al. Gut-liver axis and probiotics: their role in non-alcoholic fatty liver disease. World J Gastroenterol 2014;20(42): 15518–31.
59. Zhu L, Baker SS, Gill C, et al. Characterization of gut microbiomes in nonalcoholic steatohepatitis (NASH) patients: a connection between endogenous alcohol and NASH. Hepatology 2013;57(2):601–9.
60. Del Chierico F, Nobili V, Vernocchi P, et al. Gut microbiota profiling of pediatric nonalcoholic fatty liver disease and obese patients unveiled by an integrated meta-omics-based approach. Hepatology 2017;65(2):451–64.
61. Zhou H, Hylemon PB. Bile acids are nutrient signaling hormones. Steroids 2014; 86:62–8.
62. Legry V, Francque S, Haas JT, et al. Bile acid alterations are associated with insulin resistance, but not with NASH, in obese subjects. J Clin Endocrinol Metab 2017;102(10):3783–94.
63. Jahnel J, Zohrer E, Alisi A, et al. Serum bile acid levels in children with nonalcoholic fatty liver disease. J Pediatr Gastroenterol Nutr 2015;61(1):85–90.
64. Pacifico L, Poggiogalle E, Cantisani V, et al. Pediatric nonalcoholic fatty liver disease: a clinical and laboratory challenge. World J Hepatol 2010;2(7):275–88.
65. Kleiner DE, Brunt EM. Nonalcoholic fatty liver disease: pathologic patterns and biopsy evaluation in clinical research. Semin Liver Dis 2012;32(1):3–13.
66. Ratziu V, Charlotte F, Heurtier A, et al. Sampling variability of liver biopsy in nonalcoholic fatty liver disease. Gastroenterology 2005;128(7):1898–906.
67. Sharma P, Martin DR, Pineda N, et al. Quantitative analysis of T2-correction in single-voxel magnetic resonance spectroscopy of hepatic lipid fraction. J Magn Reson Imaging 2009;29(3):629–35.
68. Noureddin M, Lam J, Peterson MR, et al. Utility of magnetic resonance imaging versus histology for quantifying changes in liver fat in nonalcoholic fatty liver disease trials. Hepatology 2013;58(6):1930–40.
69. Middleton MS, Van Natta ML, Heba ER, et al. Diagnostic accuracy of magnetic resonance imaging hepatic proton density fat fraction in pediatric nonalcoholic fatty liver disease. Hepatology 2018;67(3):858–72.
70. St Pierre TG, House MJ, Bangma SJ, et al. Stereological analysis of liver biopsy histology sections as a reference standard for validating non-invasive liver fat fraction measurements by MRI. PLoS One 2016;11(8):e0160789.
71. Vos MB, Knight-Scott F, Konomi JV, et al. Accuracy and repeatability of magnetic resonance imaging based volumetric liver fat fraction compared to liver histology and magnetic resonance spectroscopy as reference standards. Hepatology 2017;66(Suppl 1):1108A.

72. Desai NK, Harney S, Raza R, et al. Comparison of controlled attenuation parameter and liver biopsy to assess hepatic steatosis in pediatric patients. J Pediatr 2016;173:160–4.e1.
73. Ferraioli G, Calcaterra V, Lissandrin R, et al. Noninvasive assessment of liver steatosis in children: the clinical value of controlled attenuation parameter. BMC Gastroenterol 2017;17(1):61.
74. Jackson JA, Konomi JV, Mendoza MV, et al. Performance of fibrosis prediction scores in paediatric non-alcoholic fatty liver disease. J Paediatr Child Health 2018;54(2):172–6.
75. Etchell E, Juge L, Hatt A, et al. Liver stiffness values are lower in pediatric subjects than in adults and increase with age: a multifrequency MR elastography study. Radiology 2017;283(1):222–30.
76. Mansoor S, Collyer E, Alkhouri N. A comprehensive review of noninvasive liver fibrosis tests in pediatric nonalcoholic Fatty liver disease. Curr Gastroenterol Rep 2015;17(6):23.
77. Nobili V, Vizzutti F, Arena U, et al. Accuracy and reproducibility of transient elastography for the diagnosis of fibrosis in pediatric nonalcoholic steatohepatitis. Hepatology 2008;48(2):442–8.
78. Pinto J, Matos H, Nobre S, et al. Comparison of acoustic radiation force impulse/ serum noninvasive markers for fibrosis prediction in liver transplant. J Pediatr Gastroenterol Nutr 2014;58(3):382–6.
79. Joshi M, Dillman JR, Singh K, et al. Quantitative MRI of fatty liver disease in a large pediatric cohort: correlation between liver fat fraction, stiffness, volume, and patient-specific factors. Abdom Radiol (NY) 2018;43(5):1168–79.
80. Schwimmer JB, Behling C, Angeles JE, et al. Magnetic resonance elastography measured shear stiffness as a biomarker of fibrosis in pediatric nonalcoholic fatty liver disease. Hepatology 2017;66(5):1474–85.
81. Africa JA, Newton KP, Schwimmer JB. Lifestyle interventions including nutrition, exercise, and supplements for nonalcoholic fatty liver disease in children. Dig Dis Sci 2016;61(5):1375–86.
82. Ramon-Krauel M, Salsberg SL, Ebbeling CB, et al. A low-glycemic-load versus low-fat diet in the treatment of fatty liver in obese children. Child Obes 2013;9(3):252–60.
83. Jin R, Welsh JA, Le N-A, et al. Dietary fructose reduction improves markers of cardiovascular disease risk in Hispanic-American adolescents with NAFLD. Nutrients 2014;6(8):3187–201.
84. Nobili V, Marcellini M, Devito R, et al. NAFLD in children: a prospective clinical-pathological study and effect of lifestyle advice. Hepatology 2006;44(2):458–65.
85. Koot BG, van der Baan-Slootweg OH, Vinke S, et al. Intensive lifestyle treatment for non-alcoholic fatty liver disease in children with severe obesity: inpatient versus ambulatory treatment. Int J Obes (Lond) 2016;40(1):51–7.
86. Manco M, Mosca A, De Peppo F, et al. The benefit of sleeve gastrectomy in obese adolescents on nonalcoholic steatohepatitis and hepatic fibrosis. J Pediatr 2017;180:31–7.e2.
87. Esposito E, Iacono A, Bianco G, et al. Probiotics reduce the inflammatory response induced by a high-fat diet in the liver of young rats. J Nutr 2009;139(5):905–11.
88. Gao X, Zhu Y, Wen Y, et al. Efficacy of probiotics in non-alcoholic fatty liver disease in adult and children: a meta-analysis of randomized controlled trials. Hepatol Res 2016;46(12):1226–33.
89. Alisi A, Bedogni G, Baviera G, et al. Randomised clinical trial: the beneficial effects of VSL#3 in obese children with non-alcoholic steatohepatitis. Aliment Pharmacol Ther 2014;39(11):1276–85.

90. Ceccarelli S, Panera N, Mina M, et al. LPS-induced TNF-alpha factor mediates pro-inflammatory and pro-fibrogenic pattern in non-alcoholic fatty liver disease. Oncotarget 2015;6(39):41434–52.

91. Ma Y, Huang Y, Yan L, et al. Synthetic FXR agonist GW4064 prevents diet-induced hepatic steatosis and insulin resistance. Pharm Res 2013;30(5):1447–57.

92. Makishima M, Okamoto AY, Repa JJ, et al. Identification of a nuclear receptor for bile acids. Science 1999;284(5418):1362–5.

93. Neuschwander-Tetri BA, Loomba R, Sanyal AJ, et al. Farnesoid X nuclear receptor ligand obeticholic acid for non-cirrhotic, non-alcoholic steatohepatitis (FLINT): a multicentre, randomised, placebo-controlled trial. Lancet 2015; 385(9972):956–65.

94. Pawar A, Jump DB. Unsaturated fatty acid regulation of peroxisome proliferator-activated receptor alpha activity in rat primary hepatocytes. J Biol Chem 2003; 278(38):35931–9.

95. Chen LH, Wang YF, Xu QH, et al. Omega-3 fatty acids as a treatment for non-alcoholic fatty liver disease in children: a systematic review and meta-analysis of randomized controlled trials. Clin Nutr 2018;37(2):516–21.

96. Pacifico L, Bonci E, Di Martino M, et al. A double-blind, placebo-controlled randomized trial to evaluate the efficacy of docosahexaenoic acid supplementation on hepatic fat and associated cardiovascular risk factors in overweight children with nonalcoholic fatty liver disease. Nutr Metab Cardiovasc Dis 2015;25(8):734–41.

97. Lavine JE, Schwimmer JB, Van Natta ML, et al. Effect of vitamin E or metformin for treatment of nonalcoholic fatty liver disease in children and adolescents: the TONIC randomized controlled trial. JAMA 2011;305(16):1659–68.

98. Alkhouri N, Feldstein AE. The TONIC trial: a step forward in treating pediatric nonalcoholic fatty liver disease. Hepatology 2012;55(4):1292–5.

99. Vos MB, Colvin R, Belt P, et al. Correlation of vitamin E, uric acid, and diet composition with histologic features of pediatric NAFLD. J Pediatr Gastroenterol Nutr 2012;54(1):90–6.

100. Lavine JE. Vitamin E treatment of nonalcoholic steatohepatitis in children: a pilot study. J Pediatr 2000;136(6):734–8.

101. Vajro P, Mandato C, Franzese A, et al. Vitamin E treatment in pediatric obesity-related liver disease: a randomized study. J Pediatr Gastroenterol Nutr 2004; 38(1):48–55.

102. Schwimmer JB, Lavine JE, Wilson LA, et al. In children with nonalcoholic fatty liver disease, cysteamine bitartrate delayed release improves liver enzymes but does not reduce disease activity scores. Gastroenterology 2016;151(6):1141–54.e9.

103. Rosselli MS, Burgueño AL, Carabelli J, et al. Losartan reduces liver expression of plasminogen activator inhibitor-1 (PAI-1) in a high fat-induced rat nonalcoholic fatty liver disease model. Atherosclerosis 2006;206(1):119–26.

104. Hirata T, Tomita K, Kawai T, et al. Effect of telmisartan or losartan for treatment of nonalcoholic fatty liver disease: fatty liver protection trial by telmisartan or losartan study (FANTASY). Int J Endocrinol 2013;2013:587140.

105. McPherson S, Wilkinson N, Tiniakos D, et al. A randomised controlled trial of losartan as an anti-fibrotic agent in non-alcoholic steatohepatitis. PLoS One 2017; 12(4):e0175717.

106. Dhir G, Cusi K. Glucagon like peptide-1 receptor agonists for the management of obesity and non-alcoholic fatty liver disease: a novel therapeutic option. J Investig Med 2018;66(1):7–10.

107. Armstrong MJ, Gaunt P, Aithal GP, et al. Liraglutide safety and efficacy in patients with non-alcoholic steatohepatitis (LEAN): a multicentre, double-blind, randomised, placebo-controlled phase 2 study. Lancet 2016;387(10019):679–90.

108. Spahis S, Alvarez F, Dubois J, et al. Plasma fatty acid composition in French-Canadian children with non-alcoholic fatty liver disease: effect of n-3 PUFA supplementation. Prostaglandins Leukot Essents Fatty Acids 2015;99:25–34.

UNITED STATES POSTAL SERVICE ®

Statement of Ownership, Management, and Circulation
(All Periodicals Publications Except Requester Publications)

1. Publication Title	2. Publication Number	3. Filing Date
GASTROENTEROLOGY CLINICS OF NORTH AMERICA	000 – 279	9/18/18

4. Issue Frequency	5. Number of Issues Published Annually	6. Annual Subscription Price
MAR, JUN, SEP, DEC	4	$350.00

7. Complete Mailing Address of Known Office of Publication (Not printer) (Street, city, county, state, and ZIP+4®)

ELSEVIER INC.
230 Park Avenue, Suite 800
New York, NY 10169

Contact Person
STEPHEN R. BUSHING

Telephone (Include area code)
215-239-3688

8. Complete Mailing Address of Headquarters or General Business Office of Publisher (Not printer)

ELSEVIER INC.
230 Park Avenue, Suite 800
New York, NY 10169

9. Full Names and Complete Mailing Addresses of Publisher, Editor, and Managing Editor (Do not leave blank)

Publisher (Name and complete mailing address)

TAYLOR E BALL, ELSEVIER INC.
1600 JOHN F KENNEDY BLVD. SUITE 1800
PHILADELPHIA, PA 19103-2899

Editor (Name and complete mailing address)

KERRY HOLLAND, ELSEVIER INC.
1600 JOHN F KENNEDY BLVD. SUITE 1800
PHILADELPHIA, PA 19103-2899

Managing Editor (Name and complete mailing address)

PATRICK MANLEY, ELSEVIER INC.
1600 JOHN F KENNEDY BLVD. SUITE 1800
PHILADELPHIA, PA 19103-2899

10. Owner (Do not leave blank. If the publication is owned by a corporation, give the name and address of the corporation immediately followed by the names and addresses of all stockholders owning or holding 1 percent or more of the total amount of stock. If not owned by a corporation, give the names and addresses of the individual owners. If owned by a partnership or other unincorporated firm, give its name and address as well as those of each individual owner. If the publication is published by a nonprofit organization, give its name and address.)

Full Name	Complete Mailing Address
WHOLLY OWNED SUBSIDIARY OF REED/ELSEVIER, US HOLDINGS	1600 JOHN F KENNEDY BLVD. SUITE 1800 PHILADELPHIA, PA 19103-2899

11. Known Bondholders, Mortgagees, and Other Security Holders Owning or Holding 1 Percent or More of Total Amount of Bonds, Mortgages, or Other Securities. If none, check box → ☐ None

Full Name	Complete Mailing Address
N/A	

12. Tax Status (For completion by nonprofit organizations authorized to mail at nonprofit rates) (Check one)
The purpose, function, and nonprofit status of this organization and the exempt status for federal income tax purposes:
☒ Has Not Changed During Preceding 12 Months
☐ Has Changed During Preceding 12 Months (Publisher must submit explanation of change with this statement)

PS Form 3526, July 2014 [Page 1 of 4 (see instructions page 4)] PSN: 7530-01-000-9931   PRIVACY NOTICE: See our privacy policy on www.usps.com.

---

13. Publication Title	14. Issue Date for Circulation Data Below
GASTROENTEROLOGY CLINICS OF NORTH AMERICA	JUNE 2018

15. Extent and Nature of Circulation			Average No. Copies Each Issue During Preceding 12 Months	No. Copies of Single Issue Published Nearest to Filing Date
a. Total Number of Copies (Net press run)			234	305
b. Paid Circulation (By Mail and Outside the Mail)	(1)	Mailed Outside-County Paid Subscriptions Stated on PS Form 3541 (include paid distribution above nominal rate, advertiser's proof copies, and exchange copies)	94	115
	(2)	Mailed In-County Paid Subscriptions Stated on PS Form 3541 (include paid distribution above nominal rate, advertiser's proof copies, and exchange copies)	0	0
	(3)	Paid Distribution Outside the Mails Including Sales Through Dealers and Carriers, Street Vendors, Counter Sales, and Other Paid Distribution Outside USPS®	68	80
	(4)	Paid Distribution by Other Classes of Mail Through the USPS (e.g., First-Class Mail®)	0	0
c. Total Paid Distribution (Sum of 15b (1), (2), (3), and (4))			162	195
d. Free or Nominal Rate Distribution (By Mail and Outside the Mail)	(1)	Free or Nominal Rate Outside-County Copies included on PS Form 3541	61	93
	(2)	Free or Nominal Rate In-County Copies Included on PS Form 3541	0	0
	(3)	Free or Nominal Rate Copies Mailed at Other Classes Through the USPS (e.g., First-Class Mail)	0	0
	(4)	Free or Nominal Rate Distribution Outside the Mail (Carriers or other means)	0	0
e. Total Free or Nominal Rate Distribution (Sum of 15d (1), (2), (3) and (4))			61	93
f. Total Distribution (Sum of 15c and 15e)			223	280
g. Copies not Distributed (See Instructions to Publishers #4 (page 83))			12	17
h. Total (Sum of 15f and g)			235	297
i. Percent Paid (15c divided by 15f times 100)			72.65%	69.64%

* If you are claiming electronic copies, go to line 16 on page 3. If you are not claiming electronic copies, skip to line 17 on page 3.

16. Electronic Copy Circulation	Average No. Copies Each Issue During Preceding 12 Months	No. Copies of Single Issue Published Nearest to Filing Date
a. Paid Electronic Copies	0	0
b. Total Paid Print Copies (Line 15c) + Paid Electronic Copies (Line 16a)	162	195
c. Total Print Distribution (Line 15f) + Paid Electronic Copies (Line 16a)	223	280
d. Percent Paid (Both Print & Electronic Copies) (16b divided by 16c × 100)	72.65%	69.64%

☒ I certify that 50% of all my distributed copies (electronic and print) are paid above a nominal price.

17. Publication of Statement of Ownership
☒ If the publication is a general publication, publication of this statement is required. Will be printed in the DECEMBER 2018 issue of this publication.   ☐ Publication not required.

18. Signature and Title of Editor, Publisher, Business Manager, or Owner

STEPHEN R. BUSHING - INVENTORY DISTRIBUTION CONTROL MANAGER

Date 9/18/18

I certify that all information furnished on this form is true and complete. I understand that anyone who furnishes false or misleading information on this form or who omits material or information requested on the form may be subject to criminal sanctions (including fines and imprisonment) and/or civil sanctions (including civil penalties).

PS Form 3526, July 2014 (Page 3 of 4)   PRIVACY NOTICE: See our privacy policy on www.usps.com.

Printed and bound by CPI Group (UK) Ltd, Croydon, CR0 4YY

12/10/2024

01773485-0001